Reoperative
Vascular Surgery

Science and Practice of Surgery

Consulting Editors

John F. Burke

Benedict Professor of Surgery
Harvard Medical School
Massachusetts General Hospital
Boston, Massachusetts

Peter J. Morris

Nuffield Professor of Surgery
University of Oxford
John Radcliffe Hospital
Oxford, England

Additional Volumes in Preparation

Reoperative Vascular Surgery

Edited by

HUGH H. TROUT, III
JOSEPH M. GIORDANO
RALPH G. DePALMA

Department of Surgery
George Washington University Medical Center
Washington, D.C.

Marcel Dekker, Inc.　　　　　New York and Basel

Library of Congress Cataloging-in-Publication

Reoperative vascular surgery.

   (Science and practice of surgery ; 14)
   Includes index.
    1. Blood-vessels--Surgery. 2. Surgery, operative.
3. Blood-vessels--Surgery--Complications and sequelae.
I. Trout, Hugh H. II. Giordano, Joseph M.
III. DePalma, Ralph G. IV. Series.
[DNLM: 1. Surgery, Operative. 2. Vascular Surgery.
W1 SC679 v.14 / WG 170 R4245]
RD598.5.R467 1987   617'.413   87-13458
ISBN 0-8247-7723-9

MARCEL DEKKER, INC.
270 Madison Avenue, New York, New York 10016

Current printing (last digit):
10 9 8 7 6 5 4 3 2 1

PRINTED IN THE UNITED STATES OF AMERICA

Preface

The great progress made in the specialty of vascular surgery over the last 35 years has standardized the primary operative approach to vascular disease, produced a generation of experienced vascular surgeons, and added to a knowledge of the outcome of vascular surgical procedures. This cumulative experience and the confidence derived from it now allows us to address an increasingly important problem: reoperation for complications as well as for early or late failure of vascular operative procedures.

Reoperations after initial vascular reconstruction are not uncommon. Most reoperative procedures, however, are not needed because of initial surgical misjudgments or poorly executed operations. Instead, late reoperations are most often required because of progression of vascular disease or the failure of synthetic vascular prostheses to remain patent for extended periods of time.

Reoperative vascular procedures will be increasingly performed. The reasons for this are: (1) more primary vascular procedures are being performed, (2) more aggressive attempts are being made to revascularize limbs previously considered nonsalvagable, and (3) patients with vascular disease may live longer due to better cardiac management and, possibly, due to modification and control of risk factors such as hyperlipidemia, smoking, and hypertension.

This book reviews the problems of reoperation after common vascular procedures. Few surgeons have extensive experience with vascular reoperations. Moreover reoperative vascular procedures are usually difficult: these operations often require dissections in areas of tissue scarring where landmarks are obscured; available graft options have frequently been compromised by previous use of autogenous veins; finally these patients usually present with an urgent need for reoperation due to infection, aneurysm, or limb-threatening ischemia.

Although some sections of this volume must consider operative vascular complications, its primary intent was not to focus on these complications or their etiology. Our goal was to outline approaches and technical options available to the surgeon when treating patients requiring vascular reoperations. Each topic covered has been subdivided into: incidence and etiology, preoperative evaluation, technical considerations, postoperative management, and results. This design permits quick reference when urgent vascular reoperative procedures are needed.

We have particularly emphasized technical considerations. There is often little room for error with these operations and every technical advantage possible must be used. For example, a particular principle we value is the need to avoid, whenever possible, extensive dissection within scar tissue. Such dissections are difficult, time consuming, and often further compromise reconstructive options because important vessels are damaged. Internal balloon control of vessels requires minimal dissection and causes little endothelial damage, particularly if the balloon is distended only to the point of allowing no further bleeding.

We believe that residents, vascular fellows, as well as general and vascular surgeons will find each particular topic discussed in a thorough manner by surgeons of particular expertise. Though improvisation will often be needed in reoperative vascular surgery, when the need for a vascular reoperation arises we hope this volume will substantially contribute to the care of these most difficult and challenging patients.

We are grateful to the contributing authors and coauthors for the high quality of their contributions to this project. Finally, especial thanks are extended to Paul Dolgert, Della McEneaney, and the rest of the staff at Marcel Dekker, Inc., for their steadfast support and continued patience both in starting and in finishing this book.

Hugh H. Trout, III
Joseph M. Giordano
Ralph G. DePalma

Contributors

Enrico Ascer, M.D., F.A.C.S. Head, Vascular Surgical Research Laboratory, Department of Surgery, Montefiore Medical Center-Albert Einstein College of Medicine, New York, New York

William H. Baker, M.D. Professor and Chief, Department of Surgery, Section of Peripheral Vascular Surgery, Loyola University Medical Center, Maywood, Illinois

Paul E. Collier, M.D.* Instructor in Surgery and Fellow in Vascular Surgery, Division of Vascular Surgery, Montefiore Medical Center-Albert Einstein College of Medicine, New York, New York

Fuad Joseph Dagher, M.D. Professor of Surgery, Chief, Vascular and Transplant Service, University of Maryland School of Medicine and Hospital, Baltimore, Maryland

Ralph G. DePalma, M.D. Professor and Chairman, Department of Surgery, George Washington University Medical Center, Washington, D.C.

William E. Evans, M.D. Director of Vascular Services, St. Anthony Medical Center, Columbus, Ohio

---

*Present affiliation: Staff Surgeon, Department of Surgery, Sewickley Valley Hospital, Sewickley, Pennsylvania.

Joseph M. Giordano, M.D. Professor of Surgery, Department of Surgery; Director, Division of Vascular Surgery, George Washington University Medical Center, Washington, D.C.

Edward R. Gomez, M.D. Instructor of Surgery, Uniformed Services University of the Health Sciences, Bethesda, Maryland; Fellow, Peripheral Vascular Surgery Service, Walter Reed Army Medical Center, Washington, D.C.

Sushil K. Gupta, M.S., B.S. Associate Chief of Vascular Surgery and Associate Professor of Surgery, Department of Surgery, Montefiore Medical Center, Albert Einstein College of Medicine, New York, New York

James P. Hayes, M.S. Biomedical Engineer, Supervisor, Department of Vascular Research, St. Anthony Medical Center, Columbus, Ohio

Norman R. Hertzer, M.D. Department of Vascular Surgery, The Cleveland Clinic Foundation, Cleveland, Ohio

Larry H. Hollier, M.D., F.A.C.C., F.A.C.S. Head, Section of Vascular Surgery, Mayo Clinic, Rochester, Minnesota

Said A. Karmi, M.D., F.A.C.S. Professor of Surgery and Urology, Director of Transplant Sciences, Department of Urology, George Washington University Medical Center, Washington, D.C.

Terry A. King, M.D. Assistant Clinical Professor of Surgery, Case-Western Reserve University School of Medicine; Head, Section of Peripheral Vascular Surgery, Mt. Sinai Medical Center, Cleveland, Ohio

Robert P. Leather, M.D., F.A.C.S. Professor of Surgery, Chief, Center Vascular Surgery Service, Department of Surgery, Albany Medical Center, Albany, New York

Herbert I. Machleder, M.D. Professor of Surgery, Vascular Surgery Section, Department of Surgery, UCLA School of Medicine, Los Angeles, California

Mary H. McGrath, M.D. Associate Professor of Surgery, Director, Division of Plastic and Reconstructive Surgery, Department of Surgery, George Washington University Medical Center, Washington, D.C.

Franz L. Moll, M.D.† Vascular Research Fellow, Department of Surgery, The Center for the Health Sciences, UCLA School of Medicine, Los Angeles, California

Anselmo A. Nunez, M.D.++ Fellow, Division of Vascular Surgery, Montefiore Medical Center-Albert Einstein College of Medicine, New York, New York

Patrick J. O'Hara, M.D. Staff Surgeon, Department of Vascular Surgery, The Cleveland Clinic Foundation, Cleveland, Ohio

Paul M. Orecchia, M.D. Assistant Professor of Surgery, Uniformed Services University of the Health Sciences, Bethesda, Maryland; Assistant Chief, Peripheral Vascular Surgery Service, Walter Reed Army Medical Center, Washington, D.C.

Norman M. Rich, M.D., F.A.C.S. Professor and Chairman, Department of Surgery, Uniformed Services University of the Health Sciences, Bethesda, Maryland; Peripheral Vascular Surgery Service, Walter Reed Army Medical Center, Washington, D.C.

Jeffrey R. Rubin, M.D. Assistant Professor of Surgery, Case-Western Reserve University; Chief, Section of Vascular Surgery, Veterans Administration Medical Center, Cleveland, Ohio

James M. Salander, M.D., F.A.C.S. Associate Professor of Surgery, Uniformed Services University of the Health Sciences, Bethesda, Maryland; Chief, Peripheral Vascular Surgery Service, Walter Reed Army Medical Center, Washington, D.C.

Thomas H. Schwarcz, M.D.†† Fellow in Peripheral Vascular Surgery, Section of Peripheral Vascular Surgery, Loyola University Medical Center, Maywood, Illinois

Dhiraj M. Shah, M.D. Professor of Surgery, Department of Surgery, Albany Medical Center, Albany, New York

---

Present affiliation:

† Surgeon, Department of Surgery, Medical Center Alkmaar, Alkmaar, The Netherlands

++Assistant Professor of Clinical Surgery, Department of Surgery, University of Miami School of Medicine, Miami, Florida

††Assistant Professor of Surgery, Division of Vascular Surgery, University of Illinois College of Medicine at Chicago, Chicago, Illinois

Anton Sidawy, M.D. Chief of Vascular Surgery, Veterans Administration Medical Center; Assistant Professor of Surgery, George Washington University Medical Center, Washington, D.C.

James C. Stanley, M.D. Professor of Surgery, Head, Division of Peripheral Vascular Surgery, Department of Surgery, University of Michigan Medical School, Ann Arbor, Michigan

Hugh H. Trout, III, M.D. Professor of Surgery, Department of Surgery, George Washington University Medical Center, Washington, D.C.

Frank J. Veith, M.D. Chief of Vascular Surgery, Department of Surgery, Montefiore Medical Center-Albert Einstein College of Medicine, New York, New York

J. Leonel Villavicencio, M.D., V.S., F.A.C.S. Professor of Surgery, Department of Surgery, F. Edward Herbert School of Medicine, Uniformed Services University of the Health Sciences, Bethesda, Maryland; Director of Venous and Lymphatic Surgical Clinic, Walter Reed Army Medical Center, Washington, D.C.

Contents

CONTENTS

1

Reoperative Vascular Surgery
General Considerations

RALPH G. DePALMA and HUGH H. TROUT, III
George Washington University Medical Center, Washington, D.C.

> The peculiarity of vascular surgery lies, above all, in being the surgery of ruins.
>
> *J. Cid dos Santos*

Ideal surgical interventions should achieve definitive end points or, at the least, yield long-term amelioration of symptoms or disease. One of the founders of vascular surgery (1) spoke about the unique problems of patients with vascular disease that vitiate the benefits of initially successful operations. In spite of this pessimism, DeBakey and associates (2) early grasped the segmental nature of atherosclerosis; their recognition of this pattern of atherosclerotic involvement was critical in developing elegant modern vascular surgical techniques. Vascular operations are based on the fact that proximal and distal arteries are usually sufficiently free of disease to allow reconstruction either by endarterectomy or bypass. With advances in angiography, noninvasive laboratory testing, anesthesia, and perioperative care, vascular surgeons have become less pessimistic and more aggressive. We now recognize problems predisposing to reconstructive failures and are willing to reoperate to address these problems. Recent studies (3) of the durability of vascular operations indicate qualified optimism, particularly if late mortality due to progression of atherosclerosis is to be controlled. Some vascular surgeons have developed research interests in atherosclerosis, and others have documented the late mortality of patients mainly due to coronary artery disease

(4-11). Aggressive prophylactic coronary artery surgery has been advocated in conjunction with peripheral reconstructive procedures (12,13), and strong evidence for enhanced survival with combined procedures has been summarized (14). Active risk factor intervention might ameliorate the course of atherosclerosis in indigenous vessels and possibly enhance graft durability (15). Recently, quantitative data about the cell physiology of the injured arterial wall (16,17) and vein grafts (18) promise better insight and perhaps ultimate control of processes promoting atherosclerosis or myointimal change.

Important causes for reoperations include atherosclerosis or degenerative changes in vascular grafts and indigenous arteries, either proximal or distal to reconstructed segments (3). Related, but not identical, problems are juxta-anastomotic myointimal hyperplasia and diffuse or localized myointimal hyperplasia affecting vein grafts or endarterectomy sites. We are still not clear about the etiology or the spectrum of cellular changes comprising these two entities. To minimize graft thrombogenicity, much still needs to be learned about the interaction of graft and host vessel compliance as well as understanding the mechanical and biological characteristics of different grafts. Infection and suture failure, with concomitant hemorrhage or thrombosis, are complications that require reoperative intervention both early and late. In a broad sense, organ rejection after transplantation is a vascular failure; the response is associated with platelet accumulation in the graft aggregating on vascular endothelial cells (19).

The dramatic growth of vascular surgery in the last three decades attests to its immediate efficacy for management of almost all arterial lesions. In contrast to pharmaceutical treatment, surgical interventions reconstitute normal vascular function, restoring pulsatile flow and eliminating local thrombotic or aneurysmal change. Increased life expectancy is clear, for example, after abdominal aortic aneurysm repair (20,21) or after bypass for left main coronary artery or triple vessel coronary disease (22). Though prolonged life expectancy after other arterial reconstructions is not as readily documented, it is apparent that quality of life is frequently improved. Nonetheless, there remain many challenges for study and improvement. We need to know whether or not established atherosclerosis can be ameliorated and whether or not the durability of particular reconstructions can be enhanced. Vascular surgeons are now clearly alert to the need for surgical reintervention in the same vascular bed to prolong graft function or at other sites to prolong life. The widespread application and successful results of reoperations stimulated this book, which focuses on problems presented by particular reoperative procedures. This chapter reviews the incidence of common vascular reoperations, measures that might retard atherosclerosis progression, and examines general principles that might reduce the need for reoperation.

Incidence of Reoperative Surgery

In 1975, a regional society of vascular surgery was founded in Cleveland to monitor the quality of surgical care (23). As part of an effort to achieve a high standard of surgical care for patients with vascular disease, the society required that continued membership be based on an annual review of performance and objective peer review accomplished through the use of data processed by a computer registry. Dr. Alfred W. Humphries was one of the founders and the first president of the society; his interest in computers, support by the vascular surgical community, and grants from the Cleveland Foundation resulted in a computerized registry by 1978. The founding members entered data for personal cases dating back to 1975, and this registry soon produced information summarizing a broad range of vascular experiences in the metropolitan area (24-27).

For this chapter, the registry supplied data* from 28,707 operations on 25,555 patients, performed by society members since 1975 and entered into the computer up to January 1985. These data give a first approximation of incidence of reoperative problems. There were 7054 total primary operations for carotid disease; reoperations on the same side were done in 207 patients, or 2.9%. The data for aortoiliac disease included 4697 occlusive or aneurysmal reconstructions; further refinement would be necessary to discern differences between reoperations done for each procedure. Probably, more reoperations were done for occlusive rather than aneurysmal disease. Within the interval studied, 15.7% of aortofemoral or aortoiliac bypasses required reoperation. Reoperation was needed in 28.3% of 611 femorofemoral bypasses, and among 193 axillofemoral bypasses, a startling 86% of patients required reoperation. Presumably "extra-anatomic" bypasses were done mainly in high risk patients for occlusive disease. Among 2682 femoropopliteal or profundoplasty (i.e., infrainguinal) procedures, 46.3% of patients required reoperation. Overall, among 25,555 patients undergoing primary vascular operations, 3152 (12%) required additional vascular procedures for the same problem that caused the first operation to be performed. Fully 10%

---

*We wish to thank Joseph C. Avellone for contributing data from the Cleveland Vascular Society.

(2598) of all patients required at least another additional operation; however, the reoperation rate decreased markedly after the third intervention. Only 1.7% had two additional operations, 0.3% had three additional operations, and 34 patients (0.12%) had four or more additional operations.

These incidences do not take into account differential death rates, atherosclerotic risk factors, anatomic patterns of vascular disease, or failure to detect recurrence. The data do call attention to a need to analyze further factors predisposing to reoperation (e.g., a comprehensive analysis of host risk factors, choice of graft or technique, and other variables that could be obtained from this data base). The amount of information needed to answer detailed questions often lies beyond the scope of any individual or even group practice experience, emphasizing the value of this type of registry. For example, an interesting fact is that reoperations were not always done by the same surgeon. Among the 207 carotid reoperations in the Cleveland registry, 35% were done by different surgeons; similarly, 267 (36%) of 737 of aortoiliac femoral reoperations were performed by different area surgeons.

A review of the literature dealing with recurrent disease yields rather similar reoperative incidences. Redo surgery is distinct from disease recurrence; the latter depends on the sensitivity of methods used to detect recurrence. Other factors bearing on the incidence of recurrence include the diligence with which patients are reexamined, the continuance of cigarette smoking and other atherosclerotic risk factors, and the population examined (e.g., whether predominantly private or service patients). It is useful to review selected literature dealing with the durability of three major reconstructions: carotid endarterectomy, reconstructions for aortoiliac disease, and femoropopliteal bypass.

Carotid endarterectomy is the most common operation performed by vascular surgeons; it is estimated that 90,000 to 100,000 of these procedures are performed each year (28). In reports describing recurrent lesions detected by angiography, three large series (29-31) revealed incidences ranging from 1.2 to 3.6% with similar reoperation rates. All of these patients were symptomatic, and angiograms were obtained in response to recurrent symptoms. All underwent reoperation. Later studies (32-38) using noninvasive testing reported recurrence rates ranging from 8.8 to 14.8%. Interestingly, in these series, when reported, the reoperative rate ranged from 2.3 to 2.6%, similar to both the Cleveland Registry data and the other operative series (29-31). In general, the reoperative mortality (3.1%) and stroke (1.5%) rate are similar to those observed after the patient's first carotid endarterectomy. Early recurrences (i.e., within the first 2 postoperative years) were more likely to be due to myointimal hyperplasia, whereas the pathology of late recurrences was more likely to be characteristic of atherosclerosis (39). In a review of 29 patients, Claggett and associates (40) showed that continued cigarette smoking was associated with recurrence of carotid lesions, while O'Donnell and co-workers (41) linked noninvasively discovered carotid lesion recurrences to hyperlipidemia in 276 carotid bifurcations followed up to 15 years. Duplex scanning has shown a startlingly high incidence of recurrent or residual lesions (42); some recurrent lesions occurring early in the postoperative period appeared to regress when observed by serial duplex scanning (43). Reoperation, therefore, was not based on noninvasive observations alone. Rather, recurrent symptoms dictated a need for reoperation after carotid endarterectomy.

Studies of the natural history of bilateral aortoiliac or aortofemoral reconstructions for lower extremity ischemia revealed cumulative 10 year patency rates ranging from 66 to 79% in two large series (44,45). A morphologic determinant of failure of aortofemoral bypass was simultaneous lesions, producing stenoses of the profunda femoris artery and tibial trifurcation vessels (44). Recent operative mortality of this procedure ranged from 2.5 to 3%, with a cumulative lower extremity salvage rate of 85%. Crawford and associates (45) noted the long-term survival of these patients in contrast to patients with femoropopliteal disease. This phenomenon perhaps indicates a difference in cardiac prognosis for those patients in whom the aorta is the major locus of atherosclerotic disease compared with those with involvement of the trifurcation of the popliteal artery (46). After 10 years, half of the patients in Crawford's series (45) were alive. The most common cause of reconstructive failure in these patients was downstream atherosclerosis, and this resulted in reoperation rates of 8 to 10%. The most important risk factor associated with thrombosis of an aortofemoral limb was shown to be continued cigarette smoking (47-49). This risk factor appears to be particularly potent in patients with occlusive as opposed to aneurysmal disease.

The limits of effectiveness of femoropopliteal bypass are difficult to assess for several reasons. Atherosclerotic involvement of the infrainguinal arteries is quite varied, and continued evolution of new techniques of revascularization and new grafts render concurrent comparison of these procedures difficult. It has become apparent, however, that in situ vein bypass grafting below knee to tibial vessels yielded cumulative long-term patency results up to 70.4% at 3 years (50). The limits of conventional autogenous reverse grafting were estimated in 1975 by Szilagyi and associates (51). Structural quality of vein grafts was found to be of decisive importance. A patency half-life of 10.5 years was found with good and excellent grafts; with fair and poor veins, the patency half-life was 6 months. With femoral-femoral or femoral-popliteal above knee operations, 5 year patency rates of 56 to 58% were obtained; 10 year patency rates were 48 and 44%, respectively. Cumulative patency rates of infrapopliteal bypasses were 37% at 5 years and 28% at 8 years. Though it is too soon to be certain, these long-term results appear to be substantially poorer than those anticipated with in situ vein bypasses. Late cumulative patency in diabetic and nondiabetic patients was equal. Review of autogenous venous bypass grafts 5 and 10 years later by DeWeese and Rob (7.8) exemplify studies of the natural history of patients with this distribution of disease. Mortality rates at 5 and 10 years were 48 and 73%, respectively, with 36% of deaths due to myocardial infarction. Actual patency of survivors was 59% at 5 years and 38% at 10 years.

The introduction of expanded polytetrafluoroethylene (PTFE) grafts and other venous substitutes extended the range of revascularization of the lower extremity, as did techniques of sequential grafting. In a randomized trial (52), PTFE grafts above the knee yielded results up to 30 months quite comparable with those from vein grafts. The use of PTFE grafts in selected cases to preserve autogenous venous tissue for coronary reconstruction or for more distal bypass became a provocative issue, as did treatment of claudication by femoropopliteal bypass. This operation is usually done for "critical ischemia," which requires a rigorous definition (53). It is difficult in a heterogeneous group of infrainguinal procedures to determine a single reoperative rate; however, 35 to 45% in 5 years is a reasonable estimate, which also correlates with the Cleveland experience. Overall, the femoral-popliteal or femorotibial reoperations restore patency in about half of the patients (54-56).

Each of these three vascular reconstructions (i.e., carotid, aortic, and infrainguinal) exhibit unique characteristics related to the graft choice, technical factors, and the natural history of atherosclerotic disease involving both the arteries, which prompted the initial reconstruction, as well as the remote vessels. The patterns of atherosclerotic involvement, the age of the patient, and an estimate of the rate of atherosclerosis progression are important in determining priorities for each individual. For example, the use of prosthetic grafts above the knee or extra-anatomic bypass grafts is perhaps more applicable to older or high risk patients. Risk factor intervention may be beneficial in minimizing carotid and aortoiliac reoperations, while failing infrainguinal procedures have not been as clearly linked to continued atherosclerotic risk factors (3).

Risk Factor Control After Vascular Reconstruction

Risk Factors

A "risk" factor for a disease exhibits a statistical and biologically plausible relationship to the disease in question. The risk factor almost always precedes the disease, but may coexist as well. The association will have a strong graded relationship to disease production and be related independently and directly to its onset. For example, there exist predictable quantitative relationships with the amount of cigarette smoking and cholesterol elevation to onset of symptomatic atherosclerotic disease. Along with hypertension and diabetes, these comprise the major risk factors exhibiting consistent and reproducible effects on atherosclerotic disease in western society (57).

It would appear logical to assume that risk factors are the same as etiologic or pathogenetic factors in disease production in a given individual, but this is not necessarily scientifically rigorous. Further, on the surface, it would appear that amelioration of risk factors might render atherosclerotic disease less severe and arterial reconstructions more durable. In fact, except for cessation of smoking (58,59), there is little clinical evidence showing that efforts to alter other risk factors enhances cumulative patency of peripheral reconstructions. Possible reasons for this discrepancy relate to the time frame in which peripheral reconstructions are viewed. In the main, older people undergo peripheral vascular reconstructions, and only modest reductions in risk factors (e.g., serum cholesterol level) were actually achieved clinically.

Cigarette Smoking

Cigarette smoking is the most pervasive risk factor predisposing to postoperative reconstructive failures after operations done for peripheral occlusive disease. This can be most clearly demonstrated in aortofemoral grafts (47,48). Aortofemoral graft failure is usually associated with progression of downstream atherosclerosis leading to sudden unilateral graft limb occlusion. Other factors include presence of false aneurysm, infection, and occasionally mechanical prosthetic failure (59), now fortunately rare. It is important to convince the patient to give up cigarette smoking before any reconstruction; compliance with this advice can be assessed by measurement of blood thiocyanate (60) or carboxyhemoglobin levels. Cigarette smokers changing to cigar or pipe smoking tend to inhale; if they are unable to discontinue smoking completely, they should at least not resume cigar or pipe smoking until the habit of smoke inhalation is under control. Biochemical testing will also aid in detecting whether the patient has adopted a pattern of inhaling tobacco smoke or continues to smoke cigarattes.

In a study of biochemical factors after peripheral reconstructions, Greenhalgh (59) concluded that there was little evidence to warrant dietary advice to enhance graft patency. It is clear, however, that elevated levels of low density lipoprotein (LDL) cholesterol cause progression of coronary disease, are associated with increased mortality and morbidity (61), and clearly affect 10 year survival after coronary bypass (62). In addition, hypercholesterolemia predisposes to clamp atheroma experimentally (63) and accelerates atherosclerosis after endothelial injury due to balloon embolectomy in humans (64). Since peripheral grafts are most often performed in the sixth and seventh decades of life, the majority of patients presenting for peripheral reconstruction do not exhibit frank lipid abnormalities and offer less opportunity for extended follow-up study. It is not known whether or not dietary intervention would have value in the late stages of disease while blood lipid levels are normal. Early cessation of smoking is most important, but hyperlipidemia should be detected and treated in younger persons (usually the fourth to fifth decades of life) who require reconstruction (65).

Lipid Reduction

When patients exhibit hypercholesterolemia or hypertriglyceridemia, dietary alterations are recommended as a first step. These dietary alterations consist of the following:

Meat: Only three meals a week or fewer should contain lean beef or lamb. Meat should be trimmed of visible fat. Pork and other fatty meats such as hot dogs, canned processed meats, cold cuts, and sausages should be eliminated completely.

Chicken without skin, veal, turkey, or fish is permitted in any amount. Shellfish of all kinds (shrimp, lobster, crab, etc.) are allowed. Even though they are high in cholesterol, these apparently do not elevate blood cholesterol.

Carbohydrates: Foods such as rice, potatoes, pasta, bread, and popcorn are allowed in moderation. The major concern with these is weight gain. There are two restrictions: (a) bread should be as high in fiber content as possible, thereby eliminating many commercial brands; (b) popcorn should be made at home with margarine flavoring (that served at the movies is not allowed because it usually is made with peanut or coconut oil).

Vegetables: A liberal intake of all kinds of vegetables is encouraged.

Dairy Products: No butter, eggs, or whole milk is allowed. "Second Nature" or "Eggbeaters" may be substituted for eggs.

Margarine and skim milk are allowed. Cheeses are limited to skim milk products such as cottage, ricotta, Greek or feta cheese.

Sugar: Sugar should be eliminated from the diet as much as possible. No desserts, candy, or soft drinks that contain sugar are allowed. The most common form of hyperlipidemia is related to sucrose intake.

Fruit: Whole natural fruits are recommended as substitutes for desserts high in sucrose content. Canned fruits that have been canned in sugar syrup are not permitted.

Beverages: Coffee is permitted in moderation. Tea and alcohol in moderation are permitted. Wine is allowed.

Cooking Oil: Oils such as olive, corn, or safflower are to be used for salad dressings and for cooking, instead of shortening.

Vitamin Supplements: A daily vitamin supplement containing 300 mg of ascorbic acid, vitamin A (5000 USP units), and vitamin B complex is advised.

A novel dietary approach recently reviewed (66) involves intake of fish and fish oils that supply eicosapentanoic acid and docasahexaenoic acids. Eskimos consume such diets and are apparently much less susceptible to vascular disease. Supplementation with fish oil fatty acids reduces total serum cholesterol and favorably increases high density lipoprotein fraction. These fats also appear to replace platelet membrane arachidonic acid, causing decreased platelet aggregation and increased bleeding time (67). The effects of such dietary alteration on the prevention and treatment of atherosclerosis require clinical trials.

In addition, there is popular interest among the lay public in intensive dietary and exercise programs to treat ischemic heart disease. One radical program is Pritikin's, which consists of a 10% fat diet, rigorously excluding salt, sugar, alcohol, and caffeine. Dietary protein is derived from plant sources, with the addition of skim milk and small amounts of fish or fowl. This diet minimizes fat consumption to 10% or less of the calories and is taught in a center. Smoking is not allowed. Reductions in average serum cholesterol levels from 236+9 to 179+6 mg/dl have been obtained with increased maximal work capacity in patients with ischemic heart disease (68). Combined with intensively supervised exercise programs, this regimen exerted a favorable effect on noninsulin-dependent diabetics (69). The long-term effects of aggressive dietary interventions on survival of grafts, surgical patients, and influence on the arterial wall need prospective evaluation. There are, however, experimental and epidemiologic data showing that reduction of lipid levels below certain thresholds (e.g., total cholesterol 140 mg/dl, which is much lower than the accepted normal level in the United States) is related to arrest and occasionally regression of atherosclerotic lesions (70).

Drug therapy with cholestyramine and/or lovastatin has also been shown to be effective in lowering low-density lipoprotein (LDL) cholesterol. Treatment with lovastatin and its analogs appears to offer considerable promise because of the few side effects and the substantial lowering of LDL cholesterol attained with their use (70a).

Antiplatelet Therapy

Aspirin and dipyridamole reduce platelet adherence to prosthetic vascular grafts (71-73). In only one study (74), however, has this phenomenon been related to enhanced prosthetic graft survival in man, and that study only reported a 12 month lifetable follow-up. Experimentally, inhibition by anti-platelet drugs of juxta-anastomotic intimal hyperplasia has been described in some animal models (75). Aspirin has a potential beneficial effect because it inhibits production of thromboxane A_2, a platelet aggregator, RDP Unfortunately, aspirin has a potentially deleterious effect in that it also inhibits endothelial cell production of prostacyclin. Prostacyclin is postulated to protect the intima by preventing further platelet adherence. The dosage and combination of aspirin and dipyridamole employed clinically have not been rationally based, but rather were chosen empirically. Experimental work in monkeys and rabbits in the senior author's laboratory showed that aspirin and dipyridamole in dosages of 13.5 mg/kg per day of aspirin and 15 mg/kg per day of dipyridamole accelerated development of dietarily induced atherosclerosis in rhesus monkeys (76,77) and inhibited the rate of endothelial regrowth on balloon-injured rabbit aortas (78). When endothelial regrowth was slowed, increased arterial wall thickening occurred beneath the more slowly growing endothelium (79). In fact, dipyridamole is mainly a coronary vasodilator and also has been shown to promote the proliferation of smooth muscle cells (80). Aspirin and dipyridamole did not appear to alter indium-111-labeled platelet adherence in recently endarterectomized carotid artery segments (81), but this negative study might have had methodologic problems. These experimental data indicate that much needs to be learned about the proper indications, choices, and doses of antiplatelet agents.

In one influential study (82-83), aspirin-dipyridamole, when initiated before operation, were shown to prolong coronary vein bypass patency. On the other hand, Mannick (84) reported no prolongation of femoral popliteal vein graft survival with aspirin-dipyridamole, although others (85) described an improved PTFE patency. A recent prospective study (86) using 650 mg of aspirin begun only 2 to 3 days postoperatively revealed no effect in prolonging patency of either vein or PTFE grafts. Key problems are consistent measurement of drug effects and dosage as well as timing in relation to use of antiplatelet agents. Measurement of changed platelet function during administration of platelet inhibitory drugs in human patients is difficult, and considerable individual variation exists. Aspirin affects platelet aggregation, bleeding time, and mediator release, but not platelet survival or adhesion. Dipyridamole affects platelet adhesion and survival, but not aggregation, bleeding time, or mediator release. Wecksler (87,88) and co-workers and Hirsch (89) provided illuminating summaries of the effects of these agents, which should be considered when long-term therapy is to be recommended. Recent data suggest that low daily doses of aspirin, in the range of 40 to 80 mg, selectively inhibit platelet function without impairing vascular prostacyclin synthesis. Dipyridamole appears to add nothing to measured platelet responses. In patients undergoing coronary bypass, there now exists a physiologic basis for advocating low dose aspirin in the prevention of arterial thrombotic events that might be generalized to patients receiving peripheral grafts. Determining the rationale and proper dosage of antiplatelet agents requires clinical trials in patients selected to control the variables of age, sex, graft placement, type of graft, and extent of atherosclerotic involvement.

Hypertension

Among all the risk factors, hypertension is most closely associated with carotid disease (90): more widespread treatment of hypertension has apparently resulted in a considerable reduction in the risk of stroke. Because patients with carotid disease and stroke are frequently hypertensive, it is important to treat hypertension after carotid endarterectomy. Hypertension is an important factor associated with late strokes after carotid endarterectomy (5), as well as in nonoperated patients with unoperated carotid stenoses (91). Elevated diastolic pressure is one also of the factors correlated with rupture of small abdominal aneurysms (92). It is rare for hypertension per se to cause graft failure, though occasionally severe hypertensive episodes (e.g., in excess of 250 mmHg) cause graft-suture line leaks or dehiscence of newly formed anastomoses.

Diabetes Mellitus

There is no evidence to suggest that rigid control of diabetes affects graft patency after successful infrainguinal reconstructions (50,51). Diabetics have a much-shortened life span, however, with a mortality rate of 92% compared with 65% in nondiabetic patients 10 years after femoropopliteal bypass (8). Diabetes exerts an unfavorable effect on the long-term patency of aortofemoral bypass (44) and seems to be associated with extensive atherosclerotic involvement of the profunda femoris artery and its branches (93). Diabetics also exhibit enhanced adherence of red cells to endothelium and other abnormalities that might lead to vascular complications (94). Compelling evidence for diabetic control comes from the transplantation experience where renal transplants done in poorly controlled diabetics deteriorate due to recurrence of the original small vessel renal disease. Pancreatic transplantation with physiologic regulation of blood sugar levels appears to prolong the life of renal transplant recipients, and regression of diabetic nephropathy has been documented (95).

Cardiac Transplants

After cardiac transplantation, control of risk factors predisposing to coronary atherosclerosis has been long recognized as a valid therapeutic objective. In 1968, Barnard (96) described severe coronary atherosclerosis in the cardiac allograft recovered after the death of his first patient who received a cardiac transplant. His patient had been hyperlipidemic with cholesterol levels ranging over 300 mg/dl. Shumway's group (97) has been among the leaders in recognizing graft coronary arteriosclerosis in human heart transplant recipients. The initial adverse event in this setting is postulated to be immune injury to the arterial endothelium, resulting in loss of endothelial integrity and exposure of thrombogenic surfaces. Griepp and associates (98) published a plan for the control of graft arteriosclerosis in human heart transplant patients, employing anticoagulation and antiplatelet measures, weight control, and a low cholesterol, low saturated fat diet. These efforts have resulted in significantly decreased incidence of arteriosclerosis in the coronary arteries of the transplanted hearts in the treated group.

Choice of Graft and Operative Technique

In 1973, Szilagyi and associates (99) described degenerative changes in femoropopliteal reversed saphenous vein grafts. At that time, he concluded that: "Atherosclerosis, in particular, appears to be an inevitable ultimate abnormality that overtakes these implants commonly and perhaps universally if they stay in situ long enough." Accrued statistical evidence of graft deterioration of 33% for reverse saphenous veins grafts at that time warranted this conclusion. Currently, with improved methods of vein preparation and harvesting (18) and the in situ vein bypass technique that minimizes both endothelial and adventitial damage (50), there might be a greater durability of saphenous vein grafts. Whether the in situ technique is absolutely necessary for enhanced vein graft patency or whether implantation in the subcutaneous position with optimal handling of reversed saphenous vein grafts will suffice is an important future issue.

In carotid reconstruction, a key question is whether or not patch angioplasty decreases the incidence of late occlusion due to myointimal fibrous change or recurrent atherosclerosis. As mentioned previously (39,40), continued cigarette smoking and hyperlipidemia are the most frequent risk factors associated with recurring carotid lesions. The long-term durability of patched versus nonpatched reconstructions, the optimal patch material, and the use of antiplatelet agents before and after carotid reconstruction are unresolved issues.

With aortoiliac or femoral reconstruction, technical factors in tissue handling of the large indigenous arteries are less demanding in the aorta than, for example, the distal reaches of the arteries of the lower extremity. In operations on the aorta and its major branches, high flow and relative lack of vascular myointimal responses are advantages. Infection is a lethal threat, and some experimental evidence (100) has indicated that Dacron velour knitted grafts were incorporated better and were more resistant to infection by bacterial challenge than were woven grafts. Knitted grafts, however, tend to bleed more at operation. In terms of long-term patency, grafts with knitted versus woven limbs implanted in the groin probably exhibit no difference. Woven Dacron grafts work well for reconstructions within the abdomen; when groin implantation is needed, the senior author prefers a knitted prosthetic limb to minimize the possibility of infection. Postoperative antibiotic therapy can be continued until graft incorporation has occurred. A recent report (101), as well as the data from the Cleveland registry, show that femorofemoral and axillofemoral bypasses more commonly require reoperations than do aortofemoral reconstructions. These bypasses should be selected for patients with aortic sepsis or who are inordinate risks for conventional reconstruction. An externally supported prosthesis may offer an advantage in the axillofemoral position, though this has not yet been proved.

The key element for long-term reconstructive durability is proper graft selection for particular patients and operative sites. Vascular conduits behave uniquely in different sites. As mentioned previously, polytetrafluorethylene grafts above the knee approximate vein grafts in durability. For coronary reconstruction, saphenous vein or internal mammary artery conduits are both durable, but there is a dominant advantage to the internal mammary artery. This choice was the most influential factor in long-term patient survival, preceded only by advanced age and impaired left ventricular function as reported in a recent 10 year survival study of primary myocardial revascularization (102). Vein graft atherosclerosis occurs in almost half of patients with coronary artery bypass grafts by the 10th postoperative year (103). Saphenous vein grafts in the aortorenal position sometimes present special problems and occasionally become aneurysmal, particularly when used in young people (15). When applicable, autogenous arterial grafts obtained from the internal iliac arteries or transaortic endarterectomy as recommended by Stoney and associates (104) may be better substitutes. Arterial autografts from endarterectomized occluded superficial femoral artery segments are also valuable options. This autogenous patch is particularly suitable for profundoplasty, and succeeds even in the presence of infection.

Finally, intelligent operative choices related to the pattern of atherosclerotic disease and age are critical. Patients with aneurysms or predominantly dilating large vessel disease offer much latitude in graft choice. With infrainguinal occlusive disease, the choice of an above-knee reconstruction versus a below-knee reconstruction or sequential grafting depends on whether or not ischemic tissue must be healed at the foot. Plantar ulcerations require distal delivery of pulsatile flow, while bypass to an isolated popliteal segment probably suffices in cases without tissue loss. In the lower extremity and elsewhere, graft length is important. Given adequate inflow and outflow, the shorter the graft, the greater the likelihood of long-term patency.

The surgeon must strive to minimize trauma to the arterial wall as well as to autogenous conduits. The muscular arteries of the extremities are particularly prone to development of surgically induced atheromatous lesions. The gentlest possible occlusive techniques should be employed to minimize damage to the endothelium and media of these highly reactive vessels. Indigenous arteries can be atraumatically occluded using vessel loops, gentle clamps, and internally inflated balloons. Even tourniquet occlusion of the entire limb has been suggested. Gentle occlusion of vein grafts can be obtained with finger pressure. Diseased arteries need to be opened precisely without disrupting tenuous intimal-medial attachments. Suture choice must be appropriate; the evolution of fine monofilament sutures has been an important advance. Anastomoses of the abdominal aorta, iliac arteries, and common femoral arteries require generous bites of arterial tissue through the healthy areas to fashion secure, hemodynamically efficient anastomoses. The graft can be tailored when aneurysmal or diseased tissue needs to be excluded. The inlay suture technique, using generous bites of 00 or 000 prolene, to ridges of aortic tissue as described by Crawford and Snyder (105) is advantageous. This method minimizes operating time and blood loss and provides secure immediate and long-term results. In contrast, smaller vessels and distal infrainguinal reconstructions often require magnification, micro-surgical technique, and axial illumination.

Atherosclerosis is the most common vascular disease encountered; how-ever, the surgeon should be alert for abnormalities in blood clotting (e.g., antithrombin-III deficiency (106) and other hypercoagulable states (107). Subsets of patients exist with connective tissue disorders needing accurate diagnosis and control to prevent progression of ischemic complications (108,109). The long-term management of aortoarteritis, giant cell arteritis, and Takayasu's disease requires periodic monitoring of sedimentation rate and steroid treatment to keep sedimentation rate near normal. These patients often die of complications related to carotid occlusion and hypertension, which might be postponed by surgery and meticulous medical control (108). It is also important to recognize that giant cell arteritis is associated with thoracic aortic aneurysms (110). To manage such patients, a diagnosis of the underlying disease must be obtained by arterial biopsy and appropriate im-munologic studies.

Whatever the etiology of vascular disorders, vascular surgeons recognize an obligation to treat and monitor for the duration of their life all patients with chronic vascular disease. For example, the most common associated factor in aneurysm formation is the history of another aneurysm (111). Many patients require another vascular operation for occlusive or embolic complications secondary to coronary or carotid atherosclerosis, especially carotid or coronary revascularization. In the first year after surgery, provision should be made for quarterly follow-up examinations to detect early technical problems. Annual examinations should then be arranged. At these exami-nations, inquiries are made about control of atherosclerotic risk factors, principally cigarette smoking, and new symptoms related to other vulnerable arterial segments are investigated. Routine noninvasive examinations include peripheral Doppler pressures and waveform analyses for extremity grafts. Probably all atherosclerotic patients would benefit from serial duplex carotid scans. Ultrasound and computerized axial tomography are noninvasive and useful to reexamine aortic reconstructions. If a new lesion is found, arterio-graphy should be recommended to delineate the extent of the new lesion and its relationship to a previously placed graft.

These follow-up examinations do not require inordinate time or complex arrangements. The patient is asked to report annually on the anniversary of his or her operation, a date that is usually remembered. Vascular surgeons performing annual postreconstructive examinations learn much about the durability of the reconstruction and disease progression. Most importantly, he or she will be able to intervene preemptively when objective evidence of deteriorating graft function is obtained, notably, a decrease in ankle pressure after a femoropopliteal bypass. Preemptive interventions in infrainguinal reconstructions promise better results than secondary operations after thrombosis has occurred (56,112,113). It is a simple matter to maintain a card file listing the names, addresses, and phone numbers of all patients operated by month. The patient or the referring physician is contacted when there is failure to report during an anniversary month. If the patient required reoperation elsewhere, a written follow-up may be obtained. As a result of conscientious efforts, vascular surgery during its brief history has become quite refined. Vascular surgeons enjoy a unique opportunity for lifelong study of innovative reconstructions and the efficacy of interventions to control a crippling and lethal disease.

References

1. Quoted by H.H.G. Eastcott, MB, FRCS, FACS Hon.
2. DeBakey ME, Crawford ES, Cooley DA, Morris GC Jr: Surgical considerations of occlusive disease of the abdominal aorta and iliac and femoral arteries: analysis of 302 cases. Ann Surg 148:306-324, 1958.
3. DePalma RG, Clowes AW: Intervention in atherosclerosis: a review for surgeons. Surgery 84:175-189, 1978.
4. DeBakey ME, Crawford ES, Cooley DA, Morris GC, Garrett HE, Fields WS: Cerebral arterial insufficiency: one to 11 year results following arterial reconstructive operations. Ann Surg 161:921-945, 1965.
5. Hertzer NR, Avison R: Cumulative stroke and survival ten years after carotid endarterectomy. J Vasc Surg 2:661-668, 1985.
6. Brown DW, Hollier LH, Pairolero PC, Kazmier FJ, McCready RA: Abdominal aortic aneurysm and coronary artery disease. Arch Surg 116:1484, 1981.
7. Deweese JA, Rob CG: Autogenous venous bypass grafts five years later. Ann Surg 174:346-356, 1971.
8. DeWeese JA, Rob CG: Autogenous venous grafts ten years later. Surgery 82:755-784, 1977.
9. Hertzer NR: Fatal myocardial infarctions following abdominal aortic aneurysm resection: three hundred and forty-three patients followed 6-11 years postoperatively. Ann Surg 192:667-673, 1980.
10. Hertzer NR: Fatal myocardial infarction following lower extremity revascularization; two hundred seventy three patients followed 6 to 11 postoperative years. Ann Surg 193:492, 1981.

11. Hertzer NR, Lees CD: Fatal myocardial infarction following carotid endarterectomy; 335 patients followed 6-11 years after operation. Ann Surg 194:212-218, 1981.

12. Hertzer NR, Loop FD, Taylor PC, Beven EG: Combined myocardial revascularization and carotid endarterectomy. J Thorac Cardiovasc Surg 84:572-589, 1983.

13. Hertzer NR, Beven EG, Young JR, O'Hara PJ, Ruschhaupf WF III, Graor RA, Dewolfe VG, Maljovec LC: Coronary artery disease in peripheral vascular patients. A classification of 1000 coronary angiograms and results of surgical management. Ann Surg 199:223-233, 1984.

14. DeBakey ME, Lawrie GM; combined coronary artery and peripheral vascular disease: recognition and treatment. J Vasc Surg 1:605-608, 1984.

15. DePalma RG: Atherosclerosis in vascular grafts. In: Paoletti and Gotto (Eds): Atherosclerosis Reviews, Volume 6. New York, 1979, Raven Press, pp. 147-177.

16. Clowes AW, Reidy MA, Clowes MM: Mechanisms of stenosis after arterial injury. Lab Invest 49:208-215, 1983.

17. Clowes AW, Clowes MM: Kinetics of cellular proliferation after arterial injury. II. Inhibition of smooth muscle growth by heparin. Lab Invest 52:611-616, 1985.

18. LoGerfo, FW, Haudenschild CC, Quist WC: A clinical technique for prevention of spasm and preservation of endothelium in saphenous vein grafts. Arch Surg 119:1212-1214, 1984.

19. vonWillebrand, E, Zola H, Hayry P: Thrombocyte aggregates in renal allografts. Transplantation 39:258-263, 1985.

20. Steinberg I, Tobier N: Study of 200 patients with abdominal aneurysms diagnosed by intravenous aortography; comparative longevity with and without aneurysmectomy. Circulation 35:630-535, 1965.

21. Szilagy DE, Smith RF, DeRusso FJ, Elliot JP, Sherrin FW: Contribution of abdominal aortic aneurysmectomy to prolongation of life. Ann Surg 164:678-699, 1966.

22. Takaro T, Hultgren HN, Lipton MJ, Detre KM: The V.A. Cooperative Randomized Study for Coronary Artery Occlusive Disease II. Subgroup with significant left main lesions. Circulation 54:107-117, 1976.

23. Avellone JC, Beven EG, Hertzer NR, Humphries AW, Plecha FR, Pories WJ, DePalma RG: A regional specialty as a model to monitor surgical care. JAMA 240:2177-2180, 1978.

24. Plecha RF, Avellone JC, Beven EG, DePalma RG, Hertzer NR: A computerized vascular registry: experience of the Cleveland Vascular Society. Surgery 86:826, 1979.

25. Hoffman M, Avellone JC, Plecha FR, Rhodes RS, Donovan DL, Beven EG, DePalma RG, Frisch JUA: Operation for ruptured abdominal

aortic aneurysms: a community-wide experience. Surgery 91:597-602, 1982.

26. Hertzer NR, Avellone JC, Farrell CJ, Plecha FR, Rhodes RS, Sharp WV, Wright GF: The risk of vascular surgery in a metropolitan community. J Vasc Surg 1:13-21, 1984.

27. Plecha FR, Bertin VJ, Plecha EJ, Avellone JC, Farrell CJ, Hertzer NR, Mayda J, Rhodes RS: The early results of vascular surgery in patients 75 years of age and older: an analysis of 3259 cases. J Vasc Surg 2:769-774, 1985.

28. Baker WH: 1984: Newspeak, doublethink, and vascular surgery. J Vasc Surg 2:745-748, 1985.

29. Cossman D, Callow AD, Stein A, Matsumoto G: Early restenosis after carotid endarterectomy. Arch Surg 113:275-278, 1978.

30. Stoney RJ, String ST: Recurrent carotid stenosis. Surgery 80:701-710, 1976.

31. Hertzer NR, Martinez BD, Beven EG: Recurrent stenosis after carotid endarterectomy. Surg Gynecol Obstet 149:360-364, 1979.

32. Baker WH, Hayes AC, Mahler D, Littooy FN: Durability of carotid endarterectomy. Surgery 94:112-115, 1983.

33. Cantelmo NL, Cutler BS, Wheeler HB, Herrmann JB, Cardullo PA: Noninvasive detection of carotid stenosis following endarterectomy. Arch Surg 116:1005-1008, 1981.

34. Coban MP, Kingston V, Shanik G: Stenosis following carotid endarterectomy. Arch Surg 119:1033-1035, 1984.

35. Kremen JE, Gee W, Kaupp HA, McDonald KM: Restenosis or occlusion after carotid endarterectomy. Arch Surg 1143:608-610, 1979.

36. Thomas M, Otic SM, Rush M, Zyroff J, Dilley RB, Bernstein EF: Recurrent carotid artery stenosis following endarterectomy. Ann. Surg. 200:74-79, 1984.

37. Turipseed WD, Berkoff HA, Crummy A: Postoperative occlusion after carotid endarterectomy. Arch Surg 115:573-574, 1980.

38. Zierler RE, Bandyk DF, Thiele BL, Strandness E, Jr: Carotid artery stenosis following endarterectomy. Arch Surg 117:1408-1415, 1982.

39. Das MB, Hertzer NR, Ratliffe NB, O'Hara PJ, Beven EG: Recurrent carotid stenosis: a five-year series of 65 reoperations. Ann Surg 202:28-35, 1985.

40. Claggett GP, Rich NM, McDonald PT, Salander JM, Youkery JR, Olson DW, Hutton JE: Etiologic factors for recurrent carotid stenosis. Surgery 93:313-318, 1983.

41. O'Donnell TF, Callow AD, Scott G, Shepard AD, Heggerick RUT, MacKey WC: Ultrasound characteristics of recurrent carotid artery disease: hypothesis explaining the low incidence of symptomatic recurrence. J Vasc Surg 2:26-41, 1985.

42. Keagy BA, Edrington RD, Poole MA, Johnson G: Incidence of recurrent or residual stenosis after carotid endarterectomy. Am J Surg 149: 722-725, 1985.

43. Nicholls SC, Phillips DJ, Bergelin BS, Beach KW, Priimozich BS, Strandness DE: Carotid endarterectomy: relationship of outcome to early restenosis. J Vasc Surg 2:375-381, 1985.

44. Malone JM, Moore WS, Goldstone J: The natural history of bilateral aortofemoral grafts for ischemia of the lower extremities. Arch Surg 110:1300-1306, 1975.

45. Crawford ES, Bomberger RA, Glaeser DH, Saleh SA, Russell WL: Aortoiliac occlusive diseases: factors influencing survival and function following reconstructive operation over a twenty five year period. Surgery 90: 1055-1067, 1981.

46. Kallero KS, Berquist D, Cederholm C, Jonsson D, Olsson PO, Takolander R: Late mortality and morbidity after arterial reconstruction: the influence of arteriosclerosis in popliteal artery trifurcation. J Vasc Surg 2:541-546, 1985.

47. Wray R, DePalma RG, Huban CA: Late occlusion of aortofemoral bypass grafts: influence of cigarette smoking. Surgery 70:969-973, 1971.

48. Robicsek KF, Daugherty HK, Mullen DC, Masters TNB, Narbay D, Sanger PW: The effect of continued cigarette smoking on the patency of synthetic grafts in Leriche syndrome. J Thorac Cardiovasc Surg 70: 107-113, 1975.

49. Hyde GL, McCready RA, Schwartz RW, Mattingly SS, Ernst CB: Durability of occluded aortofemoral limbs. Surgery 94:748-759, 1983.

50. Corson JD, Karmody AM, Shah DM, Naraynsingh MB, Young HL, Leather RP: In situ vein bypasses to distal tibial and limited outflow tracts for limb salvage. Surgery 84:756-763, 1984.

51. Szilagyi DE, Hageman JH, Smith RF, Elliot MP, Brown F, Dietz P: Autogenous vein grafting in femoropopliteal atherosclerosis: the limits of its effectiveness. Surgery 86:836-851, 1979.

52. Bergan JJ, Veith FJ, Bernhard VM, Yao JST, Flinn WF, Gupta SK, Scher LA, Samson RH, Towne JB: Randomization of autogenous vein and PTFE grafts in femoral distal reconstruction. Surgery 92:921-929, 1982.

53. Bell PRF, Charlesworth D, DePalma RG, Eastcott HHG, Ekloff B, Gruss JD, Jamieson CW: Editoral. The definition of critical ischemia of a limb. Br J Surg 69(suppl):S3-S5, 1982.

54. Veith FJ, Gupta S, Daly V: Management of early and late thrombosis of expanded polytetrafluoroethylene (PTFE) femoropopliteal bypass grafts: favorable prognosis with appropriate reoperation. Surgery 87: 581-587, 1980.

55. Flinn WR, Harris JP, Rudo ND, Bergan JJ, Yao JST: Results of repetitive distal revascularization. Surgery 91:566-572, 1982.

56. Whittemore AD, Clowes AW, Cough NP, Mannick JA: Secondary femoropopliteal reconstruction. Ann Surg 193:35-42, 1981.

57. Gordon T, Kannel WB: Predisposition to atherosclerosis in the head, heart and legs. The Framingham Study. JAMA 221:661-666, 1972.

58. Greenhalgh RM, Laing SP, Cole PV, Taylor GW: Smoking and arterial reconstruction. Br J Surg 68:605-607, 1981.

59. Greenhalgh RM: Mechanical and biochemical factors influencing arterial reconstruction. Ann R Coll Surg Engl 63:399-404, 1981.

60. Bujtts WC, Kuehneman M, Widdowson GM: Automated method for determining thiocyanate to distinguish smokers from nonsmokers. Clin Chem 20:1344-1348, 1974.

61. Gordon T, Castelli WP, Hjortand MC, Kannell WB, Dawber TR: Predicting coronary heart disease in middle aged and older patients. JAMA 238:497-499, 1977.

62. Cosgrove DM, Loop FD, Lytle BW, Gill CC, Golding LAR, Gibson C, Stewart RW, Taylor PC, Goormastic M: Determinants of 10-year survival after primary myocardial revascularization. Ann Surg 202:480-490, 1985.

63. DePalma RG, Chidi CC, Sternfeld WC, Koletsky S: Pathogenesis and prevention of trauma provoked atheromas. Surgery 82:429-437, 1977.

64. Chidi CC, DePalma RG: Atherogenic potential of the embolectomy catheter. Surgery 84:175-189, 1978.

65. Rosen AB, DePalma RG, Victor Y: Risk factors in peripheral atherosclerosis. Arch Surg 107:303-307, 1973.

66. Gotto AM: Lipids, lipoproteins and apoliproproteins: biological endpoints and means of intervention. In: Hegyeli RJ (Ed.): Atherosclerosis Reviews Volume 12, New York, Raven Press, 1984, pp. 87-101.

67. Lorenz R, Spengler U, Fischer S, Duhon J, Weber PC: Platelet function, thromboxane formation and blood pressure control during supplementation of the western diet with cod liver oil. Circulation 67:504-511, 1983.

68. Barnard RJ, Weber F, Weingarten W, Bennett CM, Pritikin R: Effects of intensive short term exercise and nutrition programs on patients with coronary heart disease. J Cardiac Rehab 1:99-103, 1981.

69. Barnard RJ, Lattimore L, Holly RG, Cherny S, Pritikin N: Response of noninsulin dependent diabetic patients to an intensive program of diet and exercise. Diabet Care 5:370-373, 1982.

70. DePalma RG: Management of atherosclerotic vascular disease. In: Wilson SE, Veith FJ, Hobson RW II, and Williams RA (eds.): Vascular Surgery: Principles and Practice. New York, McGraw-Hill (in press).

70a. The Lovastatin Study Group II: Therapeutic response to lovastatin

(Mevinalin) in nonfamilial Hypercholesterolemia, a multicenter study. JAMA 256: 2829-2834, 1986.

71. Oblath RW, Buckley FO Jr, Green RM, Schwartz SI, Deweese JA: Prevention of platelet aggregation and adherence to prosthetic vascular grafts by aspirin and dipyridamole. Surgery 84:37-44, 1978.

72. Feins RH, Roedersheimer R, Green RM, Deweese JA: Platelet aggregation inhibition in human umbilical vein grafts and negatively charged bovine heterografts. Surgery 85:395-399, 1979.

73. McCollum CN, Kester RC, Rajah SM, Learoyd P, Pepper M: Arterial graft maturation: the duration of thrombotic activity in Dacron aortobifemoral grafts measured by platelet and fibrinogen kinetics. Br J Surg 68:61-64, 1981.

74. Goldman M, Hall C, Dykes J, Hawker RJ, McCollum CN: Does ^{111}indium platelet deposition predict patency in prosthetic arterial grafts? Br J Surg 70:635-638, 1983.

75. Hagen P, Wang Z, Mikat EM, Hackel DB: Antiplatelet therapy reduces aortic intimal hyperplasia distal to small diameter vascular prostheses (PTFE) in nonhuman primates. Ann Surg 195:328-329, 1982.

76. DePalma RG, Bellkon EM, Manalo PM: Failure of antiplatelet agents to control dietary atherosclerosis. J Cardiovasc Surg 22:445-446, 1981.

77. Manalo-Sears P, DePalma RG, Bellon EM: Effect of antiplatelet agents on morphology of dietary induced atherosclerosis in rhesus monkeys. Am J Clin Pathol 78:280, 1982.

78. Bomberger RA, DePalma RG, Ambrose A, Manalo P: Aspirin and dipyridamole inhibit endothelial healing. Arch Surg 117:1459-1464, 1982.

79. Bomberger RA, Wilburn J, DePalma RG: Aspirin and dipyridamole increase intimal thickening after injury. Surg Forum 34:471-473.

80. Morisaki N, Stitts JM, Bartels-Tomei L, Milo GE, Panganamala RV, Cornwell DG: Dipyridamole: an antioxidant that promotes the proliferation of smooth muscle cells. Artery 11:88-107, 1982.

81. Lusby RJ, Ferrell LD, Englestad RL, Price DC, Lipton MJ, Stoney RJ: Vessel wall and indiuim-111-platelet response to carotid endarterectomy. Surgery 93:424-432, 1983.

82. Chesebro JH, Clements IP, Foster V, Elveback LR, Smith HC, Bardsley WT, Frye RI, Holmes DR Jr, Vlietstra RE, Pluth JR, Wallace RB, Puga FJ, Orszulak TA, Peihler JM, Schaff HV, Danielson GK: A platelet-inhibitor-drug trial in coronary artery bypass operations. N Engl J Med 307:73-78, 1982.

83. Chesebro JH, Foster V, Elveback LR, Clements IP, Smith HC, Holmes DR Jr, Bardsley WT, Pluth JR, Wallace RB, Puga FJ, Orszulak TA, Piehler JM, Danielson GK, Schaff HV, Frye RI: Effect of dipyridamole and aspirin on late vein graft patency after coronary bypass operations. N Engl J Med 310:209-214, 1984.

84. Mannick JA: Discussion of a paper. Surgery 92:1024, 1982.

85. Green RM, Roedersheimer LR, Deweese JA: Effects of aspirin and dipyridamole on expanded PTFE graft patency. Surgery 92:1016-1025, 1982.

86. Satiani B: A prospective randomized trial of aspirin in femoral popiteal and tibial bypass grafts. Angiology 36:608-616, 1985.

87. Wecksler BB: Arterial thrombosis, atherosclerosis and platelet activity: a reassessment of antiplatelet therapy. In: Hegyeli RJ (eds.): Atherosclerosis Reviews Volume 12, New York, Raven Press, 1984, pp. 39-50.

88. Wecksler BB, Kent JL, Rudolph D, Scherer PB, Levy DE: Effect of low dose aspirin on platelet function in patients with recent cerebral ischemia. Stroke 16:5-9, 1985.

89. Hirsch J: Progress review: the relationship between dose of aspirin, side effects and antithrombotic effectiveness. Stroke 16:1-4, 1985.

90. Nicholls ES, Johansen HL: Implications of changing trends in cerebrovascular and ischemic heart disease mortality (editorial). Stroke 14:153-156, 1983.

91. Moore DJ, Miles RD, Gooley NA, Sumner DS: Noninvasive assessment of stroke risk in asymptomatic and nonhemispheric patients with suspected carotid disease. Ann Surg 202:491-503, 1985.

92. Cronenwett JL, Murphy TF, Zelenock GB, Whitehouse WM, Lindenauer SM, Graham LM, Quint LE, Silver TM, Stanley JC: Actuarial analysis of variables associated with rupture of small abdominal aneurysms. Surgery 98:472-483, 1985.

93. King TA, DePalma RG, Rhodes RS: Diabetes mellitus and atherosclerotic involvement of the profunda femoris artery. Surg Gynecol Obstet 159:553-556, 1984.

94. Wautier JL, Paton RC, Wautier MP, Pintigny D, Abadie E, Passa P, Caen JP: Increased adherence of erythrocytes to epithelial cells in diabetes mellitus and its relation to vascular complications. N Engl J Med 305:237-242, 1981.

95. Sutherland DER, Goetz FC, Najarians JS: One hundred pancreas transplants at a single institution. Ann Surg 200:414-440, 1984.

96. Barnard CN: What have we learned about cardiac transplants? J Thorac Cardiovasc Surg 56:457-468, 1968.

97. Copeland JG, Griepp RB, Bieber CP, Billinghaus M, Schroeder JS, Hunt S, Mason J, Stinson EB, Shumway NE: Successful retransplantation of the human heart. J Thorac Cardiovasc Surg 73:242-247, 1977.

98. Griepp, RB, Stinson EB, Bieber CP, Rietz BA, Copeland JG, Oyer PE, Shumway NE: Control of graft arteriosclerosis in human heart transplant recipients. Surgery 81:202-219, 1977.

99. Szilagyi DE, Elliott JP, Hageman JH, Smith RF, Dalliolmo CA: Biologic fate of autogenous vein implants as arterial substitutes: clinical, angiographic and histopathologic observations in femoropopliteal operations for atherosclerosis. Ann Surg 178:232-246, 1973.

100. Roon HJ, Malone JM, Moore WS, Bean B, Campagna G: Bacteremic infectability: a function of vascular material and design. J Surg Res 22:489-498, 1977.

101. Donaldson MC, Louras JC, Bucknam CA: Axillofemoral bypass: a tool with a limited role. J. Vasc Surg (in press).

102. Cosgrove DM, Loop FD, Lytle BW, Gill CC, Goldring LR, Stewart RW, Taylor PC, Goormastic M: Determinants of 10 years survival after primary myocardial revascularization. Ann Surg 202:480-490, 1985.

103. Campeau L, Enjalbert M, Lesperance J, et al.: Atherosclerosis and late closure of aortocoronary saphenous vein grafts. Circulation 68 (suppl):1-7, 1983.

104. Stoney RJ: The arterial autograft. In: Rutherford RB (ed.): Vascular Surgery, Philadelphia, WB Saunders Company, 1985, pp. 378-381.

105. Crawford ES, Snyder DM: Thoracoabdominal aneurysm. In: Rutherford RB (ed.): Vascular Surgery, Philadelphia, WB Saunders Company, 1985, pp. 772-785.

106. Flinn WR, McDaniel MD, Yao JST, Fahey VA, Green D: Antithrombin III deficiency as a reflection of dynamic protein metabolism in patients undergoing vascular reconstruction. J Vasc Surg 1:888-895, 1984.

107. Towne JB, Bandyk DF, Hussey A, Tollack VT: Abnormal plasminogen: a genetically determined cause of hypercoagulability. J Vasc Surg 1:896-902, 1984.

108. DePalma RG, Moskowitz RW, Holden WD: Peripheral ischemia and collegen disease: clinical manifestations, diagnosis and management. Arch Surg 105:313-318, 1972.

109. Baker WH, Potthoff WP, Biller B, McCoyd K: Carotid artery thrombosis associated with lupus anticoagulant. Surgery 98:612-615, 1985.

110. Spence RK, Estella F, Gisser S, Schiffman R, Camision RC: Thoracic aortic aneurysm secondary to giant cell arteritis: a reappraisal of etiology, treatment and possible prevention. J Cardiovasc Surg 26: 492-495, 1980.

111. Crawford ES: Aortic aneurysm: a multifocal disease. Arch Surg 117: 1393-1400, 1982.

112. O'Mara CS, Flinn WR, Johnson ND, Bergan JJ, Yao JS: Recognition and surgical management of patent but hemodynamically failed arterial grafts. Ann Surg 194:467-476, 1981.

113.   Veith FJ, Weiser RK, Gupta SK, Ascer E, Scher LA, Samson RH,
       White-Flores JA, Sprayregen S: Diagnosis and management of failing
       lower extremity arterial reconstructions prior to graft occlusion. J
       Cardiovasc Surg 25:381-384, 1984.

2

Management of False Aneurysms in the Groin After Previous Vascular Procedures

WILLIAM E. EVANS and JAMES P. HAYES
St. Anthony Medical Center, Columbus, Ohio

The occurrence of anastomotic aneurysms after vascular reconstructive procedures continues despite the technical advances of the past two decades. The potential causative factors include suture (1,2) and graft materials, anastomatic tension (3), compliance mismatch (4), and healing complications (5). Endarterectomy, profundoplasty, or a combination of both procedures at the anastomotic site may further aggravate these factors (6).

Incidence and Etiology

The reported incidence of anastomotic aneurysms varies considerably (7-9). Anastomotic aneurysms most frequently occur in the femoral artery after reconstructive procedures in which the femoral artery is either the inflow or outflow site (7-9). In a recent review of 2500 femoral anastomoses (10), 72 (2.8%) anastomotic aneurysms were discovered in 57 patients (Table 1).

The time from initial reconstruction to anastomotic aneurysm occurrence varies with the presence or absence of sepsis (11). Generally, with sepsis, the aneurysm will occur in a few weeks to months, whereas in nonseptic cases, the interval can range from 1 to 16 years.

A pulsatile groin mass is the most common sign of a femoral anastomotic aneurysm (9,11). In 67% of our patients, this was the initial presentation of the aneurysm. Symptoms of graft occlusion were found in 8% and infection in 5%. The aneurysm was asymptomatic and found incidentally on physical examination at operation, or by angiography in 20% of the cases (Table 2) (10).

Table 1 Prior Arterial Reconstruction in 57 Patients

Procedure	No. of Patients
Aortofemoral bypass	
Occlusive disease	30
Aneurysmal disease	15
Femoral-popliteal tibial	8
Aorto-profunda-anterior tibial	1
Iliac-common femoral	1
Femoral embolectomy X 3	1

Source: From Ref. 10, used with permission

The primary causes of anastomotic aneurysm formation are arterial wall failure, suture failure, graft failure, and infection. Arterial wall failure is indicated by dehiscence of the anastomosis, with suture material being free of the host artery. Graft failure is indicated by a recognizable flaw in the graft material or by the suture material being free of the graft. Arterial wall failure was the finding in 71%, graft failure in 14%, suture failure in 7%, and infection in 7% of our cases in which a cause of aneurysm formation could be determined (10).

Table 2 Initial Presentation of 72 Aneurysms

Presentation	Number (%)
Pulsatile groin mass	48 (67)
Symptoms of graft occlusion	6 (8)
Infection	4 (5)
Asymptomatic (found at physical exam, angiography, or at operation)	14 (20)

Source: From Ref. 10, used with permission.

Arterial Wall

Arterial wall weakness is the leading cause of anastomotic aneurysm formation (9). It has been suggested (12) that disruption of the vasa vasorum may cause degenerative changes in the arterial wall leading to aneurysmal formation. Disruption of the vasa vasorum occurs in all types of vascular reconstructive procedures, and the overall incidence of anastomotic aneurysms is low. Therefore, vasa vasorum disruption must be questioned as a significant causative factor.

Collagen, which is the primary structural component responsible for arterial wall tensile strength, is reduced in true aneurysmal disease (13). In addition, the wall of the aneurysm is weakened by fragmentation and other changes within the fibrous network. For these reasons, it might be expected that more anastomotic aneurysms occur after reconstruction for aneurysmal rather than occlusive disease. However, no statistically significant difference in the rate of anastomotic aneurysm occurrence after reconstruction for occlusive or aneurysmal disease could be demonstrated in our patients (10).

Endarterectomy may weaken the arterial wall due to a reduction in tensile strength (3-6). The degree of arterial wall weakness caused by endarterectomy is difficult to assess (3). In general, the deeper the plane of dissection is, the weaker the wall will be (14). Care should be taken to ensure proper suture placement when constructing an anastomosis after endarterectomy (3,6,15).

Suture Junction

In the immediate postoperative period, all vascular anastomoses are entirely dependent on suture line integrity. In later years, the graft-artery junction is maintained by the suture line and by external fibrous bonding due to scarring. This fibrous tissue is not capable of resisting the stresses of pulsatile blood flow without the suture material.

The use of silk as a suture material has been implicated as a major cause of anastomotic disruption leading to aneurysm formation (8). This is due to the fact that the tensile strength of silk is reduced by 10 to 20% after 1 month and by almost 100% at 2 years (3). Although the use of silk as a suture material has been abandoned, anastomotic aneurysms continue to occur.

Prosthesis

Factors associated with the prosthesis contributing to aneurysm formation include compliance mismatch (14) between the graft and host artery, increased anastomotic tension due to insufficient graft length, uneven tension on the anastomosis as a result of beveling the graft, prosthetic deterioration, or an actual flaw in the graft material (3).

Infection

Infection and its effects on wound healing are potential causative factors in anastomotic aneurysm formation. The necrotizing effect of the septic process will eventually cause disintegration of the arterial wall, resulting in suture line disruption, bleeding, and eventual anastomotic aneurysm formation. Manifestations of a septic anastomotic aneurysm include intermittent bleeding from the groin area, hematoma formation, pus drainage, and lymphorrhea (11).

Technical Considerations

Surgical intervention is aimed at resection of the aneurysm and restoring the circulation to the affected extremity via repair of the defective anastomosis or bypassing the aneurysm. Elective repair before complications occur provides for the best result. In 72 cases of anastomotic aneurysm occurrence, repair was accomplished by the use of an interposition graft between the old graft and the profunda femoris artery in 57 patients (79%), ligation only in 7 (10%), anastomotic revision in 3 (4%), and resection and distal reconstruction in 2 (3%) (Table 3).

Table 3   Repair Technique

Technique	No. (%)
Interposition graft	57 (79.0)
Ligation only (unreconstructable vessels)	7 (10.0)
Anastomotic revision	3 (4.0)
Resection with femoral popliteal limb	2 (3.0)
Exision infected graft limb	1 (1.3)
Femoral-femoral crossover graft	1 (1.3)
Aortofemoral bypass graft replacement	1 (1.3)

Source: From Ref. 10, used with permission.

In those cases where an aortofemoral bypass (AFB) is the primary procedure, the preferred technique for aneurysm repair is the use of an interposition graft between the graft limb proximally and the profunda femoris artery distally. The old groin incision is used. The aneurysm is located by a combination of sharp and blunt dissections, and the aortofemoral limb is isolated (Fig. 1). After systemic heparinization, the graft limb is cross-clamped. The aneurysm is then opened, and the thrombus removed. Back-bleeding from the superficial femoral and profunda femoris arteries is controlled by the use of balloon catheters. Because the distal anastomosis is the most technically demanding, it is completed first. An appropriately sized, preclotted graft is slid over the occlusion catheters, and the distal anastomosis is completed (Fig. 2). If the superficial femoral and profunda orifices are both open, their common orifice can be incorporated in a single anastomosis. Once the distal anastomosis is completed, the catheters are removed and distal control is obtained by clamp placement above the anastomosis.

Attention is next turned to the proximal anastomosis. The limb of the AFB graft is trimmed, and the graft is sewn end-to-end (Fig. 3). Before completing the anastomosis, air and debris are blown free of the graft by backbleeding from the distal site and antegrade flushing from above. The anastomosis is then completed and flow to the extremity is reestablished.

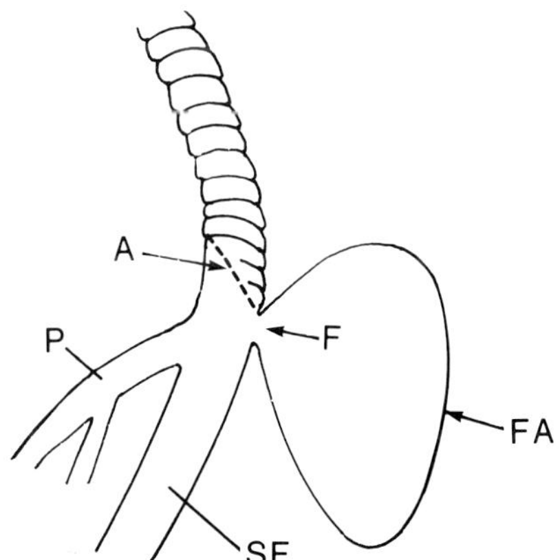

Figure 1 Breakdown at site of old anastomosis. (A) with development of fistula (F) and a false aneurysm (FA) at the level of the profunda (P) and superficial femoral (SF) arteries.

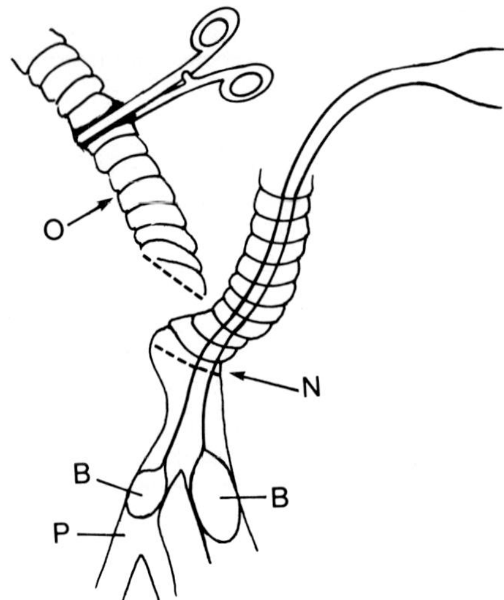

Figure 2 Disconnection of old graft (0) and anastomosis (N) of new graft over balloon catheters (B).

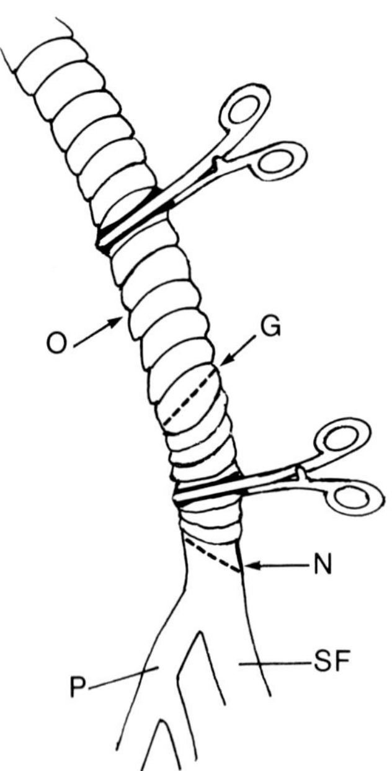

Figure 3 Old graft (0) trimmed and proximal anastomosis (G) constructed.

Graft infection should be ruled out as a cause of aneurysm formation. If graft infection is identified, then management should proceed appropriately. The safest course of action is removal of the infected graft and debridement of the infected and devitalized tissue. If revascularization is required, this can be accomplished by grafting through uninfected planes.

Results

Two (3.5%) patients died after aneurysm repair, both as a result of myocardial infection. Two amputations were required, one below the knee in a patient with no improvement of an ischemic extremity, and one above the knee in a patient developing ischemia after removal of an infected AFB graft limb. The 5 year survival rate after anastomotic repair is 49%.

Aneurysm recurrence has been a problem in only seven (9.7%) instances at times ranging from less than 1 month to up to 66 months after initial repair. Arterial wall failure was implicated as the cause in five and infection as the cause in two. Two patients died after secondary repair, both due to sepsis. The other five continue to be followed up and have had no further recurrence at up to 42 months after secondary repair (10%).

Conclusion

Many of the factors associated with anastomotic aneurysm formation are controllable by the surgeon. These include ensuring sufficient graft length, surgical asepsis to ensure wound healing, ligation of all transected lymphatics, and possibly limiting the use of endarterectomy (9). Compliance mismatch between the prosthesis and host artery is minimized when the graft/artery diameter ratio is about 1.4 (16).

Factors such as a structural defect in the native arterial wall are uncontrollable. Due to such uncontrollable factors, avoidance of all anastomotic aneurysms is probably not possible. However, successful treatment of them is.

References

1. Reul GJ Jr: The role of sutures in complications in vascular surgery and their relationship to pseudoaneurysm formation. In Bernhard VM, Towne JB (Eds): Complications in Vascular Surgery. New York, Grune & Stratton, 1980, pp. 615-638.

2. Starr DS, Weatherford SC, Lawrie GM, et al: Suture material as a factor in occurrence of anastomotic false aneurysms: an analysis of 26 cases. Arch Surg 114:412-415, 1979.
3. Courbier R, Larranaga J: Natural history and management of anastomotic aneurysms. In Bergan JJ, Yao JST (Eds): Aneurysms: Diagnosis and Treatment. New York, Grune & Stratton, 1982, pp. 567-580.
4. Sumner DS: Hemodynamics and pathophysiology of arterial disease. In Rutherford RB (Ed): Vascular Surgery. Philadelphia, WB Saunders, 1984, pp. 19-41.
5. Agrifoglio G, Costantini S, Zanetta M, et al: Infections and anastomotic false aneurysms in reconstructive vascular surgery. J Cardiovasc Surg 20:25-32, 1979.
6. Moore WS: Anastomotic aneurysms. In Rutherford RB (Ed): Vascular Surgery. Philadelphia, WB Saunders, 1984, pp. 821-827.
7. Satiani B, Kazmers M, Evans WE: Anastomotic arterial aneurysms: a continuing challenge. Ann Surg 192:674-682, 1980.
8. Stoney RJ, Albo FJ, Wylie EJ: False aneurysms occurring after arterial grafting operations. Am J Surg 110:153-161, 1965.
9. Szilagyi DE, Smith FR, Elliott JP, et al: Anastomotic aneurysms after vascular reconstruction: problems of incidence, etiology and treatment. Surgery 178:800-816, 1975.
10. Evans WE, Hayes JP, Vermilion BD: Anastomotic femoral false aneurysms. In Bernhard VM, Towne JB (Eds): Complications in Vascular Surgery, 2nd Edition. New York, Grune & Stratton, 1985, pp. 205-211. 205-211.
11. Haimovici H: Anastomotic aneurysms. In Haimovici H (Ed): Vascular Surgery Principles and Techniques, 2nd Edition. Norwalk, Connecticut, Appleton-Century-Crofts, 1984, pp. 745-762.
12. Benjamin HB: The importance of the vasa vasorum of the aorta. Surg Gynecol Obstet 110:224-230, 1960.
13. Sumner DS, Hokansen DE, Strandness DE Jr: Stress-strain characteristics and collagen-elastic content of abdominal aortic aneurysms. Surg Gynecol Obstet 130:459-466, 1970.
14. Stoney RJ: The technique of thromboendarterectomy. In Rutherford RB (Ed): Vascular Surgery. Philadelphia, WB Saunders, 1984, pp. 357-360.
15. Ochsner JF: Management of femoral pseudoaneurysms. Surg Clin North Am 62:431-440, 1982.
16. Paasche PE, Kinley CE, Donald FG, et al: Consideration of suture line stresses in the selection of synthetic grafts for implantation. J Biomech 6:253-258, 1973.

3

Graft Infections and Graft Enteric Fistulas and Erosions

HUGH H. TROUT, III
George Washington University Medical Center,
Washington, D.C.

When arterial prosthetic grafts become infected or communicate with the gastrointestinal tract (fistulas or erosions), their removal is almost always required. Three major problems, however, must be addressed in devising surgical treatment for these conditions. First, recurrent infection is common unless autogenous tissue is employed in the infected field or a remote prosthetic bypass is inserted in an uncontaminated field. Second, severe metabolic disturbances result when the lower extremities are rendered ischemic for prolonged intervals. Finally, days to months after the operation, the oversewn stump of the aorta may rupture into the duodenum or peritoneal cavity. This late rupture may relate to continued periaortic infection, aortic wall weakness caused by the earlier infection, or unfavorable hemodynamic stresses on the aortic stump below the renal arteries.

Most reports about patients with infected prostheses, prosthetic enteric erosions, or fistulas in the medical literature describe small numbers of patients with a multiplicity of problems, treatments, and results. Sufficient anecdotal data have now been accumulated, however, to make it possible to outline prudent management guidelines for these serious problems.

Definition of Terms

Infections of prosthetic grafts can be restricted to the body of the graft itself or can involve suture lines as well as the prosthesis. When suture lines are involved, there may be a fistula to overlying bowel, usually duodenum, at the proximal suture line of an abdominal aortic graft. These *graft enteric fistulas (GEF)* (also called *prosthetic enteric fistulas* or *secondary aortoenteric fistulas*) (Fig. 1) may result from pressure necrosis of overlying bowel, rupture of a pseudoaneurysm into adjacent bowel, or infection of the proximal prosthetic suture line with fistula formation into adjacent bowel.

Erosions of bowel next to vascular prostheses without suture line involvement have been called *paraprosthetic fistulas* (1). The term *graft enteric erosion* (GEE) (Fig. 2) succinctly describes the communication between the lumen of the bowel and the lumen of the prosthesis via the interstices of the prosthetic graft (2). This term will be used henceforth.

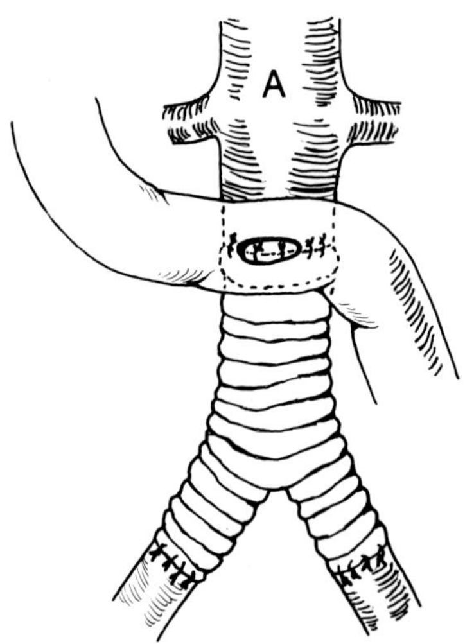

Graft Enteric Fistula

(G E F)

Figure 1   Graft enteric fistula. A communication between bowel and the arterial circulation at the level of an arterial prosthetic suture line. (Reproduced with permission from Ann Surg 199:669-683.)

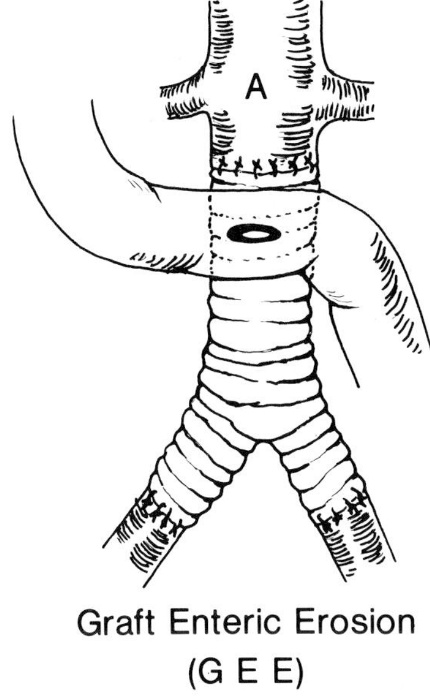

Graft Enteric Erosion
(G E E)

Figure 2   Graft enteric erosion. A communication between bowel and the interstices of an arterial prosthetic graft. The suture line is not involved. (Reproduced with permission from Ann Surg 199:669-683, 1984.)

Infected aortic grafts, graft enteric fistulas, and graft enteric erosions each are serious conditions that are usually treated similarly. In each instance, the graft is infected and acts as a foreign body. Treatment by any modality other than graft removal is unduly hazardous.

Incidence

As experience has been gained with improved operative techniques and use of perioperative systemic antibiotics (3-5), the incidence of arterial prosthetic infection has decreased to about 2%. Although groin incisions were formerly a frequent site of infection, with increasing experience in the proper techniques of groin incision and closure, there seems to be less of a difference in the incidence of graft infection between those with an aortoiliac graft and those with an aortofemoral graft (4,5). Nonetheless, the earlier experience with frequent groin infections should remind surgeons of the considerable care necessary when placing a graft in the groin.

Etiology

Patients with infected arterial prostheses or prosthetic enteric erosions or fistulas frequently have identifiable predisposing factors. These include multiple vascular procedures, wound complications, emergency aneurysmectomy, and technical problems (6).

Controversy exists about whether bacteremia with seeding of the intimal surface of the prosthesis is a frequent cause of graft infection. In dogs, systemic injection of bacteria is a common method of establishing an experimental model of prosthetic graft infection (7). The circumstantial evidence that systemic seeding of a prosthetic graft also can occur in human patients is the occasional prolonged interval between graft insertion and graft infection. Direct evidence is anecdotal, but convincing, in the rare graft infection caused by an unusual organism that had been earlier cultured from a remote site such as the urinary tract (8).

The most common etiology of graft infection, however, is believed to be local contamination at the time of graft insertion. Several factors contribute to this belief. First, many patients with graft infection had associated wound or technical problems at the time of graft insertion. Second, there does not seem to be a difference in the rate of infection in humans with knitted prosthetic grafts that are designed to allow tissue ingrowth and those with woven grafts that allow considerably less ingrowth. In humans, neither woven nor knitted grafts, however, will achieve complete endothelialization of the prosthetic inner surface (9). In contrast, in the experimental dog model when the graft lumen was reendothelialized, grafts were resistant to systemic bacteremic challenge, whereas grafts without extensive tissue ingrowth were susceptible to systemic bacterial (10). Third, the incidence of graft infection after procedures known to cause bacteremia (e.g., dental, colon, or urologic manipulations) is quite low. Finally, although infections of a recently inserted remote prosthetic bypass sometimes occur after removal of an infected graft (6-11), this occurrence is rare, even when systemic antibiotics are not used (12).

The debate as to whether bacteremia or technical factors account for the majority of graft infections is probably not important. Both obviously can be incriminated on occasion, and measures that are designed to prevent either should be aggressively employed. Great care should be given to maneuvers designed to prevent graft infection at the time of original graft insertion. In addition, in patients with prosthetic arterial grafts, prophylactic antibiotics should be used when bacteremia is anticipated.

Location

With infected aortic prostheses, there is a predilection for suture line involvement, but the graft itself may be the sole site of infection or present in combination with an enteroprosthetic erosion. Also, as noted, the groin is a common site of graft infection, and most often seems related to early postoperative wound complications including hematomas, infection, or seromas at this site.

Organisms

Staphylococcus aureus is cultured in amost 50% of patients with prosthetic graft infections. *Escherichia coli, S. albus, Pseudomonas, Klebsiella,* and *Proteus* account for most of the remainder, and range from 18% for *E. coli* to 4% for *Proteus* (2). The enteric prosthetic erosions and fistulas usually culture enteric pathogens such as *E. coli, Enterococcus, Bacteroides,* and *Streptococcus* (13). These data suggest that the prophylactic antibiotic to be administered before prosthetic graft insertion should be selected to be effective against both gram-positive and gram-negative organisms. Particular attention should be given to choosing a drug with effective staphylococcal prophylaxis.

Diagnosis

Most prosthetic graft infections in the groin present with a mass, erythema, or spontaneous drainage (6). Infections involving the proximal portions of prosthetic bifurcation grafts may present with pseudoaneurysm formation, local hemorrhage, or silent graft occlusion (6,14). Systemic sepsis can also occur, though most often it is associated with graft enteric erosions or fistulas. The most frequent mode of presentation in patients with a graft enteric erosion or fistula is either hematemesis or melena followed by sepsis, abdominal pain, or hematochezia (13).

Diagnosis of a superficial infected prosthetic arterial graft is usually apparent by simple physical examination. When the suprainguinal portion of an aortic bifurcation graft is solely involved, however, the diagnosis of an infected prosthesis can be difficult. Gallium scanning (15), labeled leukocyte scanning (16,17), computed tomographic (CT) scanning (18,19) and magnetic resonance imaging (MRI) have all been occasionally useful. Unfortunately, no diagnostic test has yet proved to be highly sensitive in detecting these proximal aortic graft infections. Accordingly, patients with arterial prostheses who develop unexplained fever must be repeatedly retested in a search for an occult graft infection. Occasionally, the definitive diagnosis can only be made by exploratory celiotomy.

Patients with graft enteric fistulas (GEF) involving the proximal suture line often present initially with an episode of brisk upper gastrointestinal (GI) bleeding, which tends to slow or stop for a short period. This presents a serious problem. If untreated, the GEF will enlarge and massive uncontrollable bleeding will occur. Accordingly, after the "herald bleed," the diagnostic test of choice is endoscopy in an attempt to visualize the graft or suture line as well as to rule out other causes of upper GI bleeding such as varices, Mallory-Weiss tears, and gastric and duodenal ulcerations. In contrast, patients with graft enteric erosions (GEE) present with sepsis, hematochezia, melena, or anemia, but not with massive hemorrhage (13). The differentiation between a GEF and a GEE is important only in that patients with GEE will not have sudden massive blood loss; thus, a carefully planned and executed operative procedure may be possible in contradistinction to the hurried procedure necessary in the patient with continued rapid blood loss through a GEF.

The diagnosis of GEF or GEE may be obscure even after the full range of diagnostic tests have been performed; abdominal exploration may be required when diagnostic uncertainty remains (see the section on "Modest Bleeding from Prosthetic Enteric Erosion or Fistula"). All patients with arterial prosthetic grafts who exhibit evidence of sepsis or bleeding should be suspected of having a graft infection, a graft enteric fistula, or a graft enteric erosion. If abdominal exploration is performed, all bowel must be dissected away from the entire length of the prosthetic graft before the diagnosis of infection, fistula, or erosion can be excluded. This is particularly so in patients with graft enteric fistula or erosion because obvious inflammation or a mass rarely exists. Only after the duodenum is dissected free will the communication be recognized.

Prevention

Most prosthetic infections, fistulas, and erosions can be attributed to multiple or emergent vascular procedures or to technical problems during the operative procedure. General preventive measures that have been demonstrated to be beneficial include preoperative showering with an antiseptic soap (20), not shaving rather than shaving the operative site the night before operation (20), and avoidance, when possible, of operating on patients with remote sites of

infection such as urinary or respiratory tract (21). Brief preoperative hospital-
ization (20), use of porvidine-iodine scrub for operative preparation (22), and
use of prophylactic antibiotics (22) have also proved beneficial.

Bunt (2) discussed operative preventive measures that have been advocated
but not yet proven. Among those I think important are closure of the old
aneurysmal aortic wall over a newly inserted graft and careful closure of the
retroperitoneum to separate bowel from the prosthetic graft. An end-to-end
anastomosis at the proximal suture line is usually the preferred technique
because the flow characteristics may be slightly better. Also, the proximal
suture line can then be covered with a cuff of the Dacron graft. This step may
lessen the incidence of GEF; if complications occur, perhaps a more easily
controllable GEE will develop rather than a GEF. These views are strictly
impressions, however. No convincing data exist that imply that a Dacron cuff
is beneficial or that the end-to-end approach confers any substantial
advantage over an end-to-side anastomosis—either hemodynamically or in
reducing the incidence of subsequent prosthetic infection, erosion, or fistula
(23). When an end-to-side anastomosis is performed, the angle of the
anastomosis should be acute so as to minimize hemodynamic disturbances
and the amount of anterior bowing of the prosthetic graft. In some cases,
omentum may be placed around the proximal suture line, but this should not
be routinely necessary provided that the anastomoses and retroperitoneal
flaps are fashioned with care. Finally, when treating aneurysmal disease, distal
anastomoses are constructed within the abdomen unless there is substantial
external iliac occlusive disease. In patients with occlusive disease, however,
the distal limbs of the aortic bifurcation graft are usually attached to the
femoral arteries due to the distribution of atherosclerosis.

Though some have reported an increased incidence of graft infection when
groin incisions are used, that has not been my experience. Groin infections
can be markedly reduced by not using an electrocautery, by dividing and
ligating all structures below Scarpa's fascia, by the frequent use of antibiotic
irrigation during the operation, and by careful closure using three layers of
absorbable synthetic sutures in the subcutaneous tissues in a running fashion
followed by a subcuticular skin closure and an occlusive dressing left in place
at least 72 hours. These are all anecdotal impressions, and one or more of
these measures may not be necessary. From this experience and that of
others, however, one fact seems indisputable: groin incisions, if cavalierly
approached, can result in tragedy. Accordingly, the senior surgeon should be
intimately involved both in the making as well as the closing of these
incisions.

General Principles

Management

Treatment of patients with infected arteries or arterial prostheses should be tailored to the location and type of infection as well as to the condition of the patient. In devising a management plan, however, the three principles mentioned earlier should be observed.

Aortic Stump Disruption

This is a major cause of death in patients with infected prostheses or prosthetic enteric fistulas. It usually occurs within 2 to 3 weeks after the operative procedure and is almost always fatal. The best way of protecting the aortic stump is not yet known. Varying techniques of closure have been advocated using monofilament sutures (24), staples (25), omentum (26), prevertebral fascia (27), reshaping of the distal aorta by means of an inverted V closure (28), or covering of the aortic stump with a jejunal patch (29). This last technique consists of stripping the mucosa from a short segment of isolated and well vascularized jejunum. The remaining seromuscular jejunum is then sutured over the aortic stump, providing a well vascularized seromuscular covering for the weakened and possibly still infected distal aortic stump. Though I have not had experience with this technique, the experimental and few clinical results have been sufficiently impressive to warrant expanded investigation of this method. To achieve stump closure, Reilly and co-workers (6) suggest that transient clamping of the aorta above the renal or celiac arteries might occasionally be necessary. They indicated that reimplantation of the renal arteries to a higher aortic level or hepato-right renal or spleno-left renal anastomoses may be required to allow aortic closure up to the level of the superior mesenteric artery. Regardless of the methods employed, adequate debridement of all infected tissue in the area of the infrarenal aorta is mandatory if aortic stump disruption is to be avoided.

Choice of Graft Material

There are experimental data in dogs that suggest that when prophylactic antibiotics are not used, Dacron grafts resist infection induced by intravenous bolus injections of *S. aureus* better than do polytetrafluoroethylene (PTFE) grafts (10). Similarly, investigative studies (30) show a superiority of knitted and velour Dacron grafts over woven Dacron grafts when challenged with percutaneous *S. aureus* 1 month after insertion in dogs.

In contrast, however, there are no human clinical data to suggest that any differences exist among woven, knitted, velour, or PTFE grafts in their propensity to become infected. Moreover, there are numerous anecdotal human clinical reports (31,32) of infected and exposed PTFE grafts healing with local treatment; this is only occasionally reported with Dacron.

In the future, bonding of antibiotics or bacteria-resistant surfaces to prostheses may prove beneficial (33,34). At present, in all likelihood, choice of graft material at the primary operation should be based on patency data rather than theoretical concerns about possible subsequent graft infection. In secondary operations, when choosing the type of graft to be used in the setting of prosthetic infection, erosion, or fistula, if an in situ graft is preferred, then autogenous material is the only acceptable option (see the following discussion). If a remote bypass is planned, good results can be anticipated with Dacron or PTFE. My current choice is PTFE because of its tendency to heal local subcutaneous infections and because it will remain hemostatic, whereas Dacron may become porous if coagulopathies develop during or after subsequent infected graft removal.

Treatment Options

No Treatment

Regardless of whether the patient has a prosthetic infection, erosion, or fistula, the decision not to treat is almost always fatal because of eventual exsanguination.

Local Treatment

Local antibiotic irrigations may be of value when the infection is localized to subcutaneous areas (such as the groin) where local care can be easily directed and rupture can probably be controlled (24,35). Others (36) have successfully used muscle flaps to cover exposed grafts in the groin. With intra-abdominal arterial or graft infections, however, it seems unduly dangerous to rely on local treatment measures alone. Despite rare anecdotal reports of success, most patients with aortic graft infections, enteric erosions, or fistulas have died when local treatment has been employed.

Graft Excision and Drainage

Bunt (2,13) summarized most of the cases reported in the English literature treated by graft excision and drainage. This treatment resulted in a 37%

mortality rate and a 28% amputation rate in patients with aortoiliofemoral graft infections, and a 73% mortality rate in patients with graft enteric erosion or fistula (2,13). Only two reports (4,37) of better results with graft excision without immediate reconstruction exist. Nonetheless, one of these still reported unacceptably high mortality and amputation rates (37). Graft excision and drainage may occasionally be of value in patients with end-to-side aortic prosthetic grafts placed for claudication, who develop active bleeding from a prosthetic duodenal fistula. In most situations, however, better options are usually available.

Graft Excision and In Situ Prosthetic Graft Replacement

Though occasional successes have been reported with in situ prosthetic graft replacement for infected primary aortic aneurysms, there are few reports of aortoiliac or aortofemoral bifurcation prosthetic grafts that had infection of the tube portion of the graft successfully treated by in situ replacement. Among 70 patients with graft enteric erosions or fistulas treated by in situ replacement 41 died, yielding a mortality of 59% (13).

Autogenous Replacement

Use of autogenous vein in infected arterial wounds in dogs resulted in a high incidence of arterial disruption similar to that seen when PTFE or Dacron was used (38). One center (39) has expressed a preference for PTFE as a replacement graft for traumatized and contaminated vessels. The results reported elsewhere (40) have been considerably less enthusiastic.

There are only a few reports of the use of autogenous material such as saphenous vein or endarterectomized artery in treating graft infections. Two reports (41,42), however, have been encouraging. Long-term patency may be poor, but if the infection has been eliminated, then reinsertion of prosthetic material in the area of previous infection is possible (42). The technical problems in obtaining satisfactory size and length of the autogenous vascular tissue can be formidable. Nonetheless, this approach fulfills the treatment criteria mentioned earlier in that it: (a) removes the foreign body, thus reducing the incidence of recurrent infection; (b) establishes perfusion to the lower extremities relatively promptly; and (c) reduces the likelihood of proximal aortic disruption because aortic continuity is maintained. In one study (6), the mortality using this approach was 14%, which was similar to the 13% mortality the same authors achieved by remote prosthetic bypass followed by graft removal 4 to 6 days later. Given these data, the use of autogenous reconstruction should be one of the treatment options considered when treating patients with arterial prosthetic infections, erosions, or fistulas.

Graft Excision and Remote Prosthetic Bypass

Currently, graft excision and remote bypass with a prosthetic graft are the treatments most often employed in managing patients with arterial prosthetic graft infections, erosions, or fistulas. The question arises as to whether the remote bypass should be performed first (3,6,43-47) or only, if necessary, after the infected graft is removed (4,14,48-51).

The two theoretical objections to performing the remote bypass first are: (a) that competitive, though transient, parallel flow will be established, making early thrombosis of the remote bypass likely; and (b) that the remote bypass will become secondarily seeded with bacteria when the infected graft is removed. Because of a small pressure differential, thrombosis of the remote bypass could occur before the infected graft or artery is removed. The likelihood, however, is probably quite small because the arrival of the pulse wave at the groin from a remote bypass would almost certainly be out of phase with the pulse wave from the in situ graft or artery. Ernst (52) reported a patient whose axillofemoral artery bypass remained patent until removal 123 days after insertion, despite the fact that it existed in parallel with a patent aortofemoral autogenous arterial system. None of the patients my colleagues and I have treated with remote bypass prior to graft excision has had early occlusion. Moreover, in the unlikely event that a previously inserted remote bypass did thrombose during an operation to remove an infected graft, at the completion of the infected graft removal, a thrombectomy of the remote bypass could then be easily performed.

When the few cases that have been reported are compared with the total number of remote bypasses inserted before infected graft or artery removal, the incidence of remote prosthetic grafts becoming secondarily infected is probably about 5%. Methods of reducing this incidence should include high systemic levels of appropriate broad spectrum antibiotics both at the time of remote graft insertion as well as when the infected material is removed. The incisions should be carefully planned so that infected areas can be adequately walled off from the operative field during remote bypass. These incisions and the course of the remote bypass should also be designed so that they remain unsullied when the infected artery or prosthesis is removed.

Performing a remote bypass *after* the infected graft is removed avoids possible bacteremia associated with infected artery or prosthesis removal. The overwhelming disadvantage of this approach, however, both with infected prostheses as well as with slow-leaking graft enteric erosions or fistulas, is the prolonged distal ischemia that obligatorily exists between the time the involved graft is clamped and the remote bypass is inserted. The complications of prolonged lack of perfusion of the lower extremities include distal gangrene, acidosis, hypothermia, bleeding disorders, compartment syndromes, myoglobinemia, renal failure, myocardial infarction, and death. These are markedly diminished if a remote bypass is inserted before removal of a prosthesis that is infected or involved with a GEE or GEF. The cases of infected aortic prosthetic grafts, erosions, or fistulas reported in the English literature have been reviewed (53). Patients with infected grafts identified as having been treated by aortic graft excision followed by remote bypass had a mortality of 71% (10 of 14 patients). Those with infected grafts who were treated by remote bypass followed by aortic graft excision had a mortality of 26% (6 of 23 patients). Similarly, by eliminating those patients who were bleeding briskly at the time of operation, patients with GEF or GEE who could be identified as having been treated by aortic graft excision followed by remote bypass had a mortality of 53% (40 of 75 patients). Those with GEE or GEF who were treated by remote bypass followed by aortic graft excision had a mortality of 17% (5 of 29 patients). For these reasons, when at all feasible, remote bypasses should be inserted prior to removal of infected arteries or arterial prostheses (53).

Once the decision has been reached to perform the remote bypass first, one must decide if the entire procedure of revascularization and removal of the infected artery or graft will be done sequentially during one operation or whether staged procedures will be performed. Revascularization can be followed by infected graft removal 1 to 6 days later. In patients with groin infections, it seems reasonable to perform the entire procedure sequentially in one operation. In other situations in which the infection, erosion, or fistula (providing the bleeding episodes have been modest and chronic) was intraabdominal, staging by 1 or 2 days appears to be better tolerated. Others (6) also have described the benefits of staged procedures.

Each of the problems involving infected grafts requires a variety of complex treatment decisions. These include whether to attempt partial graft excision, how to handle the patient with an aortic prosthesis who has had a recent brisk upper GI bleed, or what to do about the patient in whom the diagnosis of prosthetic enteric erosion is suspected but cannot be confirmed. These problems will be considered based on my clinical experience and experiences reported in the medical literature.

Because infections, erosions, and fistulas involving aortic bifurcation prostheses are among the most difficult to manage, the discussion that follows will emphasize treatment of groin and intra-abdominal arterial and vascular graft infections. Regardless of where the infection occurs, the principles of treatment remain constant: (a) prevent later arterial disruption; (b) perform remote bypass in uncontaminated fields or use autogenous material in contaminated fields; and (c) avoid prolonged lower extremity ischemia.

Specific Management Goals

Prosthetic Infections

Prosthetic Infection Restricted to the Groin

When a single groin infection occurs in a patient with an aortobifemoral graft, the question arises as to whether the infection is restricted solely to the groin or whether it extends up the iliac limb to the tube portion of the graft. If a draining sinus is present, the question may be answered by a gentle sinogram. When the limb is thrombosed or if both groins are infected, then it is likely that the entire graft is infected. When only one groin is involved with no obvious extension above the inguinal ligament, then a reasonable approach would include walling off the infected area with plastic adhesive drapes and making a suprainguinal curvilinear incision, similar to that used for kidney transplants, to expose the limb of the graft retroperitoneally at about the level of the internal iliac artery, taking care not to injure the ureter. This incision should be positioned so that if perigraft infection is found at this level, the incision can be promptly closed and an axillodistal superficial femoral artery bypass can still be constructed in an uncontaminated field (as discussed in the following section on infection involving an entire aorto-bifemoral prosthesis). If the tissue surrounding the graft is healthy appearing and well incorporated into the graft interstices, another incision should be made in the distal thigh and an obturator bypass (54) or a lateral subcutaneous bypass (55,56) should be constructed, taking care to avoid the contaminated area. Proximally, the graft-graft anastomosis should be end-to-end. The divided distal end of the original graft is trimmed and oversewn, and healthy autogenous tissue is closed over this stump, separating it from the newly constructed bypass. All incisions are then carefully closed in multiple layers using running sutures of synthetic absorbable suture, and occlusive dressings are applied. A groin incision can then be made to remove the infected graft completely, including the recently oversewn covered stump.

Any infected tissue is debrided, the femoral arteriotomy site oversewn, and the wound left open and drained. If the iliac portion of the graft was not involved with infection and care was exercised in all of the steps outlined, relatively prompt and uncomplicated wound healing should be anticipated.

Prosthetic Infection Involving Suprainguinal Portions of Aortofemoral Bifurcation Grafts

The diagnosis of infection restricted to the suprainguinal portion of an aortobifemoral graft can be difficult to make. When the diagnosis is certain, bilateral groin incisions should be made. If no infection is present, then an axillobifemoral bypass can be connected end-to-end to the short distal stumps of the previously inserted graft. The proximal limbs of the old aortobifemoral graft are then trimmed, oversewn, tucked beneath the inguinal ligament into the suprainguinal area, and covered with autogenous tissue. All wounds should be closed, and several days later the infected graft can be removed through a midline incision. The extent of the lower incision should be limited to avoid contaminating the femoral-femoral portion of the newly inserted axillobifemoral graft. Also, great care should be directed to closing and reinforcing the aorta in an effort to prevent aortic stump disruption.

If the diagnosis of an infected graft cannot be made preoperatively, abdominal exploration may be necessary. The diagnosis is confirmed by direct inspection of the graft, the area of infection irrigated thoroughly, and the incision closed without abdominal or wound drains. High doses of systemic antibiotics should be administered, all instruments, gowns, gloves, and drapes changed, and an axillobifemoral graft promptly constructed. Several days later, the abdominal incision can be reopened and the graft removed as previously outlined.

The alternative is to use autogenous tissue in the contaminated field (41, 42). Difficulties in obtaining adequate size and length of autogenous material and the incidence of later thrombotic complications (42), however, probably make remote bypassing with prosthetic material the preferred procedure when feasible. Nevertheless, autogenous tissue reconstruction fulfills the goals of reducing recurrent infection, preventing prolonged distal ischemia and aortic stump disruption, and should be employed when remote bypassing seems difficult or contraindicated.

The issue of whether to construct a remote bypass before or after infected graft removal was addressed earlier. All reported cases of infected aortic prostheses were reviewed, and those reports in which it could be determined in what order the bypass was performed were analyzed (53). Though the numbers were small, it was reasonably clear that insertion of a remote bypass prior to removal of an infected aortic prosthesis gives better results. In a larger number of patients with prosthetic enteric erosions and fistulas, this same conclusion appeared valid. Similarly, a report (6) that grouped patients with infected prostheses with those with prosthetic enteric erosions and fistulas noted good results when remote bypassing preceded infected graft removal.

The timing of staging is unresolved. Several of the patients our group treated had remote bypass grafting followed 24 to 48 hours later by graft removal (53). Reilly and her group (6) inserted a remote bypass and then immediately removed the involved prosthesis in 70 patients (infection, GEE, or GEF) with a mortality of 26%. Recently, this same group delayed graft removal for 4 to 6 days after insertion of a remote bypass in 15 patients with two deaths (13% mortality). Many patients can tolerate the one stage approach of remote bypassing followed immediately by infected graft removal; however, better results might be obtained by the two stage approach of insertion of a remote bypass followed, if the patient's condition permits, within 1 week by removal of the infected aortic graft. Patients suspected of having a graft enteric fistula (with a history of recent brisk gastrointestinal bleeding) probably should not be staged. In this situation, a remote bypass followed immediately by abdominal exploration and graft removal appears more appropriate.

Prosthetic Infection Involving Aortoiliac Bifurcation Grafts

These can be treated in the same manner as previously outlined for the management of suprainguinal aortofemoral bifurcation infections. The absence of a groin anastomotic site simplifies management considerably.

Prosthetic Infection Involving the Tube Portion and One Groin in a Patient with an Aortobifemoral Graft

When the prosthetic limb to the infected groin is thrombosed and that distal extremity is viable, one approach would be a contralateral axillofemoral bypass followed by complete removal of the infected bifurcation graft. When both prosthetic limbs are patent, however, a useful treatment plan is: a unilateral axillofemoral bypass on the side opposite the groin infection (the groin incision should be made first to confirm the absence of apparent infection on that side), closure of the incisions, and application of occlusive dressings. The prosthetic limb to the infected groin should then be ligated. If collateral circulation is adequate with no distal limb ischemia, the operation should be terminated; several days later, the entire aortic bifurcation prostheis should be removed. If the distal extremity becomes ischemic with ligation of the involved prosthetic limb, all gowns and instruments should be changed, the patient should be reprepared and draped, and an immediate revascularization procedure performed. Options for this procedure include: a remote ipsilateral axillodistal superficial femoral or popliteal artery bypass (57,58), or an autogenous femoral-femoral bypass from the previously inserted contralateral axillofemoral bypass to the femoral artery on the infected side (41,42). Several days later, the entire aortic bifurcation prosthesis can then be removed.

Prosthetic Infection Involving an Entire Aortobifemoral Graft

The choice here is an autogenous bypass (41,42) or bilateral axillodistal superficial femoral or popliteal bypasses. Though bilateral axillary popliteal bypasses may seem quite tenuous in this setting, I had one such patient who had no evidence of ischemia in the postoperative period. Others (58) have also reported acceptable results with these long remote bypass grafts. When severe distal occlusive disease is present, an autogenous bypass is probably preferable. Otherwise, bilateral axillary popliteal bypasses should be satisfactory for the short period necessary to clear the infection, at which time another aortobifemoral bypass could be inserted if necessary (59).

Arterial Enteric Erosions and Fistulas

Secondary Aortoduodenal Fistulas

Erosions occur between the prosthetic graft and overlying bowel. The bleeding that ensues is usually slow and intermittent and is caused either by bleeding from the eroded mucosa of the bowel or by bleeding through the interstices of the prosthetic graft. *Fistulas* occur at suture lines and can cause intermittent slow bleeding or, more ominously, a substantial "herald" bleed followed by massive bleeding and exsanguination. Preoperative differentiation between *erosion* and *fistula* is important only in that erosions will cause slow bleeding that allows treatment with remote bypass first, whereas rapid bleeding associated with fistulas may require abdominal exploration first. The diagnosis of *fistula* must be suspected if a large gastrointestinal bleed has occurred; however, some fistulas can present with only modest blood loss, making the preoperative differentiation between erosion and fistula difficult. Although the treatment goals for the two conditions are the same, management is predicated on the manner of clinical presentation.

Modest Bleeding from Prosthetic Enteric Erosion or Fistula

If the diagnosis of aortoenteric erosion or fistula is reasonably certain, the procedure of choice is either autogenous reconstruction (41,42) or insertion of a remote prosthetic bypass followed immediately or several days later by removal of the involved abdominal graft (53). Either approach is appropriate in those patients with a history of modest or chronic bleeding who have had a graft or suture line visualized by endoscopy, in those who have had a positive MRI, CT, gallium, or leukocyte scan, in those with a history of previous prosthetic aortic graft infection who were previously treated by less than complete prosthetic graft removal, and in those with abdominal aortic prosthetic grafts who have had a prolonged history of repeated septic episodes with chronic anemia with no discoverable source for these episodes despite repeated evaluations and diagnostic tests.

If the original bleeding was rapid but then stopped or slowed markedly and the diagnosis of GEF is confirmed, a remote bypass should be inserted followed immediately by removal of the abdominal prosthesis and closure of the fistula. A groin incision over the graft should be made first so that a large occlusion balloon catheter can be inserted retrograde into the aorta if the anesthesiologist reports a large amount of bright red blood in the nasogastric tube or a sudden decrease in the patient's blood pressure.

The most difficult management problems involve patients harboring a prosthetic aortic graft who exhibit brisk or modest upper gastrointestinal bleeding. Endoscopy reveals blood in the third portion of the duodenum, with no evidence of an exposed graft, varices, mucosal tears, or duodenal or gastric ulcerations. If bleeding persists at a modest rate, angiography may be helpful in making the diagnosis. If the bleeding has slowed or stopped, then questions arise as to whether a graft enteric fistula is present and whether a remote bypass should be performed immediately in preparation for subsequent abdominal exploration and graft removal.

One treatment plan is predicated on the fact that a graft enteric fistula may not necessarily be the cause of bleeding in patients with abdominal aortic prostheses. Other common causes of gastrointestinal bleeding can be missed by experienced endoscopists. Accordingly, patients with an abdominal prosthesis with recent modest to moderate upper gastrointestinal bleeding, in whom the cause of bleeding is not clearly identified by endoscopy, should be explored promptly to rule out a prosthetic enteric fistula. At this operation, the duodenum and all other overlying bowel must be completely dissected free of the graft and the anastomotic suture lines. Without this step, an erosion or fistula will be easily missed; often no mass or signs of inflammation exist around prosthetic enteric erosions or fistulas. Once an erosion or fistula is identified, the bowel is repaired, the fistula controlled locally if possible, and the abdominal incision closed. A remote bypass can then be followed by reexploration of the abdomen and graft removal. This procedure can be done in one stage, as was reported by Spanos and co-workers (45), or in multiple stages, depending on the patient's overall condition and the security of the earlier fistula closure. When the fistula cannot be securely controlled, then autogenous reconstruction can be attempted if satisfactory bypass material can be obtained. When the fistula cannot be locally controlled and autogenous bypassing is not possible, graft removal followed by remote bypass is necessary. In this situation, high amputation and mortality rates can be predicted.

Another view, and one I now hold, is that graft enteric fistulas are frequently difficult to control locally. Because the mortality and morbidity is so high when graft removal precedes remote bypass (53) and because GEF is the most likely cause of upper gastrointestinal bleeding in patients with prosthetic aortic grafts in whom endoscopy has not revealed another cause of bleeding (60), maximal expeditious efforts must be made to establish preoperatively the diagnosis of GEF. These measures include, in the following sequence: (a) complete and extremely thorough endoscopy in a stomach lavaged free of blood and clots with an Ewald tube (the endoscope should be introduced as far as possible into the duodenum in an effort to visualize the fistula) (61,62); (b) aortography with the patient in the prone position in an attempt to demonstrate a small false aneurysm at the level of the proximal aortic suture line (63); (c) computed tomography of the abdomen (64,65); and, (d) if available, magnetic resonance imaging (66). Once a reasonably firm diagnosis of GEF is made, one should stop testing. A prompt remote bypass followed by removal of the abdominal prosthesis should then be performed.

When none of those tests is positive, the source of bleeding becomes a matter of an informed clinical guess. If the previous operation was performed by an experienced vascular surgeon with an end-to-end proximal anastomosis covered by a Dacron cuff, another cause of GI bleeding might be suspected. In that situation, I would proceed first with abdominal exploration. This operation should consist of a long midline abdominal incision, careful inspection of the stomach and duodenum looking for ulcer scarring, and meticulous dissection of the third and fourth portion of the duodenum of the aortic graft pseudocapsule. If the duodenum is markedly adherent the diagnosis of GEE or GEF is highly probable. At this point, the abdominal portion of the operation should cease, the abdominal wall should be towel-clipped or stapled closed and an axillobifemoral graft constructed. With the bypass in place and those incisions closed and protected, the abdomen is re-opened to close the fistula and remove the prosthetic graft.

If the third or fourth portion of the duodenum is not densely adherent to the graft pseudocapsule, enterotomies are made to investigate other causes of GI bleeding. If no cause of GI bleeding is found, the entire third and fourth portion of the duodenum should be dissected away from the aortic graft to make absolutely sure no communication exists.

I would assume that the correct diagnosis was GEF if: (a) the previous operation was performed emergently, or by an occasional vascular surgeon, (b) there were operative complications at the time of the insertion of the aortic prosthesis, (c) the graft was inserted in an end-to-side fashion (my bias, without confirming data) so that the proximal suture line could not be covered by a Dacron cuff or (d) the upper GI bleed was quite brisk and the endoscopist was one I thought was highly skilled who could be reasonably sure the common causes of upper GI bleeding were not present. It would be best then to proceed with remote bypass followed promptly by aortic graft removal. It would be a catastrophe to construct a remote bypass followed by aortic graft removal in a patient with a bleeding duodenal ulcer. Unfortunately, sufficient anecdotal data suggest it is perhaps even more catastrophic to explore the aortic graft of a patient with a graft enteric fistula without the protection of a previously inserted remote bypass.

Rapid Bleeding from Prosthetic Enteric Fistula

Abdominal exploration and prompt exposure of the suspected suture line (usually proximal aortic) are essential. If the bleeding can be controlled by local sutures or patching, this should be done. Once bleeding is controlled, remote bypassing, reexploration, and graft removal in one or multiple stages can be accomplished. If the bleeding cannot be controlled by local sutures or patching, autogenous reconstruction should be attempted. If insufficient autogenous vascular material exists, graft removal, careful aortic stump closure, and remote bypass construction should be attempted. In this circumstance, however, the prognosis is guarded and the results may well be poor.

Operative Technique for Treating GEE or GEF

1. First, construct an axillobifemoral graft.

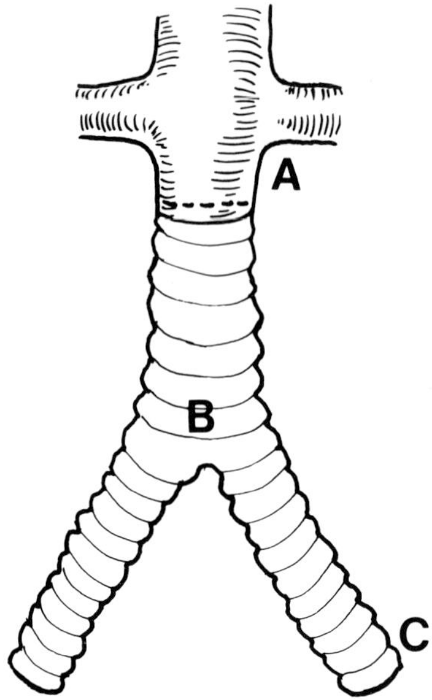

Figure 3   End-to-end aortic bifurcation graft.

2. If the previously inserted aortic graft was aortobifemoral, divide the graft and sew the new graft into the distal prosthetic limbs end-to-end.
3. Close all wounds in layers.
4. Protect all wounds with plastic adhesive.
5. Open the abdomen from the xyphoid to the pubis.
6. Do not attempt to expose the proximal aortic suture line at first.
7. Expose the graft at B (Fig. 3) or H (Fig. 4).
8. Pull the distal limbs of the aortic bifurcation graft into the abdomen, and obliterate the tracts from the abdomen to the groins with monofilament sutures.
9. Dissect the duodenum up until it becomes markedly adherent to the pseudocapsule covering the aortic graft, then stop.
10. Have the anesthesiologist give mannitol intravenously to protect the kidneys.
11. Slowly cut the pseudocapsule along the graft at B to A (Fig. 3) or at H to E (Fig. 4) until hematoma or modest bleeding is encountered.

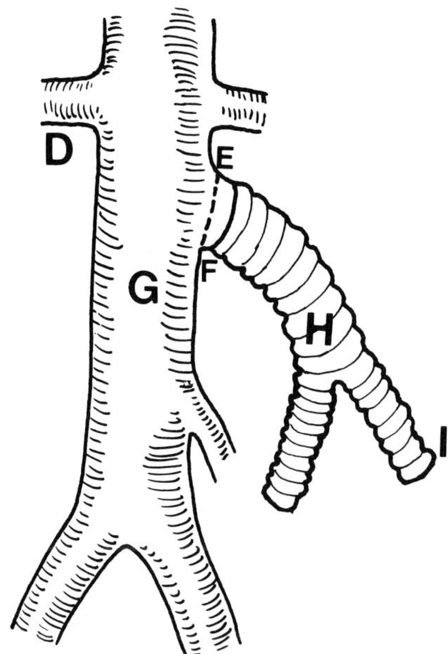

Figure 4   End-to-side aortic bifurcation graft.

12. Control any bleeding with direct pressure, make an incision in the graft at C (Fig. 3) or I (Fig. 4), and insert a 30 cc balloon catheter in the graft, advance it to A (Fig. 3) or D (Fig. 4), and inflate it.
13. Continue to dissect the pseudocapsule away from the graft and expose the proximal suture line and the fistula. If the aortic graft was inserted in an end-to-side fashion, insert another 30 cc balloon into the aorta at G (Fig. 4) to control backbleeding.
14. If the proximal anastomosis of the aortic graft was constructed in an end-to-end fashion (Fig. 3), dissect the duodenum up, disconnect the aortic graft and then dissect down both sides of the aorta just below the left renal vein (level A), place a clamp on the aorta (level A) as the balloon is removed, and close the aorta carefully using whatever technique seems most appropriate (see the section on "Management" under "General Principles").
15. If the proximal anastomosis of the aortic graft was constructed in an end-to-side fashion (Fig. 4), dissect the duodenum up, disconnect the

aortic graft, and then dissect down both sides of the aorta just below the left renal vein (level D) and place a clamp on the aorta (level D) as the proximal balloon is removed. Two options are now available.

The first, and preferred, is to close the aorta (E to F) with heavy (O-Prolene) monofilament suture, removing the distal balloon just prior to final closure. (Note: This suture line is *not* likely to remain intact for more than a week or two in the presence of the recent contamination, and dense scarring that requires closure under tension. As a consequence, it cannot be relied upon.) The aorta should then be sutured with interrupted mattress monofilament sutures or stapled closed at *both* level D and level G (Fig. 4). Presumably the aorta between levels D and G underneath the E to F suture line would then thrombose with little likelihood of subsequent exsanguinating breakdown of the E to F suture line.

The other option is to debride the aorta (E to F) and then close the aortic wall defect using autogenous patch material (such as an endarterectomized segment of a previously thrombosed superficial femoral artery harvested at the time of insertion of the remote bypass). This latter approach depends on continued integrity of the E to F patched suture line under direct arterial pressure, but if the contamination from the aortoenteric fistula was not great and the edges are adequately debrided, this patch technique may be sufficient (67).

Summary

The principles of surgical management for treating patients with infected arterial prostheses, prosthetic enteric erosions, or prosthetic enteric fistulas are as follows:

1. Prevent aortic stump disruption.
2. Place remote bypass prosthetic grafts in uncontaminated tissue planes or use autogenous bypass material.
3. Avoid prolonged lower limb ischemia.

Sequential techniques for diagnosis and treatment of the varying manifestations of infected grafts or graft enteric erosions or fistulas have been described under the heading *Specific Management Goals*. A salient point is that when graft excision precedes insertion of a remote bypass, the mortality rate with infected grafts, graft enteric fistulas, or graft enteric erosions is 50% to 75%. In contrast, if remote bypass precedes graft excision, the mortality rate is 15 to 25% (53). Whenever possible, infected arterial prostheses, prosthetic enteric erosions, or prosthetic enteric fistulas are best managed by insertion of a remote prosthetic bypass followed immediately or several days later by removal of the involved artery or prosthesis. Autogenous tissue reconstructions are another option if the diagnosis cannot be made preoperatively and adequate donor autogenous tissue exists. The perioperative diagnosis and management of infected prosthesis, graft enteric erosions, and fistulas require familiarity with the diagnostic and therapeutic options available and refined judgment as to which should be used as well as the order in which they are employed.

References

1. Elliot JP, Smith RF, Szilagyi DE: Aortoenteric and paraprosthetic-enteric fistulas. Arch Surg 108:479-490, 1974.
2. Bunt TJ: Synthetic vascular graft infections: I. Graft infections. Surgery 93:733-746, 1983.
3. Szilagyi DE, Smith RF, Elliott JP, Vrandecic MP: Infection in arterial reconstruction with synthetic grafts. Ann Surg 176:321-333, 1972.
4. Goldstone J, Moore WS: Infection in vascular prostheses: clinical manifestations and surgical management. Am J Surg 128:225-233, 1974.
5. Jamieson GG, DeWeese JA, Rob CG: Infected arterial grafts. Ann Surg 181:850-852, 1975.
6. Reilly LM, Altman H, Lusby RJ, et al: Late results following surgical management of vascular graft infection. J Vasc Surg 1:36-44, 1984.
7. Malone JM, Moore WS, Campagna G, Bean B: Bacteremic infectability of vascular grafts: the influence of pseudointimal integrity and duration of graft function. Surgery 78:211-216, 1975.
8. Moore WS: In Najarian JS, Delaney JP (Eds): Advances in Vascular Surgery. Chicago, Year Book Medical Publishers, 1983, pp. 338-339.
9. Stanley JC, Lindenauer SM, Graham LM, et al: Vascular grafts. In Moore WS (Ed): Vascular Surgery: A Comprehensive Review. New York, Grune & Stratton, 1983, pp. 245-268.
10. Moore WS, Malone JM, Keown K: Prosthetic arterial graft material: influence on neointimal healing and bacteremic infectibility. Arch Surg 115:1379-1183, 1980.
11. Yashar JJ, Weyman AK, Burnard RJ, Yashar J: Survival and limb salvage in patients with infected arterial prostheses. Am J Surg 135:499-504, 1978.

12. Stoney RJ. In Najarian JS, Delaney JP (Eds): Advances in Vascular Surgery. Chicago, Year Book Medical Publishers, 1983, p. 340.
13. Bunt TJ: Synthetic vascular graft infections: II. Graft-enteric erosions and graft-enteric fistulas. Surgery 94:1-9, 1983.
14. Liekweg WG Jr, Greenfield LJ: Vascular prosthetic infections: collected experience and results of treatment. Surgery 81:335-342, 1977.
15. Causey DA, Fajman WA, Perduc GD, et al: [67]Ga scintigraphy in post-operative synthetic graft infections. Am J Radiol 134:1041-1045, 1980.
16. Stevick CA, Fawcett HD: Aortoiliac graft infection: detection by leuko-cyte scan. Arch Surg 116:939-942, 1981.
17. Serota AI, Williams RA, Rose JG, Wilson SE: Uptake of radiolabeled leukocytes in prosthetic graft infection. Surgery 90:35-40, 1981.
18. Brown OW, Stanson AW, Pairolero PC, Hollier LH: Computerized tomography following abdominal aortic surgery. Surgery 91:716-722, 1982.
19. Mark A, Moss AA, Lusby R, Kaiser JA: CT evaluation of complications of abdominal aortic surgery. Radiology 145:409-414, 1982.
20. Cruse PJE, Foord R: A five-year prospective study of 23,649 surgical wounds. Arch Surg 107:206-210, 1973.
21. Edwards LD. The epidemiology of 2056 remote site infections and 1966 surgical wound infections occurring in 1865 patients: a four year study of 40,923 operations at Rush-Presbyterian-St. Luke's Hospital, Chicago. Ann Surg 184:758-766, 1976.
22. Kaiser AB, Clayson KR, Mulherin JL, et al: Antibiotic prophylaxis in vascular surgery. Ann Surg 188:283-289, 1978.
23. Szilagyi DE. In Najarian JS, Delaney JP (Eds): Advances in Vascular Surgery. Chicago, Year Book Medical Publishers, 1983; pp. 114-115.
24. Ehrenfeld WK: Infection in vascular surgery: surgical management and alternative routes for revascularization. In Bernhard VM, Towne JB (Eds): Complications in Vascular Surgery. New York, Grune & Stratton, 1980, pp. 503-516.
25. Stoney RJ. In Najarian JS, Delaney JP (Eds): Advances in Vascular Surgery. Chicago, Year Book Medical Publishers, 1983, pp. 331-332.
26. Goldsmith HS, de los Santos R, Vanamee P, Beattie EJ: Experimental protection of vascular prosthesis by omentum. Arch Surg 97:872-888, 1968.
27. Fry WJ, Lindenauer SM: Infection complicating the use of plastic arteri-al implants. Arch Surg 94:600-609, 1967.
28. Roy A, Hayes DF: Closure of an aortic stump. Am J Surg 145:403-404, 1983.
29. Shah DM, Buchbinder D, Leather RP, et al: Clinical use of the sero-muscular jejunal patch for protection of the infected aortic stump. Am J Surg 146:198-202, 1983.

30. Weber, TR, Lindenauer SM, Miller TA, et al: Focal infection of aorto-femoral prostheses. Surgery 79:310-312, 1976.
31. Butler HG III, Baker LD Jr, Johnson JM: Vascular access for chronic hemodialysis: polytetrafluoroethylene (PTFE) versus bovine heterograft. Am J Surg 134:791-793, 1977.
32. Tellis VA, Kohlberg WI, Bhat DJ, et al: Expanded polytetrafluoroethylene graft fistula for chronic hemodialysis. Ann Surg 189:101-105, 1979.
33. Henry R, Harvey RA, Greco RS: Antibiotic bonding to vascular prostheses. J Thorac Cardiovasc Surg 82:272-277, 1981.
34. Moore WS, Chvapil M. Seiffert G, Keown K: Development of an infection-resistant vascular prosthesis. Arch Surg 116:1403-1407, 1981.
35. Popovsky J, Singer S: Infected prosthetic grafts: local therapy with graft preservation. Arch Surg 115:203-205, 1980.
36. Fernandez MAM, Quast DC, Geis RC, Henly WS: Distally based sartorius muscle flap in the treatment of infected femoral arterial prostheses. J Cardiovasc Surg 21:628-631, 1980.
37. Turnipseed WD, Berkoff HA, Detmer DE, et al: Arterial graft infections: delayed vs immediate vascular reconstruction. Arch Surg 118:410-414, 1983.
38. Knott LH, Crawford FA Jr, Grogan JB: Comparison of autogenous vein, Dacron and Gore-tex in infected wounds. Surg Res 24:288-293, 1978.
39. Vaughan GD, Mattox KL, Feliciano DV, et al: Surgical experience with expanded polytetrafluoroethylene (PTFE) as a replacement graft for traumatized vessels. J Trauma 19:403-408, 1979.
40. Rich NM, Hughes CW: The fate of prosthetic material used to repair vascular injuries in contaminated wounds. J Trauma 12:459-467, 1972.
41. Ehrenfeld WK, Wilbur BG, Olcott CN IV, Stoney RJ: Autogenous tissue reconstruction in the management of infected prosthetic grafts. Surgery 85:82-92, 1979.
42. Seeger JM, Wheeler JR, Gregory RT, et al: Autogenous graft replacement of infected prosthetic grafts in the femoral position. Surgery 93:39-45, 1983.
43. Donovan TJ, Bucknam CA: Aorto-enteric fistula. Arch Surg 95:810-818, 1967.
44. Urdaneta LF, Visudh-Arom K, Delaney JP, Castaneda AR: Use of bilateral axillofemoral bypass prosthesis for the management of infected aortic bifurcation grafts: report of a case with extended follow-up. Surgery 65:753-756, 1969.
45. Spanos PK, Gilsdorf RB, Sako Y, Najarian JS: The management of infected abdominal aortic grafts and graft-enteric fistulas. Ann Surg 183:397-400, 1976.

46. Crawford ES, Manning LG, Kelly TF: "Redo" surgery after operations
    for aneurysm and occlusion of the abdominal aorta. Surgery 81:41-52,
    1977.
47. Perdue GD Jr, Smith RB III, Ansley JD, Costantino MJ: Impending
    aortoenteric hemorrhage: the effect of early recognition on improved
    outcome. Ann Surg 192:237-243, 1980.
48. Kleinman LH, Towne JB, Bernhard VM: A diagnostic and therapeutic
    approach to aortoenteric fistulas: clinical experience with twenty pa-
    tients. Surgery 86:868-880, 1979.
49. Buchbinder D, Leather R, Shah D, Karmody A: Pathologic interactions
    between prosthetic aortic grafts and the gastrointestinal tract: clinical
    problems and a new experimental approach. Am J Surg 140:192-198,
    1980.
50. Connolly JE, Kwaan JHM, McCart PM, et al: Aortoenteric fistula. Ann
    Surg 194:402-412, 1981.
51. Martin-Paredero V, Busuttil RW, Dixon SM, et al: Fate of aortic graft
    removal. Am J Surg 146:194-197, 1983.
52. Ernst CB: Axillary-femoral bypass graft patency without aorto-femoral
    pressure differential: disuse atrophy of ipsilateral ileo-femoral segment.
    Ann Surg 181:424-427, 1975.
53. Trout HH III, Kozloff L, Giordano JM: Priority of revascularization in
    patients with graft enteric fistulas, infected arteries or infected arterial
    protheses. Ann Surg 199:669-683., 1984.
54. Pearce WH, Ricco, JB, Yao JST, Flinn WR, Bergan JJ: Modified tech-
    nique of obturator bypass in failed or infected grafts. Ann Surg 197:344-
    347, 1983.
55. Leather RP, Karmody AM: A lateral route for extra-anatomical bypass
    of the femoral artery. Surgery 81: 307-309, 1977.
56. Trout HH III, Smith CA: Lateral iliopopliteal arterial bypass as an
    alternative to obturator bypass. Am Surg 48:63-64, 1982.
57. Kwaan JHM, Connolly JE: Extended axillopopliteal-axillotibial bypass:
    valuable adjunct to limb revascularization. Arch Surg 118:25-28, 1983.
58. Gupta SK, Veith FJ, Ascer E, Samson RH, Scher LA, White-Flores SA,
    Sprayregen S, Fell SC: Five year experience with axillopopliteal bypasses
    for limb salvage. J Cardiovasc Surg 26:321-324, 1985.
59. Reilly LM, Ehrenfeld WK, Stoney RJ: Delayed aortic prosthetic re-
    construction after removal of an infected graft. Am J Surg 148:234-239,
    1984.
60. Pelz DM, Rankin RN: Alternate bleeding sites in suspected graft-enteric
    fistula. AJR 136:707-709, 1981.
61. Brand EJ, Sivak MV Jr, Sullivan BH Jr: Aortoduodenal fistula: endosco-
    pic diagnosis. Dig Dis Sci 24:940-944, 1979.

62. Bunt TJ, Doerhoff CR: Endoscopic visualization of an intraluminal Dacron graft: definitive diagnosis of aortoduodenal fistula. South Med J 77:86-87, 1984.
63. Pingoud EG, Pais SO: Usefulness of the prone position for aortography of aortic graft-intestinal fistulae. AJR 132:836-837, 1979.
64. Ackroyd J, Williams TG, Thomas ML, Burnand KG: The diagnosis of aortic graft-enteric fistulae by computed tomography. Br J Surg 72:72-73, 1985.
65. Kay D, Kalmar JR: Computerized tomographic evaluation of aortic prosthetic graft complications. South Med J 78:296-298, 1985.
66. Justich E, Amparo EG, Hricak H, Higgins CB: Infected aortoiliofemoral grafts: magnetic resonance imaging. Radiology 154:133-136, 1985.
67. Reilly LM, Ehrenfeld WK, Goldstone J, Stoney RJ: Gastrointestinal tract involvement by prosthetic graft infection: the significance of gastrointestinal hemorrhage. Ann Surg 202:342-348, 1985.

4

Arterial Reconstruction After Failed Axillofemoral Bypass Procedures

TERRY A. KING
Case-Western Reserve University School of Medicine and Mt. Sinai Medical Center, Cleveland, Ohio

JEFFREY R. RUBIN
Case-Western Reserve University School of Medicine and Veterans Administration Medical Center, Cleveland, Ohio

Introduction

Axillofemoral bypass was first described in 1963 by Blaisdell and Hall (1) for the treatment of aortoiliac occlusive disease. The indications for selection of an extra-anatomic bypass over the "gold standard" transabdominal aorto-femoral bypass remain controversial, in part due to suboptimal patency rates when axillofemoral bypass is compared with direct aortofemoral reconstruction (2). Well accepted indications include cases of aortic graft sepsis, mycotic aneurysm, primary aortoduodenal fistula, and active intra-abdominal sepsis from other sources. Consideration of axillofemoral bypass might also be given in situations of previous aortic graft failure, a prior episode of abdominal sepsis, recent abdominal surgery for other organ systems, or an otherwise "hostile" abdominal cavity. Controversy exists over the milder indications for its use, such as for patients with an anticipated high risk of morbidity, mortality, or both, if subjected to general anesthesia and aortic cross-clamping, but there is no doubt that axillofemoral bypass has a distinct role in the salvage of life and limb.

Incidence and Etiology of Axillofemoral Graft Failure

The incidence of axillofemoral graft thrombosis in the literature is obscured by variations in the reporting of patency rates. The lifetable method of reporting graft patency determines the period from operation to graft thrombosis (2,3). The cumulative patency method does not consider graft thrombosis if it can be successfully treated by thrombectomy (4,5). Quoted patency rates for axillofemoral grafts vary from 30% at 5 years, by lifetable methods, to 74% at 5 years for cumulative patency of these grafts (2,6). Since the use of the axillofemoral bypass spans 24 years, the reports of patency are also obscured by improvements in graft materials as well as surgical technique. Although the concept of graft thrombectomy is often downplayed in the surgical literature, it may be mechanically challenging for the surgeon and stressful for patients in a relatively high risk group.

Axillofemoral graft failure can be separated into early and late causes. The perioperative problems of other vascular procedures, namely hemorrhage and thrombosis, are immediate causes of difficulty. Thrombosis may result from improper graft preparation, incorrect anastomotic site selection, and mechanical anastomotic problems, especially intimal flaps. This is more common in the diseased femoral arteries than at the axillary anastomosis. When it does occur at the proximal suture line, it places the outflow bed of the artery, the upper extremity, at risk.

Axial rotation of the graft in its relatively long tunnel may also induce an early thrombosis. An associated problem of tunneling, crossing the costal margin instead of placing the axillofemoral limb in the midaxillary line, may lead to early occlusion. Redundancy of the graft in its tunnel causes disturbances in flow, a potential source of early failure.

High outflow resistance occurs when the femoral anastomosis is placed proximal to a profunda femoris stenosis. This can also occur when the graft is placed on a diseased superficial femoral artery. An axillary anastomosis distal to an unrecognized subclavian or innominate stenosis or occlusion will limit inflow. Either situation can contribute to graft failure.

The necessity of preclotting a woven or knitted graft may lead to residual thrombus in the lumen, which can embolize when the clamps are removed and cause immediate failure.

Hemorrhage occurs at suture lines, but is usually easy to recognize. A more difficult bleeding problem may occur in the tunnels, where small subcutaneous vessels are sheared off during passage of the graft. Perigraft hematomas can compress the graft in the early postoperative period when the graft is still soft and unincorporated, but are perhaps more troublesome as sources of perigraft seromas (7). Perigraft hematomas and seromas can also result from extravasation through an improperly preclotted Dacron graft.

Late problems of axillofemoral bypass requiring reoperation include thrombosis, false aneurysm formation, infection, and perigraft seromas. The most common cause of late thrombosis is progression of atherosclerosis, both at the distal anastomosis and in the runoff bed. Other factors that can contribute to late failure include the problems already mentioned that more commonly cause early difficulties. These include anastomosis on the common femoral artery proximal to a profunda femoris stenosis or to a diseased superficial femoral artery, intimal flaps at the distal anastomosis, kinking of the graft as it passes over the costal margin instead of the midaxillary line, and axial rotation of the graft in its tunnel. Low flow rates exist in a graft segment below a high origin of a cross-femoral limb, as described elsewhere (8). Reduction of inflow can occur with progression of subclavian atherosclerosis, as well as a Y deformity of the proximal anastomosis. Figure 1 shows a schematic representation of several potential problems in axillofemoral grafting.

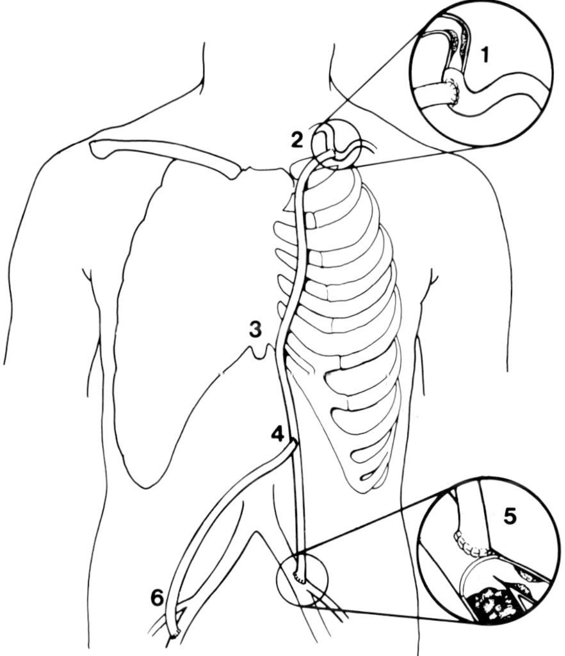

Figure 1 Schematic illustration of potential problems with axillofemoral bypass. *1*: Axillary anastomosis distal to a subclavian stenosis. *2*: Y deformity of the axillary artery. *3*: Improper tunneling causing graft to cross the costal margin. *4*: High takeoff of a cross-femoral limb. *5*:Common femoral anastomosis proximal to a profunda femoris stenosis and superficial femoral occlusion. *6*: Superficial femoral artery anastomosis. Refer to text for details.

False aneurysm formation can take place at any graft-to-artery anastomosis, but is particularly common at the femoral artery. False aneurysms at the femoral artery anastomosis will usually present early as a result of the patient's awareness of an enlarging pulsatile mass under the groin incision. The risk of rupture exists, as well as thrombosis and distal embolization. Repair of asymptomatic false aneurysms can prevent late sequelae (9).

Any prosthetic device implanted in the body is at risk for infection and sepsis, and this is also true for axillofemoral grafts. Actual rates of infection are difficult to extract from the literature, as most series are relatively small. Livesay and colleagues (10), however, noted a relatively high incidence of 6%. It is noteworthy that four of these six infections were in patients undergoing axillofemoral bypass for management of aortic graft sepsis.

A perigraft seroma is defined as a collection of clear sterile fluid within a nonsecretory fibrous pseudomembrane surrounding a vascular graft (7). It is a rare complication, and the true incidence is not known. Blumenberg and co-workers (7) reported a collected series of 279 cases. Axillounifemoral and axillobifemoral grafts accounted for 49% of all cases, with femorofemoral grafts contributing an additional 11%. With the highest incidence occurring in axillofemoral bypass, a relatively uncommon procedure, it stands to reason that the incidence is comparatively high for axillofemoral grafts.

Preoperative Evaluation

The timing of the occlusion of an axillofemoral graft with respect to the initial surgery as well as the severity of ischemia will dictate the rapidity and the extensiveness of the preoperative workup. There are, however, several aspects of the workup that are necessary for any evaluation of graft occlusion. These should include a history of past symptoms leading to the initial procedure as well as current complaints, careful physical examination, noninvasive vascular laboratory testing, and review of all prior angiograms and operative reports. This will familiarize the surgeon with the previous procedure and perhaps indicate the etiology of the thrombosis.

Several aspects of the physical examination are worth mention with regard to axillofemoral graft thrombosis. The presence or absence of pulses in both the upper and lower extremities should be noted. Absent pulses in the lower extremities would not be unexpected, but the lack of a pulse in the donor arm might indicate a proximal rather than distal problem leading to failure. This could be due to a subclavian stenosis or difficulty at the anastomosis. Acute ischemia of the lower extremities with palpable pulses in the grafts can be caused by embolization from the axillary anastomosis. A bruit in the area of the proximal incision indicates turbulence at the axillary anastomosis, another proximal disturbance.

The presence or absence of pulses in all portions of the graft should be noted. Contralateral leg ischemia with a palpable pulse in the axillofemoral segment may indicate occlusion of the cross-femoral limb of the graft.

Technical features of the previous operation must be noted. Placement of incisions may indicate an axillary anastomosis that is too far lateral on the axillary artery, which leads to a Y deformity of the axillary vessel. Small, high femoral incisions do not permit adequate exposure of the femoral bifurcation and profunda femoris artery, a technical feature just mentioned. The course of the graft must be inspected, looking for redundancy, kinking over the costal margin or inguinal ligament, perigraft seroma, or infection. Evidence of delayed wound healing might suggest a subclinical graft infection. False aneurysms can also cause occlusion, and are easily found on thorough physical examination.

Noninvasive laboratory studies should include pulse volume recordings, pulse velocity tracings, and segmental pressures of both the upper and lower extremities. Subjecting the donor vessel arm to exercise stress testing or reactive hyperemia may uncover a previously unrecognized or progressive subclavian or axillary stenosis.

Preoperative conventional angiography is probably unnecessary in instances of early axillofemoral graft occlusion and is frequently of little help in patients with late thrombosis. Standard aortography and runoff examination are limited to the translumbar approach or the Seldinger technique via the axillary artery because femoral artery access to the aorta is precluded by the presence of grafts as well as aortoiliac disease. Aortic flow is also diminished, such that adequate visualization of the femoral anastomoses is difficult. Little information, therefore, is gained that alters the surgical approach. We have had some success in obtaining meaningful preoperative information by employing intravenous digital subtraction techniques. This requires a presumptive diagnosis so that appropriate areas can be studied with the smaller fields obtained by digital angiography. This also helps to limit contrast load. Figure 2 is an example of an intravenous digital subtraction angiogram that demonstrates a Y deformity of the axillary anastomosis.

It is our standard practice to immediately heparinize and achieve therapeutic levels of anticoagulation in all patients who present with axillofemoral graft occlusion. This is accomplished with the administration of heparin sulfate, 125 mg/kg, as a bolus injection, and simultaneously beginning

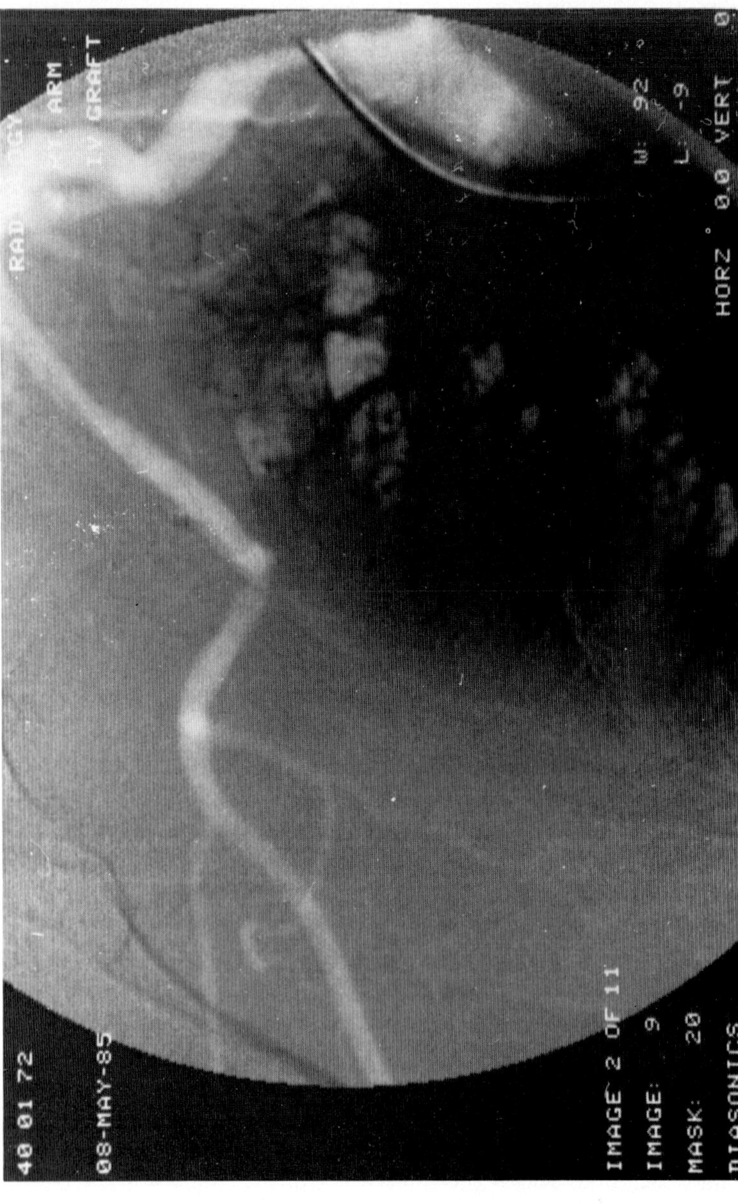

Figure 2 Intravenous digital subtraction angiogram showing a Y deformity of the axillary artery at the site of anastomosis of an occluded ® axillofemoral graft. Note the lateral placement of the anastomosis.

a heparin drip at a rate of 100 mg/hour in order to maintain a partial thromboplastin time (PTT) of 2 to 2.5 times the control value. Routine fluid resuscitation and appropriate arterial and Swan-Ganz monitoring should be carried out expeditiously in preparation for operation. In addition, a broad spectrum cephalosporin is administered intravenously immediately before surgery unless an existent infection mandates the selection of a more specific antibiotic regimen.

Operative Management

After patient stabilization and preparation, the patient is promptly taken to the operating room where skin preparation is carried out in the same fashion as for a primary procedure. This includes the preparation of a wide operative field, including both sides of the neck, the entire chest and abdomen, and both arms and both legs, including the feet. Although it is felt that local anesthesia may be employed for axillofemoral graft thrombectomy, we prefer the use of general anesthesia due to the frequent lengthy and complicated nature of these operations.

Our standard initial approach for axillofemoral thrombectomy, unless a specific etiology for the thrombosis was discovered preoperatively, includes isolation of the distal portion of the axillofemoral and the proximal portion of the femorofemoral grafts. Transverse openings are made in each graft several centimeters from the suture lines. This approach has several advantages. It limits dissection to a single groin, yet allows passage of thromboembolectomy catheters through both graft segments as well as both lower extremities. It allows angiography to be performed in a selective manner in each lower extremity, thereby limiting contrast load. Angioscopy of both distal anastomoses can also be performed through the "graftotomies." As problems are discovered, each can be approached individually.

In our experience, the most frequent etiology of both early and late graft thrombosis is related to elevated outflow resistance. The early problem is usually unrecognized profunda femoris disease, while late graft occlusion is related to progression of atherosclerosis, usually in the profunda femoris artery. Liberal use of intraoperative angiography will uncover most profunda femoris problems. This is performed by controlling inflow with a vascular clamp on the proximal graft, inserting a 10 or 12 French red rubber catheter in the distal graft via the graftotomy, and injecting 20 to 30 cc of Renograffin-60. Since the area of concern is near the injection site, exposure is immediately at the end of injection. Care should be taken to angulate the x-ray camera so that an oblique film is obtained, a method used to uncover orificial lesions of the profunda femoris artery. This can be performed with sterile cassette covers, placing the cassette under the patient, but this often results in a break in sterile technique. We have had equal success placing the film under the table, similar to methods used for intraoperative cholangiography.

When profunda femoris artery lesions are found, management consists of direct reconstruction, using extended profunda exposure, endarterectomy of the common and profunda femoris arteries, and patch angioplasty. Our preferred patch material is a segment of occluded superficial femoral artery that has been endarterectomized, saving the saphenous vein for potential distal reconstruction in the future. Vein is still preferred to prosthetics for profundoplasty, however, and in the presence of a patent superficial artery, we will use the saphenous vein (11). When profunda stenosis occurs on the side of the initial exposure, this can be performed by simple extension of the incision. A separate incision is necessary for contralateral profunda femoris reconstruction.

When profundoplasty is not sufficient for maintenance of axillofemoral patency during the period of intraoperative observation, consideration must be given to standard femorodistal reconstruction. This would require pre-bypass angiography, as described elsewhere (12). This is rarely necessary, although we have observed persistently ischemic extremities that have subsequently required distal bypass.

At the time of thrombectomy, problems with inflow can present in several ways. Difficulty in passing the thromboembolectomy catheter up the axillofemoral graft limb can indicate adherent thrombus in the graft, tortuosity of the bypass, or a Y deformity of the proximal anastomosis. Repeated thrombosis of the graft limb despite negative passes of the thromboembolectomy catheter implies aneurysmal degeneration of a Dacron graft, with residual thrombus in the aneurysms. If the adequacy of inflow is still in question, pressure is measured in the graft using an angiocatheter connected to high pressure tubing filled with heparin flush solution. The tubing is passed off the head of the table to the anesthesiologist, who then connects it to a transducer and compares it with systemic pressure. A gradient of 20 mmHg is considered a significant reduction in graft pressure.

Other mechanical factors are important in restoration of inflow. Passage of the catheter into the axillary artery is necessary to completely remove all thrombus. In certain patients, this will require a counterincision over the mid-portion of the graft and passage of the catheter from that level. The need for this can be checked by measuring the length of the catheter on the skin over the course of the graft. After the thrombectomy is completed, the graft must be completely filled with a heparinized saline solution to prevent thrombosis during the time it takes to finish the distal portion of the procedure. This is easily done with a bulb syringe filled with the flush solution inserted in the graftotomy and injecting against systemic pressure. The problem of repeat thrombosis of the axillofemoral limb while performing the distal thrombectomy can be completely averted by doing the distal portion of the procedure first. This also eliminates the need for a vascular clamp on the proximal graft, a minor but often annoying point.

Problems with inflow require surgical revision. Stenosis at the axillary anastomosis can be repaired by patch angioplasty, opening both the orifice of the graft and the axillary artery runoff. A Y deformity should be corrected by interposition grafting, allowing the axillary artery to fall back into its anatomic position. This abnormality usually occurs when the axillary anastomosis is placed too far laterally, and when corrected, should be moved to the first portion of the axillary artery, proximal to the pectoralis minor muscle insertion, as advocated by Blaisdell and Hall (1) and recently reiterated by Bunt and Moore (13).

Proximal problems, however, are rare, and most problems with inflow are related to the axillofemoral graft limb itself. Conditions such as tortuosity, kinking, axial rotation, aneurysmal degeneration, and residual pseudointima should lead to consideration of graft replacement. This can be done on the ipsilateral side, using the proximal 2 to 3 cm of the old graft at the axillary anastomosis. The old graft can be left in place, tunneling the new graft several centimeters away from it. The contralateral side should be used in situations of graft infection, and is possibly easier in the management of perigraft seroma. Both of these problems require graft removal.

An additional cause of failure already mentioned is low flow rates in the axillofemoral limb below a high takeoff of a cross-femoral limb. If this is a contributing factor to graft thrombosis, this should be replaced with a more standard suprapubic femorofemoral limb. Our preference is to use a cross-femoral graft that is 2 mm smaller than the axillofemoral limb, usually using 6 and 8 mm, respectively. This allows for an increased velocity of flow in the cross-femoral limb, thus promoting long-term patency (8).

It is still uncertain whether graft material plays a part in long-term patency (14). Recently, polytetrafluoroethylene (PTFE) has become the graft of choice because of the ease of thrombectomy (8,14). Bleeding problems are reduced as the graft requires no preclotting, and it may be more resistant to infection than Dacron (14). For these reasons, PTFE is our graft of choice, whether for primary axillofemoral bypass or thromboembolectomies that require placement of a segment of graft.

An alternative reconstructive procedure is the descending thoracic aorta to femoral bypass. Indications for this procedure are discussed elsewhere (15). This has the potential for improved long-term patency over axillo-femoral bypass, presumably on the basis of increased graft flow.

In summary, a systematic approach for the treatment of axillofemoral graft thrombosis is necessary. Our initial approach, if no specific etiology for the graft occlusion was uncovered during the preoperative evaluation, is to explore the groin ipsilateral to the axillofemoral graft. Thrombectomy of both the axillofemoral and femorofemoral components may be accomplished through a single incision using this approach, thus minimizing potential wound healing problems. Direct operative repair of lesions that may have caused the graft thrombosis may be approached through separate incisions as mandated by the clinical situation. Intraoperative angiography and/or angioscopy is a helpful adjunct for determining the possible underlying cause for graft occlusion. Finally, graft replacement should be carried out without hesitation if satisfactory results are not achieved by the measures noted.

Postoperative Management

Perioperative management of the patient with axillofemoral graft thrombectomy should include the attention to detail afforded to every vascular bypass patient. Maintenance of hydration and urine output is neces-sary to ensure adequate cardiac output, and thereby contribute to graft patency. When necessary, this is done with invasive methods, using indwel-ling arterial lines and Swan-Ganz monitoring. Broad spectrum antibiotic prophylaxis is continued for 48 hours. When documented infection is present, antibiotics are chosen on the basis of organism sensitivity and continued for longer periods. Lower extremity blood flow is documented with noninvasive testing in the operating room, and patients with marginal ischemia of the lower extremities are maintained on heparin therapy at theraputic levels of anticoagulation until the clinical result of the surgery can be ascertained. Long-term anticoagulation is reserved for patients with two or more thromboses. Aspirin, 325 mg/day, is used on a long-term basis for its anti-platelet activity. Other problems are treated aggressively as they arise.

Results

The results of reoperation for occluded axillofemoral bypass are difficult to obtain from the literature, due in part to the variability of reporting patency rates. We have already discussed the difference between lifetable patency and cumulative patency. In a recent review of 106 axillofemoral bypasses performed over 10 years, Burrell and co-workers (16) reported a thrombectomy success rate of 92%. They achieved a 97 ± 5% cumulative patency at 32 months, compared with 71 ± 8% for lifetable patency (16). They did not, however, mention the number of patients with repeat thrombosis or the morbidity and mortality of the thrombectomy. They did stress, as have others, the improved patency for the axillobifemoral bypass when compared with the axillounifemoral graft, while other factors play a lesser role (8,16).

Despite the controversies in the literature regarding indications for the procedure as well as the results, axillofemoral bypass has a definite role in the salvage of life and limb. Complications, including thrombosis, can be minimized by meticulous surgical technique. Aggressive management of graft thrombosis will maximize the functional results.

References

1. Blaidell FW, Hall AD: Axillary-femoral artery bypass for lower extremity ischemia. Surgery 54:563-568, 1963.
2. Eugene S, Goldstone J, Moore WS: Fifteen year experience with subcutaneous bypass grafts for lower extremity ischemia. Ann Surg 186: 177-183, 1976.
3. Anderson RP, Bonchek LI, Grunkemeier GL, et al: The analysis and presentation of surgical results by actuarial methods. J Surg Res 16:224, 1974.
4. Ascer E, Veith FJ, Gupta SK, Scher LA, Samson RII, White-Flores SA, Sprayregen S: Comparison of axillounifemoral and axillobifemoral bypass operations. Surgery 97:169-175, 1985.
5. Colton T: Statistics in Medicine. Boston, Little, Brown, & Co, 1976.
6. Johnson WC, LoGerfo FW, Vollman RW, Corson JD, O'Hara ET, Mannick JA, Nasbeth DC: Is axillo-bilateral femoral graft an effective substitute for aorto-bilateral femoral graft: Ann Surg 186:123-129, 1977.
7. Blumenberg RM, Gelfand ML, Dale WA: Perigraft seromas complicating arterial grafts. Surgery 194-204, 1985.
8. Blaisdell FW (moderator): Symposium on extraanatomical bypass. Contemp Surg 25:109-151, 1974.
9. Moore WS: Anastomotic aneurysms. In Rutherford RB (Ed): Vascular Surgery. Philadelphia, 1984. W. B. Saunders Co.
10. Livesay JJ, Atkinson JB, Baker JD, Bussitil RW, Barker WF, Machleder HI: Late results of extra-anatomic bypass. Arch Surg 114:1260-1267, 1979.

11. Bernhard VM: Profundaplasty. In Rutherford RB (Ed): Vascular Surgery. W. B. Saunders Co., Philadelphia, 1984.
12. King TA, Flinn WR, Yao JST, Bergan JJ: Pre-bypass arteriography. In Bergan JJ, Yao JST (Eds): Evaluation and Treatment of Upper and Lower Extremity Circulatory Disorders. New York, Grune & Stratton, 1984.
13. Bunt TJ, Moore W: Optimal proximal anastomosis/tunnel for axillo-femoral bypass. J Vasc Surg 3:673-676, 1986.
14. Bergan JJ: Complications of extra-anatomic bypass grafting to the lower extremity. In Bernhard VM, Towne JB (Eds): Complications in Vascular Surgery. New York, Grune & Stratton, 1985.
15. McCarthy W, Rubin JR, Williams L, Flinn WR, Yao JST, Bergan JJ: Thoracic aorta to femoral bypass. Arch Surg 121:681-688, 1986.
16. Burrell MJ, Wheeler JR, Gregory RT, Snyder SO Jr., Gayle RG, Mason MS: Axillofemoral bypass: ten year review. Ann Surg 195:796-799, 1985.

5

The Role of Myocardial Revascularization in Patients Requiring Peripheral Vascular Reconstruction

PATRICK J. O'HARA and NORMAN R. HERTZER
The Cleveland Clinic Foundation, Cleveland, Ohio

The material in this chapter represents the fulfillment of a request by the editors to provide a recent summary of the principal components of an ongoing study of the incidence, distribution, and treatment of associated coronary disease in patients with peripheral vascular disease at the Cleveland Clinic. This material has been published previously in a variety of sources, including both original articles and summary text book chapters and, as such, is not unique. The essential original articles are listed in the references. It is anticipated that additional results and summaries, based on this and new supplementary material, may be published in the future as needs and developments dictate.

It is generally accepted that the sequelae of coronary artery disease (CAD) comprise the leading cause of both early and late mortality in patients with peripheral vascular disease requiring arterial reconstruction, especially those with conventional clinical evidence of ischemic heart disease (1-11). This observation is not surprising since arteriosclerosis is a systemic process and most patients who require vascular reconstruction have diffuse, multisegmental arterial occlusive disease. From 1969 to 1978, myocardial infarction accounted for 45% of postoperative deaths after resection of nonruptured aortic aneurysms, and for 67% of those after elective aortic replacement for lower extremity occlusive disease at the Cleveland Clinic (6-8). A notably lower incidence of early mortality was observed among patients with no clinical evidence of coronary disease (2.9%) when compared with those clinically suspected to have CAD (9.6%). During the study period, however,

73

no deaths occurred in a group of 87 patients who had incidentally received myocardial revascularization at some time preceding their abdominal aortic operations, an observation suggesting a protective effect of coronary bypass in selected individuals (12-15).

A review of 951 patients who required surgical management of aortic aneurysms, lower extremity ischemia, and cerebrovascular disease at the Cleveland Clinic demonstrated that postoperative survival for patients with peripheral atherosclerosis is poorer than that for the normal population of the same age (7,8,16,17). Myocardial infarction caused at least 38 to 55% of all late deaths in this series. However, late survival of 331 patients who required simultaneous carotid endarterectomy and coronary artery bypass at the Cleveland Clinic was tantamount to that of the normal population and was better than that of similar patients who had carotid endarterectomy alone during the same interval (18). Because these observations suggested that myocardial revascularization might improve the operative risk and life expectancy of selected patients with peripheral vascular disease and associated CAD, preoperative coronary angiography and coronary bypass, when indicated, were recommended to all of those under consideration for elective vascular procedures beginning in 1978. "Routine" coronary angiography is not currently recommended, although it was necessary to include all patients in an initial study group in order to identify each subset having a substantial incidence of CAD (19,20).

The Incidence of Coronary Artery Disease in Patients with Peripheral Vascular Disease

Preoperative cardiac catheterization was performed in a series of 1000 patients under evaluation for elective peripheral vascular reconstruction at the Cleveland Clinic beginning in 1978 (19,20). Table 1 contains information concerning the primary peripheral vascular diagnosis at the time of the original examination, as well as the composition of this series according to sex, age, and clinical cardiac status determined by the previous history and a standard 12 lead electrocardiogram (ECG). A cardiac history of previous myocardial infarction or angina pectoris or electrocardiographic evidence of previous infarction, ST-T changes, or left bundle branch block were associated with the presence of underlying CAD. By these criteria, 446 patients had no indication of CAD, while 554 were suspected of having CAD on clinical grounds preceding coronary angiography.

While 395 patients had multiple vascular diagnoses identified during their initial evaluations, all references to the site of peripheral vascular disease

Table 1 Composition of Series According to Primary Peripheral Vascular Diagnosis

Patients	Abdominal Aortic Aneurysm (n=263)	Lower Extremity Ischemia (n=381)	Cerebrovascular Disease (n=295)	Other (n=61)	Total (n=1000)
	%	%	%	%	%
Men	84	66	59	66	68
Women	16	34	41	34	32
CAD					
No indication	48	44	43	44	45
Suspected	52	56	57	56	55
Mean age (years)	67.6	61.8	64.5	59.8	64.0

Source: From Ref. 19, used with permission.

apply to the principal diagnosis with which each patient originally presented. The miscellaneous category includes 61 patients who had other vascular diagnoses, such as visceral arterial stenosis, extremity aneurysms, or false aneurysms, and other complications of prior vascular reconstruction. Each patient underwent coronary angiography and left ventriculography using the transbrachial technique. The severity of CAD was classified according to the following guidelines (19,20):

1. Normal coronary arteries.
2. Mild to moderate CAD, with measurable disease of one or more coronary arteries, but no lesion exceeding 70% stenosis.
3. Advanced but compensated CAD, with greater than 70% stenosis of one or more coronary arteries, but no immediate indication for myocardial revascularization because of adequate intercoronary collateral circulation or because the involved vessel supplied myocardium already replaced by scar.
4. Severe, correctable, CAD, with greater than 70% stenosis of one or more coronary arteries serving unimpaired myocardium and representing immediate or foreseeable risk for myocardial infarction.
5. Severe, inoperable CAD, with greater than 70% stenosis of multiple coronary arteries, representing inadequate targets for coronary bypass because of diffuse, distal disease, or generalized ventricular impairment.

The angiographic classification of CAD and left ventricular function in this series is presented according to primary peripheral vascular diagnosis in Table 2 (19). Only 8% of the patients had normal coronary arteries, while CAD was limited to mild to moderate disease in another 32%. Advanced but compensated CAD, which did not require myocardial revascularization, was identified in 29% of patients. Severe, surgically correctable CAD was documented in 25% of the entire series, and 6% had severe CAD that was not reconstructable. The distribution of CAD and left ventricular dysfunction among the peripheral vascular diagnostic categories is nearly uniform except for a comparatively increased incidence of severe CAD among patients with aneurysm, presumably reflecting the increased mean age of this subgroup.

Left ventriculography was normal in 68% of patients, while 21% had segmental akinesia in the distribution of previous infarctions, and 11% had

Table 2   Angiographic Classification of Coronary Artery Disease and Left Ventricular Impairment According to Primary Peripheral Vascular Diagnosis

	Abdominal Aortic Aneurysm (n=263) %	Lower Extremity Ischemia (n=381) %	Cerebrovascular Disease (n=295) %	Other (n=61) %	Total (n=1000) %
CAD					
Normal	6	10	9	7	8
Mild to moderate	29	33	32	34	32
Advanced but compensated	29	29	27	34	29
Severe, correctable	31	21	26	23	25
Severe, inoperable	5	7	6	2	6
Ventricular impairment					
None	68	66	71	69	68
Segmental	24	21	18	20	21
Diffuse	8	13	11	11	11

Source: From Ref. 19, used with permission.

diffuse ventricular impairment. The objective results of ventriculography and the precatheterization assessment of cardiac status on occasion did not agree. Ventricular impairment was demonstrated only in 149 (67%) of 221 patients with a history compatible with previous myocardial infarction, and in 142 (73%) of 195 interpreted to have had prior infarction by ECG. However, ventricular impairment was documented in 168 (22%) of 779 patients with no previous symptoms of myocardial infarction, and in 175 (22%) of 805 having no evidence of infarction by ECG (19).

Factors other than the primary vascular diagnosis influenced the distribution of severe CAD, such as sex, age, and clinical cardiac status (19). Severe, correctable CAD was found in 198 (29%) of 685 men and in 53 (17%) of 315 women (p<0.001), but the difference in the incidence of nonreconstructable CAD in these two groups (6.0 and 5.4%, respectively) was not significant. Severe CAD was found in a total of 36% of patients with aortic aneurysms (mean age 67 years), in 32% of those with cerebrovascular disease (mean age 64 years), and in 28% of those with lower extremity ischemia (mean age 61 years). The influence of age on the incidence of severe, correctable and inoperable CAD is graphically depicted in Figure 1 (19). Severe CAD was present in 22% of patients younger than 50 years of age, 24% of those aged 50 to 59 years, 30% of those aged 60 to 69 years and 41% of those older than 70 years of age. A total of 323 patients were younger than 60 years of age at the time of coronary angiography, while 677 were older. Although the incidence of severe, correctable CAD in these subsets was similar (22 and 27%, respectively), nonreconstructable CAD was discovered in only 1.9% of younger patients in comparison to 7.7% of those older than 60 years of age (p<0.001).

The clinical cardiac status was the most important factor influencing the incidence of correctable and inoperable CAD in each age group (19). When suspected by conventional criteria, severe CAD was encountered in 34% of patients younger than the age of 50, 40% aged 50 to 69 years, and 51% of those older than 70 years of age (Fig. 1). Each of the features determining the clinical cardiac status was closely correlated with the results of coronary angiography. A history of angina pectoris was a reliable indication of severe coronary involvement because myocardial revascularization was warranted in half of the group of patients describing angina and another 15% had severe, inoperable CAD. A history of myocardial infarction or ischemic changes on a standard 12 lead ECG also reliably indicated underlying CAD. Severe, correctable CAD was verified by angiography in one of three patients in these groups, and another 7 to 14% had nonreconstructable lesions. By clinical

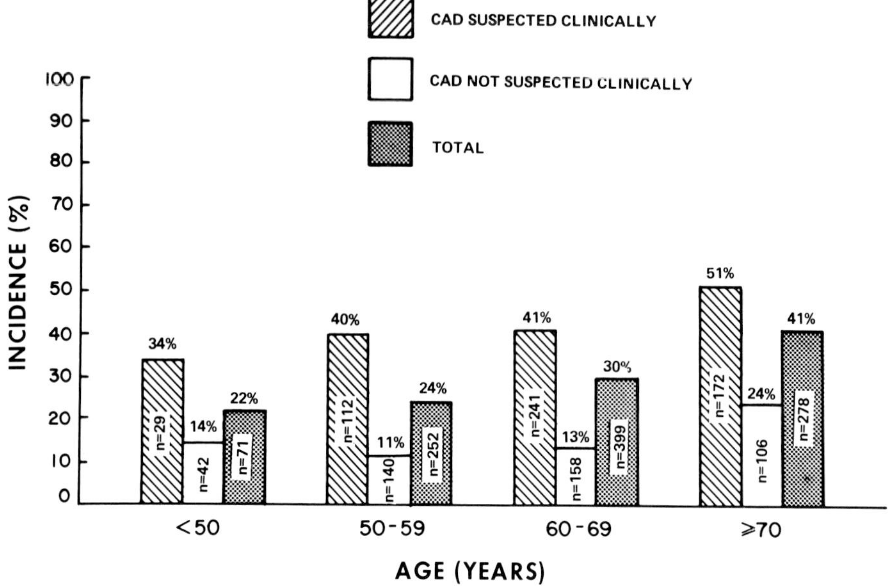

Figure 1 The incidence of severe, correctable, and inoperable coronary artery disease (CAD) according to age and clinical cardiac status at the time of coronary angiography in 1000 patients with peripheral vascular disease at the Cleveland Clinic (19).

criteria alone, coronary bypass was indicated in 34% of 554 patients who previously were suspected to have coronary disease (Fig. 2) compared with 14% of 446 who were not ($p=2 \times 10^{-13}$).

Neither hypertension nor diabetes mellitus had a meaningful influence on the incidence of severe, correctable CAD. The incidence of severe, inoperable CAD also was similar between those with and those without hypertension. However, nonreconstructable CAD was discovered in 12% of diabetics in comparison with only 4.5% of nondiabetics ($p<0.001$) (19).

Surgical Management

Based on the results of coronary angiography, 226 of the 1000 patients in this series required cardiac surgical procedures, which usually either preceded or were performed simultaneously with peripheral vascular reconstruction

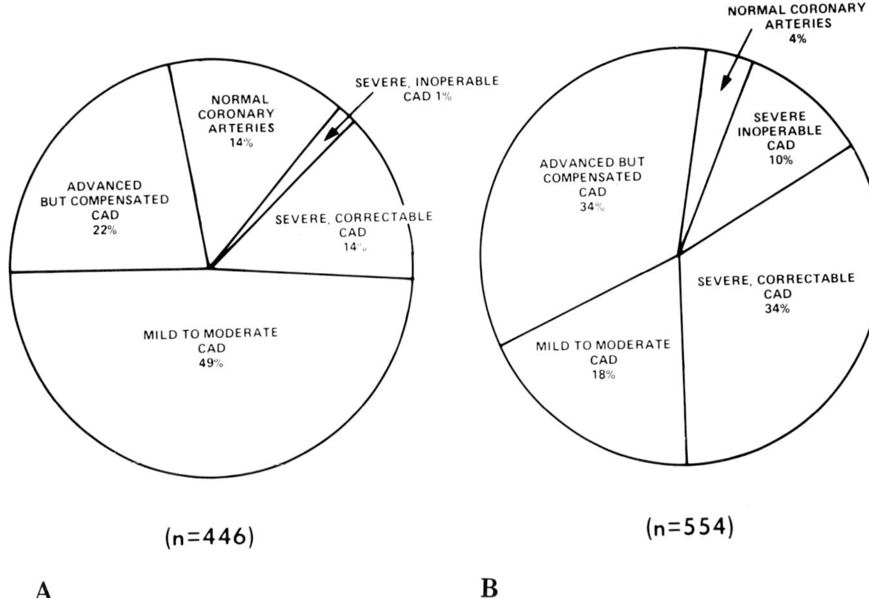

Figure 2 Angiography classification of coronary artery disease (CAD) according to clinical cardiac status at the time of coronary angiography. *A*: CAD not clinically suspected. *B*: CAD suspected clinically (19).

(19). As indicated in Table 3, 216 of these operations involved coronary bypass alone (n=212) or in conjunction with valve replacement (n=4). Another 35 patients with severe, correctable CAD also were advised to have myocardial revascularization, but either declined or never underwent treatment.

Twelve patients (mean age 65 years) died after cardiac procedures, with an operative mortality for coronary bypass (5.2%) that is similar to the results of other reports of patients in this age group (21,22). Fatalities occurred in 6 (13%) of 47 patients who required simultaneous carotid and cardiac operations, and accounted for half of all postoperative deaths. Another two patients, representing 2.9% of those who presented with aortic aneurysms and required myocardial revascularization, had ruptured aneurysms after cardiac procedures and died despite emergency repair. Severe, multivessel coronary disease, which appeared to preclude elective peripheral vascular reconstruction as well as limit life expectancy, was present in 10 of the 12 patients who died after cardiac operations (19).

Table 3 Operative Mortality for 1066 Peripheral Vascular Procedures After Elective Correction of Severe Associated Coronary Artery Disease

	Procedure	Preliminary CABG	Subsequent Peripheral Vascular Procedures	Infrarenal Aortic Aneurysm Repair	Lower Extremity Revascularization	Extracranial Reconstruction	Other	Total
Surgical management	No. of procedures	216	1066	206	335	319	206	1292
Operative mortality	No. of patients	12	21	7	6	1	7	33
		(5.5%)	(2.0%)	(3.4%)·	(1.8%)	(0.3%)	(3.4%)	(2.6%)

CABG = coronary artery bypass grafting.
Source: From Ref. 19, used with permission.

A total of 796 patients in the study group initially underwent 1066 procedures for correction of their principal peripheral vascular disease, including 130 patients advised to undergo preliminary myocardial revascularization (Table 3) (19). Overall operative mortality rates were 3.4% for elective aneurysm resection, 1.8% for lower extremity revascularization, 0.3% for extracranial reconstruction, and 3.4% for a miscellaneous group that included occasional patients with such special risks as thoracoabdominal aneurysms and infected arterial grafts. Notably, only one death (0.8%) occurred after peripheral vascular operation in the subset of 130 patients who had preliminary coronary bypass. One (1.6%) of 61 patients died after abdominal aortic aneurysm resection, and there were no deaths among 69 others who required subsequent extremity bypass or extracranial reconstruction. In summary, 33 early deaths (2.6%) occurred after the initial 1292 cardiac and vascular procedures performed in this investigation. (19)

Since these data first were reported, a total of 846 of the original 1000 patients assessed by coronary angiography now have undergone peripheral vascular reconstruction. Table 4 presents a summary of operative deaths according to age and the angiographic classification of associated coronary disease (1). As expected, surgical risk escalates with advancing age and the increasing incidence of associated severe coronary artery disease. Twenty-four deaths (2.8%) have occurred among the 846 patients, and the difference in operative mortality between those younger than 70 years of age (2.0%) and those older than 70 years (5.2%) was statistically significant (p=0.018). Early mortality also increased proportionately from 1.4% in the group with normal coronary arteries to 14% in a small subset of 28 patients who underwent peripheral vascular operation in the presence of severe, inoperable CAD. These data also suggest that preliminary coronary bypass may improve the perioperative risk of selected patients with vascular disease, especially those older than 70 years of age.

Although they previously were found to have severe CAD, the operative mortality for peripheral vascular procedures after coronary bypass in 200 patients was only 1.5%, which nearly is identical to the surgical risk among patients having normal coronary arteries. In comparison, vascular operations were performed with customary precautions in 16 of 35 patients with severe, correctable CAD who never received coronary bypass. Two (12%) of these patients died (p=0.045). A coordinated approach to associated coronary disease deters the use of age alone as a definitive contraindication to major vascular procedures, such as aortic aneurysm resection, in those who need them. Although advancing age corresponded to a higher operative mortality in some groups, none of 63 patients older than 70 years of age who received preliminary myocardial revascularization died after subsequent peripheral

Table 4   Operative Deaths After Peripheral Vascular Reconstruction in
846 Patients According to Age and Angiographic Classification of Associated
Coronary Artery Disease

Coronary Angiographic Classification	Peripheral Vascular Procedures	Peripheral Vascular Operative Deaths		
		Age <70 %	Age > 7/70 %	Total %
Normal coronary arteries	74	1.4	0	1.4
Mild to moderate CAD	278	1.4	3.1	1.8
Advanced but compensated CAD	250	2.3	6.5	3.6
Severe, correctable CAD				
With bypass	200	2.2	0	1.5
No bypass	16	11.1	14	12
Severe, inoperable CAD	28	0	25	14
Total	846	2.0	5.2	2.8

CAD = coronary artery disease.
Source: From Ref. 23, used with permission.

vascular reconstruction. Acknowledging the operative risk of coronary bypass
itself to be approximately 5%, even this figure represents an improvement in
the expected mortality rate of major peripheral vascular procedures in aged
patients with severe coronary disease.

Late Results

Of the 1000 patients with peripheral vascular disease entered into this study,
12 died after cardiac procedures and 24 have had fatal complications after
vascular reconstruction. Late information has been collected for the
remaining 964 patients during a period of 3 to 7 years (mean 4.6), with only
1.9% lost to follow-up at some interval (23). A total of 266 (28%) of these
964 operative survivors have since died, and the principal causes of late
mortality are presented in Table 5. Myocardial infarction (26%), congestive

Table 5 Primary Causes of Late Death in 964 Patients with Peripheral Vascular Disease During a Follow-up Interval of 7 years (mean 4.6)

Primary Cause of Late Death	Cardiac	Myocardial Infarction	Congestive Heart Failure	Arrhythmia	Cancer	Stroke	Ruptured Aortic Aneurysm	Renal Failure	Pulmonary Failure Or Embolism	All Other Known Causes	Sudden Death or Unknown	Total
Number of late deaths	102	68	26	8	34	21	15	14	12	20	48	266
Percent of entire series	11	7.1	2.7	0.8	3.5	2.2	1.6	1.5	1.2	2.1	5.0	28
Percent of late deaths	38	26	9.0	3.0	13	7.9	5.6	5.3	4.5	7.5	18	100

Source: From Ref. 23, used with permission.

heart failure (9%), or arrhythmias (3%) accounted for 38% of all late deaths. Fatal cardiac events have led to three times the cancer mortality (13%) and approximately four times the number of deaths caused by strokes (8%). Ruptured thoracic or abdominal arotic aneurysms occurred in 15 patients who represented 1.6% of the follow-up group and 5.6% of all late deaths.

Cardiac mortality, like operative risk, could be stratified according to age and the angiographic classification of associated coronary disease (23). In Table 6, these two factors are correlated with all operative and late deaths. Twelve percent of deaths have been associated with cardiac causes, ranging from 1.2% of patients originally documented to have normal coronary arteries to 38% of those found to have severe, nonreconstructable CAD.

Table 6   Total Cardiac Deaths in 1000 Patients with Peripheral Vascular Disease Within 7 Years (mean 4.6) of Investigation According to Age and the Angiographic Classification of Associated Coronary Disease

| | | Operative and Late Cardiac Deaths | | |
Coronary Angiographic Classification	No. of Patients	Age $<$ 70 Years %	Age $>$ 7/71 Years %	Total %
Normal coronary arteries	85	1.3	0	1.2
Mild to moderate CAD	317	3.6	7.4	4.4
Advanced but compensated CAD	289	14.6	18	16
Severe, correctable CAD				
With bypass	216	12.9	9.0	12
no bypass	35	14.3	38	26
Severe, inoperable CAD	58	46.4	30	38
Total	1000	10.2	15	12

CAD = coronary artery disease.
Source: From Ref. 23, used with permission.

Cardiac mortality has occurred in 12% of 216 patients whose severe CAD was rectified by coronary bypass, a figure transcended only by those with either normal coronary arteries or mild to moderate angiographic changes (4.4%). In comparison with the myocardial revascularization subset, cardiac deaths thus far have occurred in 9 (26%) of the 35 unoperated patients having severe, correctable coronary lesions (p=0.033). Although the overall incidence of cardiac fatalities increased from 10.2% in younger patients to 15% of those older than 70 years of age, this tendency was not observed among patients who underwent coronary bypass. In this group, only 6 (9.0%) of 67 older patients have died from cardiac complications compared with 38% of others in the same age group for whom myocardial revascularization was justified but never performed.

Cumulative Survival

Lifetable data have been computed according to Cutler and Edereer (24) and analyzed for statistical significance using the method described by Lee and Desu (25). Fatalities during the immediate postoperative period after peripheral vascular reconstruction have not been included in these calculations, but the operative mortality rate of coronary bypass is incorporated in all comparisons involving the subset with severe correctable CAD. Because myocardial revascularization was an integral feature of the coordinated treatment of associated coronary disease in this series, the importance of its surgical risk is an essential consideration.

Cumulative 5 year survival for all angiographic groups is shown in Figure 3 (23). Five year survival ranges from only 22% among patients found to have severe, nonreconstructable lesions to 85% among those having normal coronary arteries or mild to moderate CAD. Five year survival presently is 72% in patients with severe, correctable CAD who received coronary bypass. This figure exceeds that for the late results (64%) in those with advanced but compensated coronary lesions for which revascularization was not necessary, and it is surpassed only by survival in patients with normal coronary artteries or mild to moderate CAD. In comparison with the bypass group, only 43% of 35 nonoperated patients known to have severe, correctable CAD have survived 5 years since they entered this study (p=0.001).

Figure 4 illustrates actuarial data according to the clinical cardiac status at the time of coronary angiography (23). Cumulative 5 year survival currently is 63% in the group suspected to have coronary artery disease and is 81% among those who were not, but the late results for patients who underwent

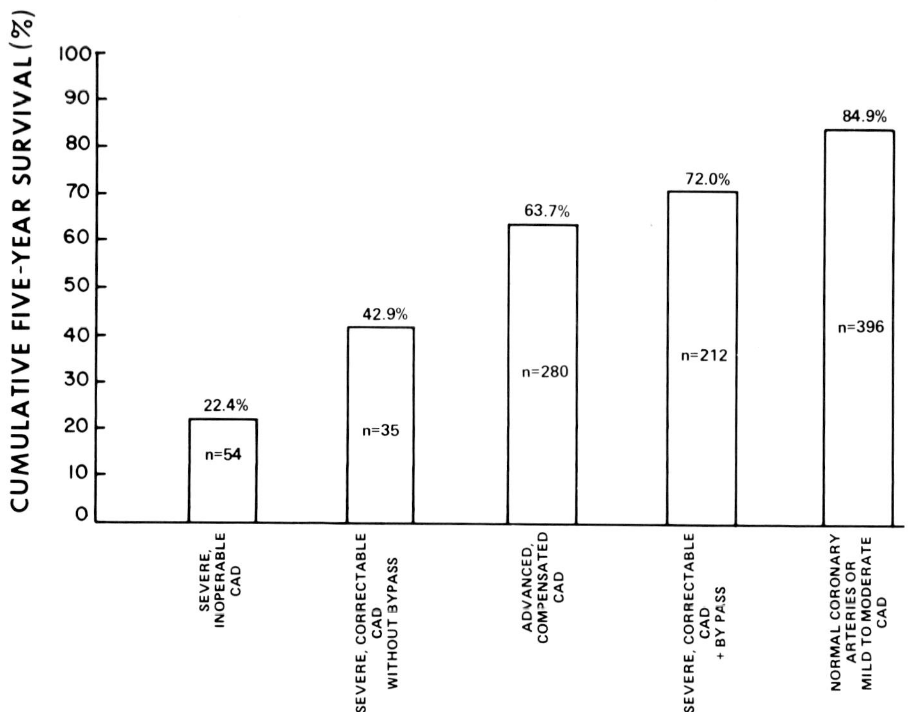

Figure 3 Cumulative 5 year survival of patients with peripheral vascular disease treated at the Cleveland Clinic, according to angiographic classification of associated coronary artery disease (CAD) (23).

coronary bypass in both groups are nearly equivalent (71 and 74%, respectively). Although 63% of the patients who had no clinical evidence of coronary disease were found to have normal coronary arteries or only mild to moderate CAD, the difference in 5 year survival between those in whom coronary bypass was necessary and all others in this group (82%) was not statistically significant (p=0.16). In comparison, 5 year survival among patients who underwent coronary bypass thus far is superior to the results (57%) for all other patients with clinical indications of associated coronary disease, although the differences have not yet achieved statistical significance (p=0.06).

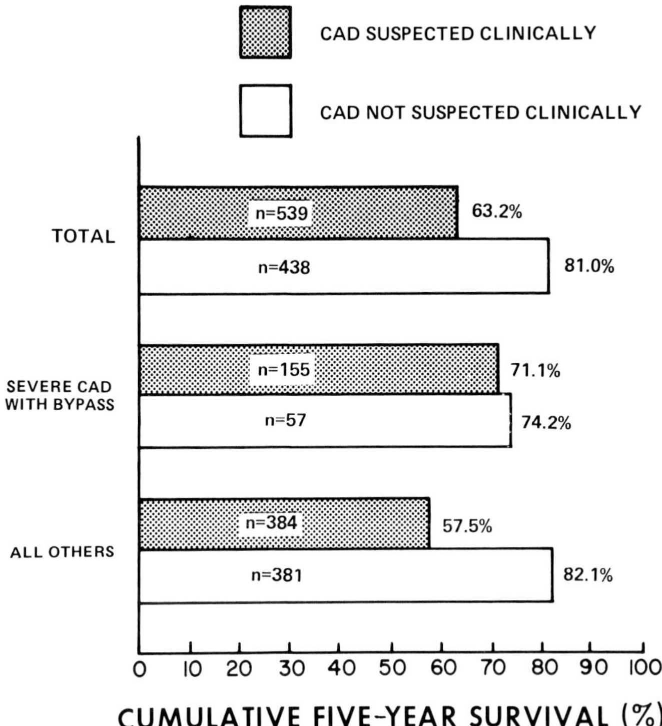

Figure 4 Cumulative 5 year survival in the total Cleveland Clinic series, according to clinical cardiac status at the time of coronary angiography with comparison of those patients managed with coronary bypass with all others in the series (23).

Less than severe coronary involvement (normal coronary arteries, mild to moderate CAD, or advanced but compensated CAD) was documented by angiography in 61% of patients younger than 60 years of age, 59% of those aged 60 to 69 years, and 49% of those older than 70 years of age who had accepted clinical indications of CAD. Cumulative 5 year survival for these three age groups is presented in Figure 5 (23). In spite of the observation that the majority of patients in the younger subsets had only a mild to intermediate degree of CAD, 5 year survival in those who underwent bypass for severe coronary lesions currently is 3 to 10% better than that of all others of similar age. A previous report from the Cleveland Clinic (26) suggested that differences in late survival in younger patients with peripheral vascular disease may not become obvious until the fifth through tenth years of follow-up. In fact, the most impressive disparities in 5 year survival within the present study have involved patients older than 70 years of age. In this group, cumulative survival is 63% after coronary bypass compared with 44% for all other patients of the same age (p=0.04).

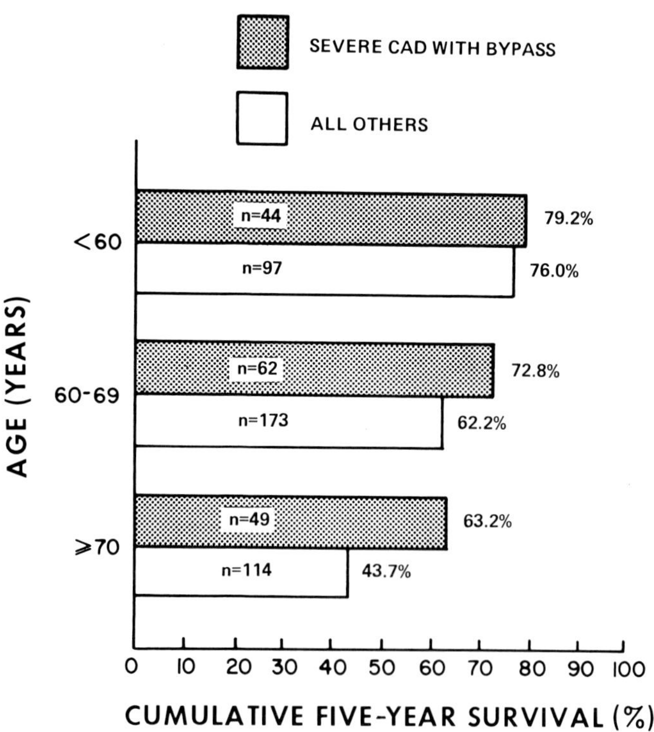

Figure 5 Cumulative 5 year survival according to age for patients with severe coronary artery disease (CAD) managed with coronary bypass compared with all others in the series (23).

Conclusions and Recommendations

Information from this prospective study of 1000 patients has led to the coordinated evaluation of associated coronary disease prior to elective peripheral vascular reconstruction at the Cleveland Clinic (Fig. 6) (27). Because 34% of vascular patients with persuasive clinical evidence of coronary involvement warranted coronary bypass (Fig. 2B), coronary angiography has remained a necessary feature of the preoperative investigation in patients suspected of having CAD, especially those who are scheduled for transabdominal aortic replacement. Although severe, correctable CAD still was identified in 14% of patients without classical evidence of ischemic heart disease (Fig. 2A), coronary bypass was a sufficiently unusual consideration in this group that stress electrocardiography or noninvasive cardiac imaging now are employed to select such patients for angiography. The algorithm in Figure 6 is a generalized guide and cannot address all clinical circumstances. Prompt surgical management of symptomatic or preocclusive carotid lesions may take priority over a time-consuming preoperative cardiac investigation, especially in patients without clinical evidence of CAD. Stress electrocardiography has clearly apparent limitations before lower extremity revascularization in patients with severe claudication or ischemic lesions, at least until the merit of nonexertional dipyridamole stress testing is established and it is released for general use (28). Nevertheless, the threat to early and late survival of associated coronary artery disease in patients with peripheral vascular disease is of such demonstrated significance that a coordinated approach to both problems is required if these patients are to receive optimal comprehensive management.

Previous experience at the Cleveland Clinic (6,18,29) has suggested that patients with severe coexisting coronary disease face a perioperative risk of approximately 10% at the time of major vascular procedures and that their 5 year survival might be augmented by as much as 29% by coronary bypass when appropriate.

Extensive studies of the first 1000 patients assessed by preoperative coronary angiography are planned to evaluate the influence of gender, diabetes, hypertension, and other factors on late results, but several preliminary conclusions may be made from the information already available. First, the operative mortality of coronary bypass (5%) in aged patients with peripheral vascular disease exceeds that anticipated for elective myocardial revascularization. Second, the risk of subsequent vascular procedures is so low that the combined mortality rate for both the cardiac and vascular operations barely surpasses that of coronary bypass alone. Despite its own intrinsic risk,

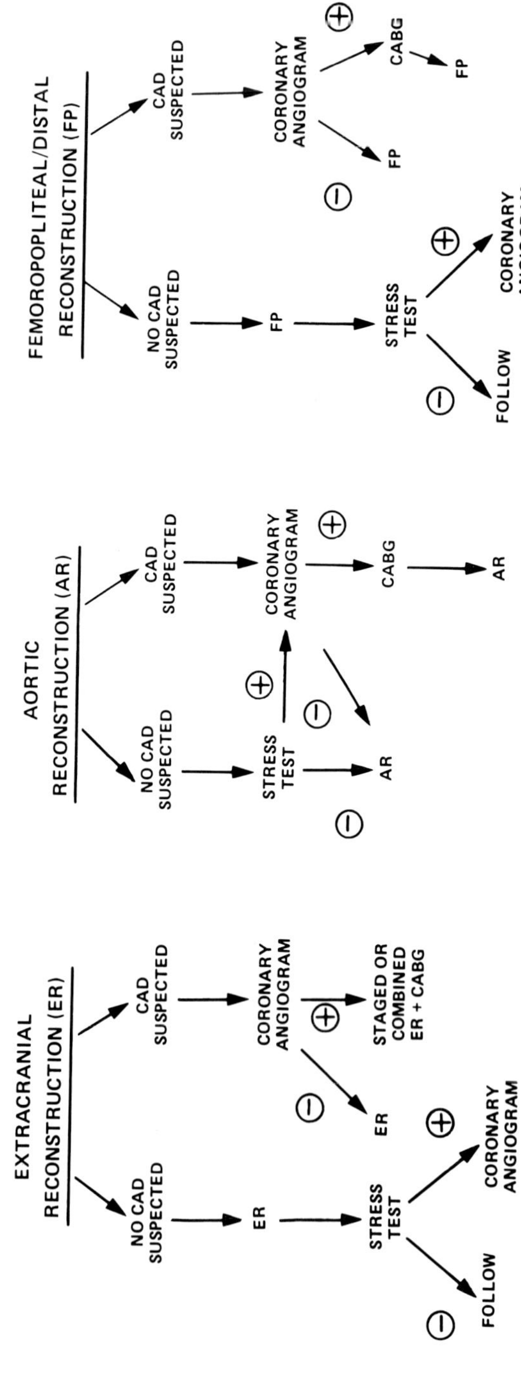

Figure 6 Current algorithm for the investigation and surgical management of associated coronary artery disease (CAD) in patients under serious consideration for elective peripheral vascular reconstruction at the Cleveland Clinic (27). CABG = coronary artery bypass grafting.

therefore, staged coronary bypass appears to reduce the overall surgical mortality in selected patients with vascular disease. Finally, the preliminary results of this prospective but nonrandomized investigation of complementary myocardial revascularization at the Cleveland Clinic demonstrates an improvement in 5 year survival in comparison with a smaller group of patients with comparable angiographic findings. Within the current study interval (mean 4.6 years), patients older than 70 years of age seem to benefit the most from the protection offered by myocardial revascularization.

References

1. DeBakey ME, Crawford ES, Cooley DA, et al. Aneurysm of the abdominal aorta. Analysis of results of graft replacement therapy one to eleven years after operation. Ann Surg 160:622-638, 1964.
2. DeBakey ME, Crawford ES, Morris GL Jr, et al. Late results of vascular surgery in the treatment of arteriosclerosis. J Cardiovasc Surg (Torino) 5:473-480, 1964.
3. DeBakey ME, Crawford ES, Cooley DA, et al. Cerebral arterial insufficiency; one to eleven year results following arterial reconstructive operation. Ann Surg 161:921-945, 1965.
4. DeWeese JA, Rob CG. Autogenous venous grafts ten years later. Surgery 82:775-784, 1977.
5. DeWeese JA, Rob CG, Satran R, Marsh DO, Joymt RJ, Summers D, Nichols C. Results of carotid endarterectomies for transient ischemic attacks — five years later. Ann Surg 178:258-264, 1973.
6. Diehl JT, Cali RF, Hertzer NR, et al. Complications of abdominal aortic reconstruction. An analysis of perioperative risk factors in 557 patients. Ann Surg 197:49-56, 1983.
7. Hertzer NR. Fatal myocardial infarction following abdominal aortic aneurysm resection. Three hundred forty three patients followed 6-11 years postoperatively. Ann Surg 192:667-673, 1980.
8. Hertzer NR. Fatal myocardial infarction following lower extremity revascularization. Two hundred seventy-three patients followed 6-11 postoperative years. Ann Surg 193:492-498, 1981.
9. Szilagyi DE, Smith RF, DeRusso FJ, Elliot JP, Sherrin FW. Contribution of abdominal aorta aneurysmectomy to prolongation of life. Ann Surg 164:678, 1966.
10. Szilagyi DE, Hageman JH, Smith RF, Elliot MP, Brown F, Dietz P. Autogenous vein grafting in femoropopliteal atherosclerosis; the limits of its effectiveness. Surgery 86:836-851, 1979.

11. Thompson JE, Austin DJ, Patman RD. Carotid endarterectomy for cerebrovascular insufficiency; long-term results in 592 patients followed up to thirteen years. Ann Surg 172:663-679, 1970.
12. Crawford ES. Material presented at the Fifteenth Annual Texas Heart Institute Symposium, Houston, Texas, September 13, 1985.
13. Crawford ES, Morris GL, Howell JF, et al. Operative risk in patients with previous coronary artery bypass. Ann Thoracic Surg 26:215-220, 1978.
14. McCollum CH, Cardia-Rinaldi R, Graham JM, et al. Myocardial revascularization prior to subsequent major surgery in patients with coronary artery disease. Surgery 81:302-304, 1977.
15. Reul GJ, Cooley DA, Duncan JM, et al. The effect of coronary bypass on the outcome of peripheral vascular operations in 1093 patients. J Vasc Surg (in press).
16. Hertzer NR. Fatal myocardial infarction following peripheral vascular operations. A study of 951 patients followed 6-11 years post operatively. Cleve Clin Q 49:1-11, 1982.
17. Hertzer NR, Lees CD. Fatal myocardial infarction following carotid endarterectomy. Three hundred thirty five patients followed 6 to 11 years after operation. Ann Surg 194:212-218, 1981.
18. Hertzer NR, Loop FD, Taylor PC, et al. Combined myocardial revascularization and carotid endarterectomy. J Thorac Cardiovasc Surg 85:577-589, 1983.
19. Hertzer NR, Beven EG, Young JR, et al. Coronary artery disease in pheripheral vascular patients. A classification of 1000 coronary angiograms and results of surgical management. Ann Surg 199:223-233, 1984.
20. Hertzer NR, Young JR, Kramer JR, et al. Routine coronary angiography prior to elective aortic reconstruction. Results of selective myocardial revascularization in patients with peripheral vascular disease. Arch Surg 114:1336-1344, 1979.
21. Gersh BJ, Kronmal RA, Frye RL, et al. Coronary arteriography and coronary artery bypass surgery: morbidity and mortality in patients 65 years or older. A report from the Coronary Artery Surgery Study. Circulation 67:483, 1983.
22. Hibler BA, Wright JO, Wright CB, et al. Coronary artery bypass surgery in the elderly. Arch Surg 118:402, 1983.
23. Hertzer NR, Young JR, Beven EG, et al. Late results of coronary bypass in selected peripheral vascular patients: five year survival according to age and clinical cardiac status. Cleve Clin Q 53:133-143, 1986.
24. Cutler SJ, Ederer F. Maximum utilization of the life table method in analyzing survival. J Chron Dis 8:688-712, 1958.

25. Lee ET, Desu MM. A computer program for comparing K samples with right-censored data. Comput Programs Biomed 2:315-321, 1972.
26. Martinez BD, Hertzer NR, Beven EG. The influence of distal arterial occlusive disease on prognosis following aortobifemoral bypass. Surgery 88:795-805, 1980.
27. Hertzer NR. Clinical experience with preoperative coronary angiography. J Vasc Surg 2: 510-514, 1985.
28. Boucher CA, Brewster DC, Darling RC, et al. Determination of cardiac risk by dipyrimadole-thallium imaging before peripheral vascular surgery. N Engl J Med 312:389, 1985.
29. Hertzer NR, Arison R. Cumulative stroke and survival ten years after carotid endarterectomy. J Vasc Surg 2:661-668, 1985.

6

Reoperation for Occluded Aortic Grafts

RALPH G. DePALMA
George Washington University Medical Center, Washington, D.C.

Aortofemoral bypass and aortoiliac reconstruction have emerged as among the more durable of peripheral vascular reconstructions. In considering reoperation for occluded aortic reconstructions, it is useful to review the history of procedures designed to bypass atherosclerosis involving the aortoiliac segment. The underlying principle is that of adequately bypassing segmental atherosclerotic disease. Some failures of these operations are caused by failure to conform to this principle and relate to common distributions of occlusive atherosclerosis. The first procedure for occlusive disease was aortoiliac in scope and was performed in 1951 by Jacques Oudot of Paris (1). He used resection and an allograft to replace the aorta and common iliac arteries. His choice of excision was influenced by Leriche's (2) concept of possible benefit from removing occluded arterial segments along with the insight some 30 years before that this operation would be feasible. Within a year, Wylie (3) successfully performed thromboendarterectomy of the aortoiliac segment, an operation still suited to selected cases of localized aortoiliac disease. DeBakey and associates (4) pioneered in treating occlusive disease of the abdominal aorta. They later emphasized the use of Dacron bifurcated grafts to bypass the involved aortoiliac segment. As a result of experience dictated by common patterns of atherosclerosis, aortoiliac and,

more commonly, aortofemoral bypass using knitted Dacron prostheses
emerged as standard vascular operations. Aortoiliac operations are more
frequently used in aneurysmal disease. This chapter examines occlusive
complications related to these reconstructions. Factors inherent in the
initial procedure predisposing to later failure will be examined, and guidelines will be suggested for preoperative management and reoperative cor-
rections.

Incidence and Etiology

Aortoiliac and aortofemoral reconstructions are durable operations. Crawford
and associates (5) showed that patients operated on for this distribution of
atherosclerotic disease have a 50% chance of being alive at 10 years. At that
time, almost 75% of them will have patent grafts. As a result of such experiences, aortofemoral bypass emerged as the preferred treatment for lower
extremity ischemia caused by proximal aortoiliac disease. It was early learned
that combined aortic bypass and femoropopliteal reconstruction using
Dacron yielded poor results. In addition, due to the frequency of involvement
of the external iliac artery by atherosclerosis, aortofemoral bypass, by
providing direct flow into the profunda femoria artery, was found to yield
slightly more favorable results than aortoiliac bypass. A precise estimate of
the incidence of rethrombosis of these grafts cannot be derived because of
the heterogeneous nature of the surgical techniques selected, technical factors
in performance of operation, variety of grafts used, and variable patterns of
host risk factors and atherosclerotic disease.

Table 1 summarizes reports dealing with late occlusion of aortofemoral
or iliac grafts in collected series (5-13) dating back to 1959. These reports,
inasmuch as they are retrospective, do not prospectively estimate possible occlusion rates of aortoiliac procedures currently performed. The data appear to
vary widely, probably because of limitations in follow-up study or varying
conventions of data presentation. Among the lowest occlusion rates reported
for bilateral aortofemoral bypass is an incidence of 3.6% by Crawford and
associates (5) compared with 12% (i.e., 44 of 360 limbs of bilateral aortofemoral knitted bifurcation grafts) described by Malone and co-workers in
1975 (9).

Due to diverse experiences and techniques of aortofemoral grafting, it is
not possible to postulate a single etiology for late occlusions. Causes of reconstructive failures are multiple. Occlusion can result from initial choice of
bypass extent (i.e., failure to perform proximal and distal anastomoses in

Table 1 Late Occlusion of Aortofemoral/Iliac Grafts

Series	Year	Time Interval	Types of Reconstruction or Graft	Incidence		Comments
Lyons and Weismann (6)	1968	1957-1965	135 Aortoiliac or Femoral Fabric Bifurcation	13/135	(13.3%)	All single limb closures-average time 17.9 months
Najafi et al. (7)	1975	1961-1971	276 Bilateral Aortofemoral (AF) 231 Aortobilat, Ext. Iliac (AI) 109 Mixed AF and AI	27/276	(7.6%)	Simultaneous sympathectomy in 301 patients
Szilagyi et al. (8)	1975	1951-1973	135 Allografts 2022 Aortoileofemoral prostheses 4 vein 172 Endarterectomy	254/2,333	(10.9%)	Overall estimate of late secondary operations, all causes
Malone et al. (9)	1975	1959-1974	130 Bilateral AF: knitted Dacron (360 limbs)	44/360	(12%)	Showed decreased cumulative patency in profunda and popliteal disease
Crawford et al. (10)	1977	1956-1976	217 Bilateral AI: knitted Dacron 357 Bilateral AF: knitted Dacron 16 Unilateral AF: knitted Dacron 12 Ileofemoral: knitted Dacron	14/217 (6.4%) 13/357 (3.6%) 3/16 3/12		Expressed preference for AF reconstruction over AI
Kanaly et al. (11)	1978	1970-1976	47 Bilateral AI 129 Bilateral AF	14/166	(8.4%)	Estimate obtained from combined data
Crawford et al. (5)	1981	1955-1981	416 Bilateral AI 396 Bilateral AF 192 other	87/949	(9.2%)	"Success Rate" increased from 88% in early years to 96% in recent years
Benhamou et al. (12)	1984	1970-1979	850 Bilateral Aortofemoral ("occasional" aortoiliac)	42/850	(4.9%)	Estimated from Text; includes Aneurysms
Deriu et al. (13)	1985	1970-1983	407 Bilateral AF (814 limbs)	46/407	(11.3%)	Estimated from Text

arteries sufficiently uninvolved or less susceptible to later progression of atherosclerosis). It is now known that the proximal aorta immediately beyond the renal arteries is much less likely to be severely involved with atherosclerosis than is distal abdominal aorta. However, inadequate thromboendarterectomy, even of the proximal abdominal aorta, predisposes to reconstructive failure due to extensive disease that has not been adequately removed. The options of proximal end-to-end versus proximal end-to-side anastomoses have yet to be characterized in terms of long-term patency. Nonetheless, the end-to-end anastomosis just below the renal arteries appears to offer favorable hemodynamic streamlining, with ease of achieving graft coverage and separation from the intestine; this option is now a more favored approach. Distally placed end-to-side anastomoses create a potentially unhealthy cul-de-sac in the distal diseased aorta, with a tendency to encroachment by atherosclerotic debris and thrombus at the proximal anastomosis. The selection and technique of prosthetic insertion are clearly important factors. Oversized prostheses will have a lower rate of flow and a greater buildup of pseudointima, which, in turn, can cause thrombosis or distal embolization. Smaller grafts, isodiametric to the femoral arteries, are preferred. Technical mishaps in graft placement such as an improper or inadequate retroperitoneal tunnel, twisting, placing the graft with too much tension (eventual pseudoaneurysm) or too little tension (anterior bowing), and creation of an intra-abdominal graft kink all predispose to late failure. Mechanical failure of graft material, usually dilation, also predisposes to thrombosis and sometimes aneurysm formation. Such instances are now rare.

Due to improved grafts as well as sound techniques of proximal anastomoses, most late graft occlusions are caused by limitations in distal outflow. In particular, the importance of the profunda femoris artery in lower limb perfusion has been recognized for years (14-17) and deserves reemphasis here. Reoperation for failed aortic grafts requires comprehensive knowledge of the anatomy (Figs. 1A and B) and reconstructive techniques (Fig. 2) applicable to the profunda femoris artery. In addition, there are certain individuals, mainly diabetics (18), in whom the profunda femoris artery may be severely diseased. In such instances, an added femoropopliteal vein graft might prolong the patency of the proximal aortic graft. For this purpose, I prefer a vein graft originating from uninvolved proximal profunda femoris artery itself (19). However, the need for ancillary femoropopliteal bypass should be rare; adequate reperfusion of the profunda femoris artery usually suffices to maintain bypass patency and eliminate major lower extremity ischemia.

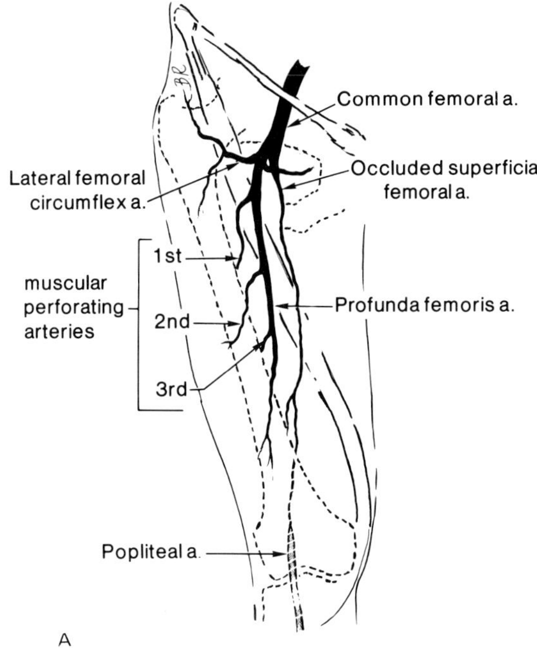

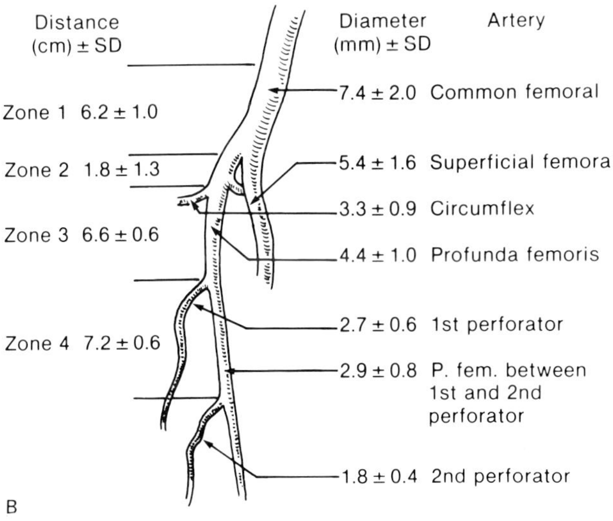

Figure 1 Anatomy of profunda femoris artery. *A*: Common anatomy of profunda femoris artery in presence of occluded superficial artery; *B*: Average diameter of profunda femoris artery and its branches. Average distance of collateral and main vessels from inguinal ligament.

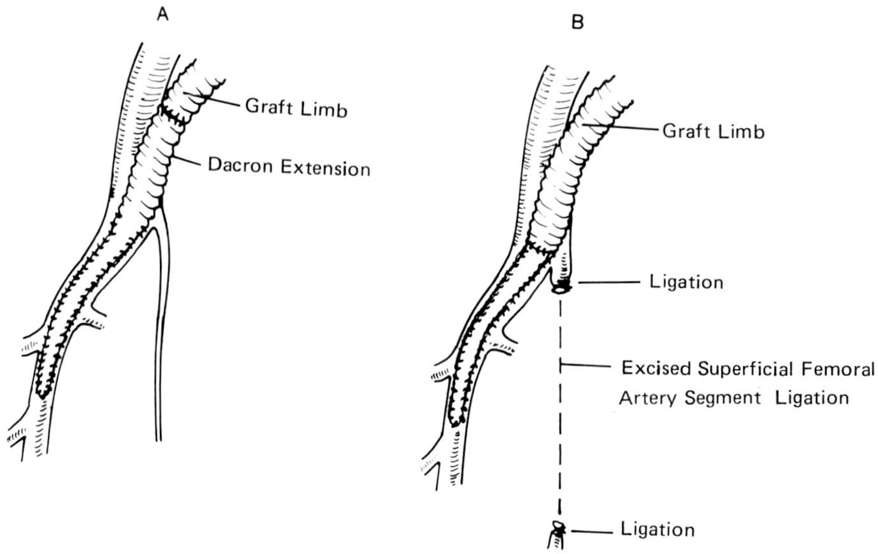

Figure 2   Two methods of profundoplasty. Endarterectomized superficial femoral artery is the preferred patch material.

In aortofemoral bypass for occlusive disease, more than in any other reconstruction, the effect of postoperative cigarette smoking is most dramatic (20,21). Sudden late occlusion of an aortofemoral limb in a nonsmoker is an exceptional event. On occasion, graft limb occlusions are silent, but clotting of one or both limbs of an aortofemoral bypass is usually a catastrophic event signaled by lower extremity ischemia, often more severe than that which prompted the first operation. Therefore, cessation of cigarette smoking should be achieved before the first operation. Continued smoking with repeated failure of redo operations is a scenario featuring elevated amputation rates, frequently proximal above the knee, and death rates up to 40% (11).

Preoperative Management

Management of thrombosed aortic grafts differs depending on whether the failure is early or late. Using the convention of Szilagyi and associates (8), an early failure can be designated as graft limb closure within 30 days of operation. In most circumstances, this event relates to technical error, commonly failure to provide adequate outflow for that limb of the graft. Graft limb occlusion in the immediate postoperative period frequently causes catastrophic ischemia of the entire lower extremity, which if not promptly corrected, causes renal failure and lower extremity gangrene. When the profunda femoris artery is compromised along with iliac collaterals, high thigh amputation or hip disarticulation can be the end result of untreated occlusion. Such early failures must be treated emergently. In most circumstances, repeat arteriography is not necessary; the patient should be taken back to the operating room immediately for exploration of the involved graft limb. Commonly, thrombectomy and revision of the distal anastomosis will be needed. The factors that predispose to thrombosis in the absence of technical failure (e.g., severe hyperglycemia or hypotension) should be corrected simultaneously. On some occasions, no technical flaw is discoverable and, in these cases, hypercoagulable states should be sought.

Late thromboses can be more benign, especially when an initial end-to-side proximal aortic anastomosis had been performed. The affected limb should be examined and Doppler pressures obtained. When no neurologic symptoms exist and if the extremity is not critically threatened, time can be taken for arteriography to assess potential proximal inflow problems as well as the configuration of the outflow vessels. Although arteriograms can be performed using a retrograde catheter technique inserted through the contralateral open graft limb, I recommend either translumbar aortography or an axillary artery approach. These arteriograms should adequately visualize the indigenous arteries proximally and distally and also afford the best possible views of the profunda femoris artery. For this purpose, oblique views are required.

With this information, the patient can be prepared for operation on an urgent basis. This preparation involves exactly the same measures necessary to replace a graft limb or, indeed, redo the original operation. Frequently though, an extensive intra-abdominal revision is not required. In assuring adequate inflow, there will be obligatory blood losses due to limb flushing to remove clot and atherosclerotic debris; therefore, the patient requires prehydration, central monitoring, as well as preoperative, intraoperative, and postoperative antibiotic prophylaxis. The latter are important to prevent graft infection, which is more common in redo operations, especially in the groin. Time must also be taken to adequately prepare the skin with preoperative antiseptic washes; the final shaving is done in the operating room.

Technical Considerations

Reoperation for Early Thrombosis

Thrombosis occurring within the immediate postoperative period requires emergency reoperation. Usually one limb of the bypass is involved. Thromboembolism into the runoff vessels, intimal flap, inadequate distal suture line, or a thrombosis due to low flow state or postoperative hypercoagulability can exist singly or in combination. Although the second operation is done as an emergency and is often limited to the groin, the same aseptic and systemic precautions are taken as with the initial operation. The steps in reexploration of early graft limb thrombosis are illustrated in Figure 3A through F.

The abdomen and both groins are prepared and draped widely. In most instances, it is possible to restore flow by thrombectomy and a limited procedure under local standby anesthesia; when abdominal reexploration is necessary, it is best to be ready with an appropriate wide field preparation. In my experience, the most common causes of early graft thrombosis are embolism, thrombosis, or dissection of a distal intimal flap. The genitalia and perineum are draped with an impermeable Steridrape cemented into place using tincture of benzoin. This precaution prevents contamination due to soaking of drapes in the groin and genital area. Skin sutures are left in place during preparation and are then removed. Subcuticular or subcutaneous sutures are cut and removed, and a self-retaining retractor is inserted.

The common femoral, the graft limb, and the outflow vessels are first controlled with vessel loops. If at the original operation it was thought that the first segment of the profunda femoris artery was more involved with atherosclerosis than usual, the lateral circumflex vein should be divided at this point. This step exposes the profunda femoris artery in its more distal reaches preparatory for possible revision of the anastomosis. An extensive revision, however, in experienced hands is usually not needed; the original anastomosis will have been performed to assure adequate distal outflow by adequate bypass of proximal atherosclerotic involvement.

The graft is then opened; distal thrombus or atherosclerotic debris are removed *before* attempting to restore proximal flow. The orifice of the profunda femoris artery is visualized and probed with a coronary dilator or small urethral sound to assess backflow. With this maneuver, a small amount of clot often escapes, thus restoring vigorous profunda backflow. When the superficial femoral artery had been patent preoperatively, a standard balloon embolectomy is then performed. Heparinization is induced either by local

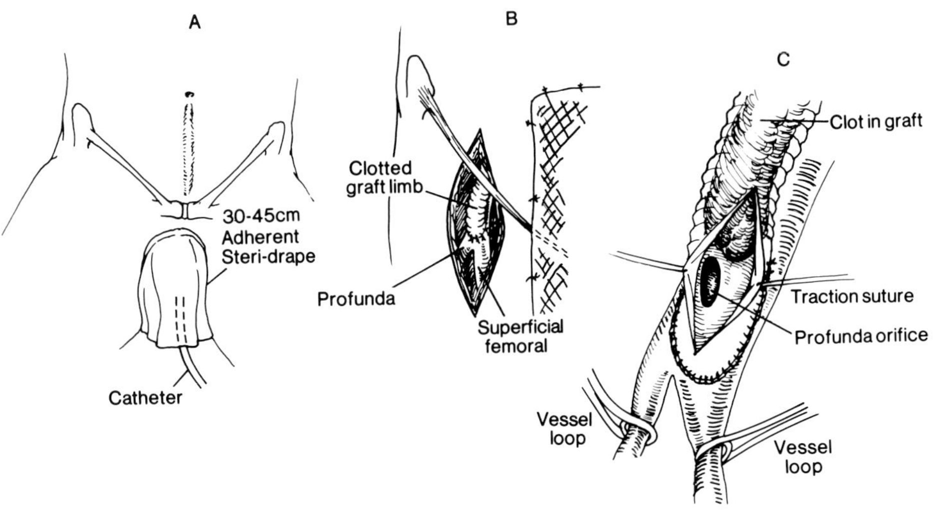

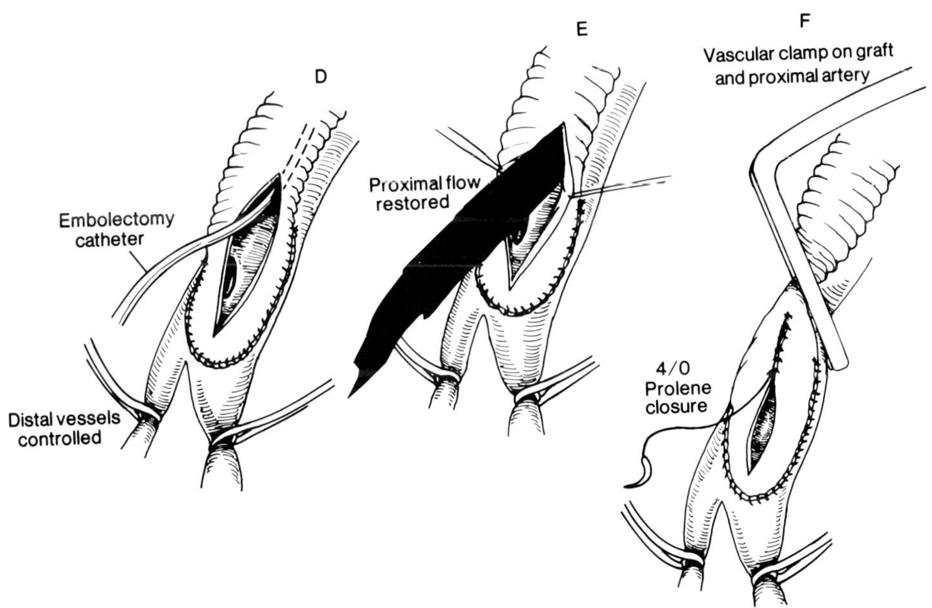

Figure 3 Thrombectomy for graft limb closure; *A*: Predrape with impermeable Steridrape before preparation of skin; *B*: Exposure of graft limb; *C*: Graft opened and local area inspected. Backbleeding from profunda orifice assessed; *D*: Distal vessels cleared; *E*: Proximal flow restored; *F*: Expeditious graft closure.

infusion or systemic heparinization using 75 to 100 units/kg weight according to the surgeon's preference. With early reoperations (i.e., thrombectomies to be performed almost immediately postoperatively), heparin should be used with caution as it can cause bleeding in the intra-abdominal portion of the graft, especially if a knitted prosthesis was used. Once backflow has been restored and the outflow defects identified and corrected, a no. 5 or 6 embolectomy catheter is passed proximally and inflated, and clot is withdrawn from the graft limb. There should be several vigorous flushes of the graft limb, yielding an audible gush of proximal inflow. Before this step, the anesthesiologist should ensure blood replacement and should also be warned to expect a sudden decrease in blood pressure when blood flow is restored to the limb. Emboli to the contralateral patent limb are not common as usually a small column of nonclotted blood exists just distal to the bifurcation in the thrombosed limb. Nonetheless, the contralateral pulse requires careful monitoring after each thrombectomy maneuver.

Retrograde perfusion through the proximal common femoral or external iliac artery is also obtained with proximal embolectomy. To avoid prolonged blood stasis in the clamped aortofemoral limb, the graft is then rapidly closed with 4-0 Prolene suture. Just before restoring flow, another brief proximal flush is carried out, assuring absence of residual clot and continued presence of inflow in the prosthetic limb. At this point, speed in closing the graft is important to prevent proximal reclotting because the graft limb is a relatively thrombogenic surface. Heparinization can then be reversed with intravenous protamine. The groin wound is then reclosed in layers after gentle irrigation with antibiotic solution. If adequate inflow cannot be obtained, a proximal technical error must be suspected. Alternatives must then be examined to obtain adequate inflow. These inevitably involve abdominal re-exploration and repositioning or replacement of the graft limb; these steps have been rarely necessary in my own experience with early occlusions of graft limbs.

Late Single Limb Thrombosis

These patients often present early with critical ischemia of the extremity and sensory paralysis, and later with varying degrees of motor paralysis. After a prolonged period of healing, dissection of the graft limb in the groin can be difficult. One dissection technique, preferred by some surgeons, entails making no attempt to identify the native vessels. The anterior surface of the distal thrombosed graft is exposed by dissection with a scalpel and promptly entered with a longitudinal incision. This incision is continued distally through the anastomosis into the patent autogenous artery. Retrograde bleeding is controlled by selective catheterization of vessel orifices with balloon occlusion catheters. Embolectomy catheters controlled with three-way stopcocks can also be used. At this point, the superficial femoral artery and/or the profunda femoris artery are further opened in preparation for subsequent patch or bypass grafting once adequate inflow is provided. Attempts to encircle vessels encased in scar can often be avoided because blood loss can be controlled with internally placed balloon catheters rather than external clamps or loops. Dissection around scarred vessels is difficult and may compromise collateral vessels as well as damage the larger vessel being dissected.

Another dissection technique, which I prefer, is to first find the profunda femoris and/or superficial femoral artery more distally in previously un-dissected areas (19). The operative exposure of the distal profunda is shown in Figure 4. The vessel or vessels are encircled at suitable sites to provide outflow in relatively undiseased zones. This technique also avoids the need to dissect vessels in densely scarred areas. A more distal bypass can then be done. Regardless of which technique is employed, the underlying strategy should be to identify adequate runoff vessels and minimize trauma to collateral vessels or the vessel being dissected. In either case, the operative approach seeks to minimize dissections of densely scarred arteries wherever possible.

There are several possible approaches for obtaining adequate inflow. Some (22,23) describe proximal balloon catheter embolectomy to restore blood flow through the thrombosed graft limb, just as is done in early cases. This maneuver might be successful, and I have often used it when late graft limb occlusion has been brought promptly to clinical notice. Bernhard and co-workers (22) and Hyde and associates (23) recommend the use of a loop stripper in the graft limb and revision of the distal anastomosis as necessary. Rarely will complete graft revision be necessary. However, with some late chronic occlusions or progressive proximal aortic disease, limited operations may not succeed. An alternative must be selected. If the etiology of occlusion is embolization of graft pseudointima or graft limb dilations, one must consider graft limb replacement. These events signify poor pseudointimal attachment or graft limb failure. Another approach, and one I prefer in chronic occlusions, is to perform a cross-femoral graft to the distal profunda femoris artery (24). Here, the status of the arterial inflow must be well delineated by preoperative arteriography. A knitted Dacron graft is sutured

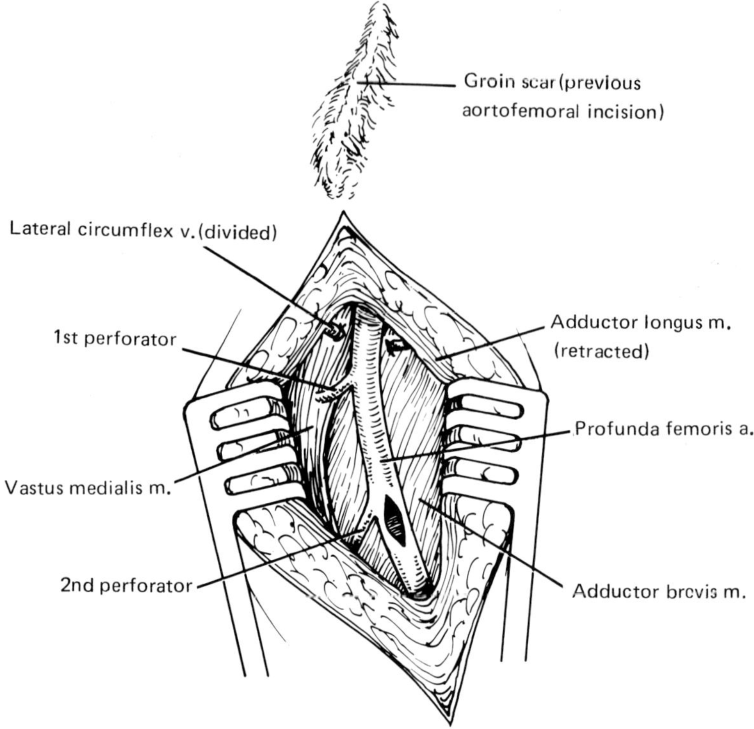

Figure 4 Exposure of profunda femoris artery at the second perforator for distal bypass.

to the contralateral donor limb. The profunda femoris artery is dissected for graft insertion in an uninvolved zone (Fig. 4), and a cross-femoral graft to the profunda is completed (Fig. 5). Another alternative involves a remote bypass such as an axillofemoral graft. The latter procedure offers the disadvantage of an intrinsically late high failure rate.

Complete Aortic Graft Thrombosis

This event is infrequent, but when it occurs, is usually catastrophic if the proximal anastomosis is end-to-end. In this circumstance, visceral ischemia, poor pelvic perfusion, renal shutdown, and impaired spinal cord perfusion can all exist. Reoperative alternatives include direct infrarenal graft revision, re-

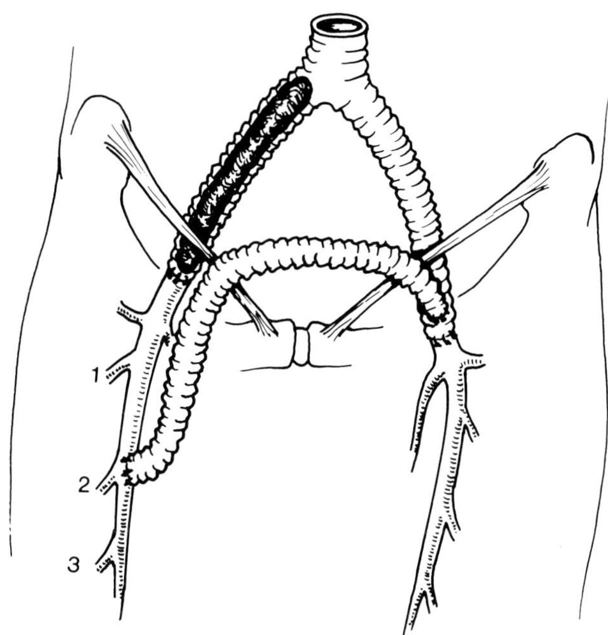

Figure 5   Femorodistal right profunda femoris artery bypass from patent left graft limb.

placement with a supraceliac graft leaving the femoral graft segments revised or attached as necessary, axillo-femoro-femoral or popliteal revision, ascending aorta to distal femoral artery bypass (25), and, finally, a procedure that appears to be quite promising, utilizing the descending thoracic aorta as an inflow site (26,27).

In general, once bilateral thrombosis of an end-to-end aortic graft anastomosis has occurred, it often becomes necessary to perform an emergency abdominal operation not only to correct lower extremity ischemia, but also to ensure visceral perfusion. In these cases, supraceliac graft replacement or intra-abdominal graft replacement should be considered. With failure of an end-to-side aortic anastomosis, the patient often returns to a preoperative state of lower extremity ischemia that, although threatening, is not as serious as complete aortic thrombosis. These patients are also suitable for elective descending thoracic aorta to femoral artery bypass.

Table 2 Results of Reoperations for Aortofemoral Graft Thrombosis

Series	Year	No. of Patients	Months to Occlusion Ave. (Range)	Operations	Host Factors	Early Results		
						Death	Major Amputation	Patency
Wray et al. (20)	1971	9	40.5 (18-72)	Thrombectomy distal revision profundoplasty	Correlation with cigarette smoking & occlusive rather than aneurysmal disease	0	2 2 reoperations successful	6
Bernhard et al. (22)	1977	38	28.6 (to 120)[a]	Thrombectomy new graft profundoplasty extraanatomic	Not described	1	3	46/50 limbs
Crawford et al. (10)	1977	79	b (44-90)	Limb replacement entire graft re-placement Thrombectomy Profundoplasty	Not described	9	5	69
Stanton et al. (28)	1977	20	Not described	Thrombectomy Limb replacement extraanatomic Profundoplasty	Not described	2	2	18
Hyde et al. (23)	1983	7	44 (9-158)	Thrombectomy Profundoplasty	All smokers	0	1	7
Benhamou et al. (12)	1984	70	Not described	Thrombectomy limb replacement new graft Partial Extra-anatomic Total extra-anatomic	Not described	6	10	54

[a]Related early case, 1 day.
[b]Not described.

Results

Table 2 summarizes the literature describing various reoperations and their results in various series of patients (10,12,20,22,23,28). The diversity of the original pathology and types of redo operations do not permit endorsement of particular options or allow projection of long-term results. However, from scrutiny of this literature, a pattern does emerge. The typical patient with occlusion of one limb of an aortofemoral bypass graft is a smoker who presents emergently with a sudden loss of one femoral pulse and severe lower extremity ischemia. He or she requires emergency reoperation 3 to 4 years after the original reconstruction. Provided there is no graft infection and the patient is seen soon after thrombosis, it is often possible to extract fresh thrombus and restore good inflow. In these cases, thrombectomy is followed by revision of the distal outflow by some form of profundoplasty. Hyde and co-workers (22) and Bernhard and associates (23) described the long-term patency for periods ranging 21 to 36 months; in this group, redo patency was about 75%. It would be desirable to express redo patency in lifetable form, but insufficient data exist to permit this depiction.

Redo abdominal aortic procedures are associated with a higher mortality (10-12) when the aorta itself is diseased and bilateral graft limb occlusion exists. In these cases using the descending thoracic aorta as the origin for the graft, originally described by Blaisdell and colleagues (29) for an infected prosthesis, is a good option. DeLaurentis (27) described his recent experience in 10 secondary revascularizations. There were no deaths, one amputation, and short-term patency existed in 9 of the 10 grafts. The only caveat when selecting this approach would involve assurance of adequate visceral and pelvic perfusion.

With the common problem of single limb occlusion in aortofemoral bypass, I have described favorable experiences (19,24) with bypasses to uninvolved distal segments of the profunda femoris artery. The limited operations completely avoid the need for dissecting the scarred groin at the site of insertion of the previously thrombosed graft limb. A femoral-femoral approach originating on the opposite patent side appears to be advantageous. As mentioned previously, axillofemoral reconstructions predispose to reoperations. Popliteal reconstruction from the axilla is also possible, but might cause impaired pelvic perfusion in certain instances. In patients with proximal patent aortic grafts but with ischemia due to progressive distal femoral atherosclerosis, profunda to popliteal bypass using a vein is useful as a secondary procedure and will relieve ischemia. This procedure also avoids the difficult groin redissection.

As with any vascular procedure, satisfactory results of redo aortic surgery for occlusion depend on appropriate choices to obtain adequate inflow and create good outflow. The same general principle applicable to all arterial surgery applies to redo surgery: adequate bypass of diseased segments. Provided host factors are favorable and technical correction is obtained, re-operations might yield immediate and long-term results approximating the original operation. Occlusion of graft limbs occurs mainly in cigarette smokers (20,21). Apart from the report of Greenhalgh and associates (30) in 1981, the current vascular surgical literature remains distressingly silent on this point. To avoid strenuous reoperations, surgeons must convince their patients preoperatively of the need to stop cigarette smoking. It is worth re-iterating that this measure, above all, is the key to improving long-term patency of primary and secondary reconstructions for aortoiliac disease.

References

1. Oudot J: La greffe vasculaire dans les thromboses du carrefour aortique. La Presse Medicale 59:234-236, 1951.
2. Leriche R: Des obliterations arterielles hautes (obliteration de la terminasion de l'aorte) comme causes des insufficances circulatoires des membres inferieurs. Bull Med Soc Chir 49:1404, 1923.
3. Wylie EJ: Thromboendarterectomy for arteriosclerotic thrombosis of major arteries. Surgery 32:275-292, 1952.
4. DeBakey ME, Crawford ES, Cooley DA, Morris GC Jr: Surgical considerations of occlusive disease of the abdominal aorta and iliac and femoral arteries: analysis of 803 cases. Ann Surg 148:306-324, 1958.
5. Crawford ES, Bomberger RA, Glaeser DH, Saleh SA, Russell WL: Aorto-iliac occlusive disease: factors influencing survival and function following reconstructive operation over a twenty-five-year period. Surgery 90:1055-1067, 1981.
6. Lyons JH Jr, Weismann RG: Surgical management of late closure of aorto-femoral reconstruction grafts. N Engl J Med 278:1035-1037, 1968.
7. Najafi H, Dye WS, Javid H, Hunter JA, Goldin MD, Serry C, Julian OC: Late thrombosis affecting one limb of aortic bifurcation graft. Arch Surg 100:409-412, 1975.
8. Szilagyi DE, Elliott JP, Smith RF, Hageman JH, Sood RK: Secondary arterial repair. The management of late failures in reconstructive arterial surgery. Arch Surg 110:485-493, 1975.
9. Malone JM, Moore WS, Goldstone J: The natural history of bilateral aorto-femoral bypass grafts for ischemia of the lower extremities. Arch Surg 100:1300-1306, 1975.

10. Crawford ES, Manning LG, Kelly TF: "Redo" surgery after operations for aneurysm and occlusion of the abdominal aorta. Surgery 81:41-52, 1977.

11. Kanaly PJ, Dilling EW, Robinson HB, Elkins RC: Discussion and management of late failures in reconstructive procedures involving the abdominal aorta. Am J Surg 136:709-718, 1978.

12. Benhamou AC, Keiffer E, Tricot JF, Maraval M, Le Thoai M, Natali J: "Redo" surgery for late aorto-femoral graft occlusive failures. J Cardiovasc Surg 25:118-125, 1984.

13. Deriu GP, Ballotta E, Grego F: Emergency surgery in late occlusion of aortobifemoral bypass reconstructions. Vasc Surg 19:329-342, 1985.

14. Leeds FH, Gilfillan RS: Revascularization of the ischemic limb. Arch Surg 82:25-31, 1961.

15. Morris GC Jr, Edwards W, Cooley DA, Crawford ES, DeBakey ME: Surgical importance of profunda femoris artery. Arch Surg 82:32-37, 1961.

16. Martin P, Renwick S, Stephenson C: On the surgery of the profunda femoris artery. Br J Surg 55:539-542, 1968.

17. Strandness DE Jr: Functional results after revascularization of the profunda femoris artery. Am J Surg 119:240-245, 1970.

18. King TA, DePalma RG, Rhodes RS: Diabetes mellitus and atherosclerotic involvement of the profunda femoris artery. Surg Gynec Obstet 159:553-556, 1984.

19. DePalma RG, Malgieri JJ, Rhodes RS, Clowes AW: Profunda femoris bypass for secondary revascularization. Surg Gynecol Obstet 151:387-390, 1980.

20. Wray R, DePalma RG, Hubay CH: Late occlusion of aortofemoral bypass grafts: influence of cigarette smoking. Surgery 70:969-973, 1971.

21. Robicsek F, Daugherty HK, Mullen DC, Masters TN, Narbay D, Sanger PW: The effect of continued cigarette smoking on the patency of synthetic vascular grafts in Leriche syndrome. J Thorac Cardiovasc Surg 70:107-112, 1975.

22. Bernhard VM, Ray LI, Towne JB: The reoperation of choice for aorto-femoral graft occlusion. Surgery 82:876-874, 1977.

23. Hyde GL, McCready RA, Schwartz RW, Mattingly SS, Ernst CB: Durability of thrombectomy of occluded aortofemoral graft limbs. Surgery 94:748-751, 1983.

24. King TA, Rhodes RS, DePalma RG: Use of the profunda femoris artery for secondary revascularization. In Bergan JJ, Yao JST (Eds). Operative Techniques in Vascular Surgery. Chicago, Grune & Stratton, 1980, pp. 233-237.

25. Wukosch DC, Cooley DA, Sandiford FY, Nappi G, Ruel GJ: Ascending aorta-abdominal bypass: indications, technique and report of 12 patients. Ann Thorac Surg 23:442-448, 1977.

26. Bowes DE, Keagy BA, Benoit CH, Pharr WF: Descending thoracic aorto-bifemoral bypass for occluded abdominal aorta: retroperitoneal route without an abdominal incision. J Cardiovasc Surg 26:41-45, 1985.
27. DeLaurentis DA: The descending thoracic aorta in reoperative aortic surgery. In Bergan JJ, Yao JST (Eds). Reoperative Arterial Surgery. Chicago, Grune & Stratton, 1986, pp. 195-203.
28. Stanton PE Jr, Lamis PA, Gross WS, McCluskey D: Correction of late aortic-bifemoral graft failures. Am Surg 43:497-502, 1977.
29. Blaisdell FW, DeMattei DA, Gauder PJ: Extraperitoneal thoracic aorta to femoral bypass graft as replacement for an infected aortic bifurcation prosthesis. Am J Surg 102:683-685, 1961.
30. Greenhalgh RM, Laing SP, Cole PV, Taylor GW: Smoking and arterial reconstruction. Br J Surg 68:605-607, 1981.

7
Reoperative Surgery of the Carotid Artery

THOMAS H. SCHWARCZ* and WILLIAM H. BAKER
Loyola University Medical Center, Maywood, Illinois

Improvement in noninvasive diagnostic methods has detected increasing numbers of patients with extracranial carotid arterial disease amenable to operation, thereby making carotid endarterectomy the most common peripheral vascular operation performed today (1). Concomitant with this increase in surgical management of carotid disease, more patients with recurrent disease as well as complications of the initial endarterectomy are being evaluated and treated. This chapter will review the incidence and pathogenesis of those lesions requiring reoperative carotid arterial surgery as well as the technical considerations in approaching these problems.

Acute Postoperative Complications

Postoperative Neurologic Deficit

Incidence and Etiology

The safety and effectiveness of carotid arterial surgery has been well established (2-5) yet the development of new neurologic impairment after surgery is a striking complication. Several large series (4-9) have demonstrated perioperative neurologic deficits in 2.5 to 4.6% of patients. Many of these

---

*Present affiliation: University of Illinois College of Medicine at Chicago, Chicago, Illinois

deficits, however, resolved without permanent neurologic sequelae. The etiology of these events varies and includes technical errors at operation such as residual intimal flaps, distal subintimal dissection, and stenoses of the arteriotomy closure resulting in acute carotid thrombosis or showering of emboli into the cerebral circulation. Additional causes include cerebral ischemia, reperfusion injury, and intracerebral hemorrhage. To some degree, these complications can be avoided with meticulous operative technique and completion assessment of the carotid artery after endarterectomy to ensure a satisfactory technical result (10-12). Unfortunately, this does not guarantee an absence of postoperative neurologic deficits, even in the most experienced centers.

Immediate Deficits

Neurologic deficits identified in the perioperative period after carotid endarterectomy can be divided into two groups. First, the management of patients waking up with an immediate acute deficit is somewhat controversial. It is presumed that an intraoperative embolism or intra-operative ischemia is responsible for the deficit rather than internal carotid occlusion. These patients are ordinarily not returned to the operating room unless carotid occlusion is strongly suspected.

The second group, those patients developing a neurologic deficit after an intervening lucid period, with a normal neurologic examination immediately after carotid endarterectomy, should be approached more aggressively. These patients are presumed to have had the ischemic insult in the recovery room (i.e., either an embolism or an internal carotid artery occlusion).

Patients experiencing a mild hemispheric transient ischemic attack (TIA) in the distribution of the operated carotid artery should be started on intravenous heparin therapy. Noninvasive testing should be utilized to evaluate the existence of total occlusion or residual stenosis. If these tests are abnormal, carotid angiography should be obtained to delineate potentially correctable lesions. If no abnormalities are identified with noninvasive testing, close observation without further surgical intervention is the most prudent approach. Any additional signs or symptoms referrable to the hemisphere of the operated carotid artery mandate angiographic evaluation.

If a substantial deficit is persistent, the patient should be returned immediately to the operating room for reexploration of the neck. Delay of less than 1 hour has been associated with complete recovery from the deficit (13,14). Delay beyond this period of time significantly decreases the likelihood of recovery for any patients with potentially reversible lesions.

Immediate Reoperation

On reexploration of the neck, if a pulsatile internal carotid artery is present, an arteriogram should be performed using direct needle puncture into the distal common carotid artery. Injection of 10 cc or less of contrast material by hand is performed. The resulting roentgenogram should demonstrate any technical errors that may require correction (Figs. 1 and 2). If the angiogram is normal, no further surgical intervention is beneficial.

If a pulseless, presumably thrombosed, internal carotid artery is palpated, the artery must be directly explored. The common carotid and external carotid arteries are cross-clamped, and the arteriotomy is reopened. The internal carotid artery is allowed to backbleed and blow out any thrombus into the operative field. If backbleeding does not occur, a no. 3 or 4 balloon catheter is passed carefully to the level of the carotid siphon. More distal passage of the catheter is usually not necessary and may cause carotid-cavernous sinus fistula. Once backbleeding from the internal carotid artery has been established, a shunt is inserted to restore cerebral perfusion immediately. Attention must then be directed to any technical faults of the endarterectomy, which should then be corrected. There will, however, be some cases in which no obvious flaw can be ascertained. Regardless, a venous patch angioplasty is performed using either external jugular vein or saphenous vein. Dacron or polytetrafluorothylene (PTFE) prosthetic patches are acceptable alternatives. Intraoperative assessment of the corrective carotid surgery is useful in selected cases to avoid further complications. Completion arteriography is a standard technique and is effective and useful in these instances (10). A few centers (12) have also reported use of B-mode ultrasound as well as pulsed Doppler probes with real-time spectral analysis in the intraoperative evaluation of carotid surgery. The technique most familiar to the surgeon should be used to assure the best possible technical result.

Postoperative care is routine. The efficacy of treatment with various anticoagulants has not been clearly established, and both heparin and warfarin predispose the patient to significant hemorrhagic complications. Aspirin and dipyridamole may play an important role in these patients, but have not been adequately evaluated in clinical trials of carotid endarterectomy.

Results

Fortunately, no large experiences have been reported. Several centers (7-9, 13,15) have described their results with smaller groups of such patients. Most patients with focal or minor deficits go on to recover substantial neurologic

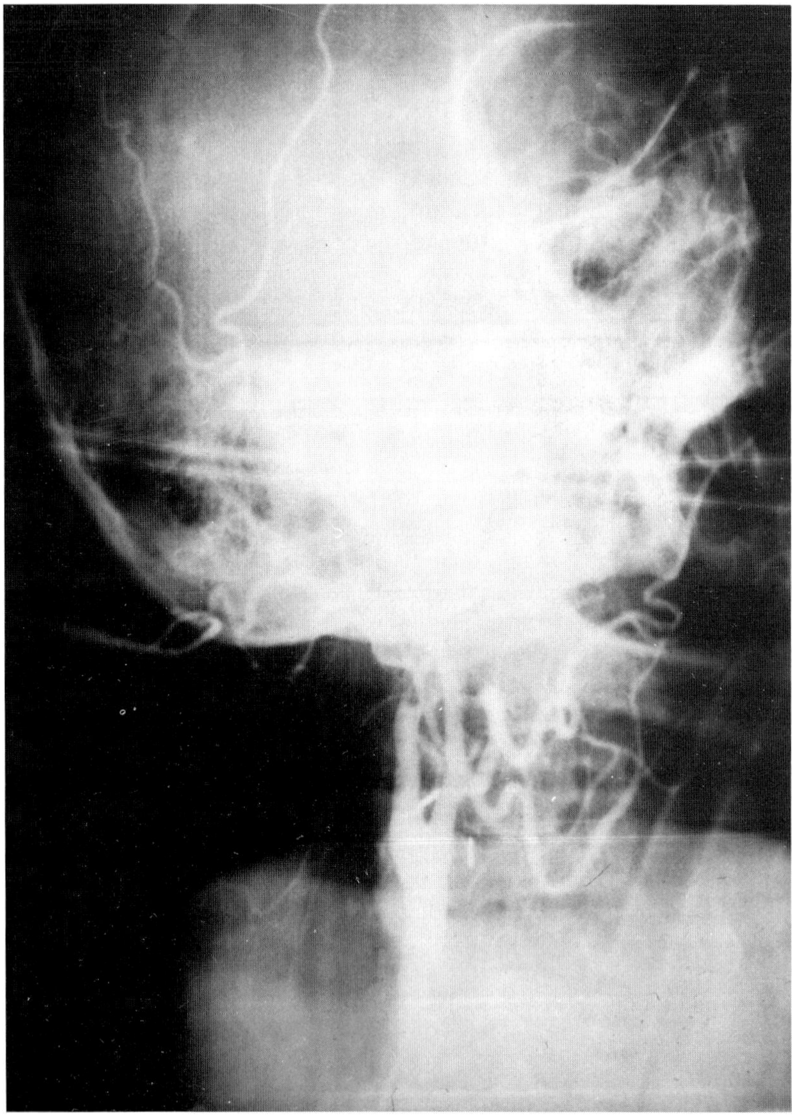

Figure 1 *Operative angiogram*: At reexploration an excellent internal carotid pulse was palpated. Angiography revealed a total occlusion at the distal end point. (From Ref. 43, p. 487, used with permission.)

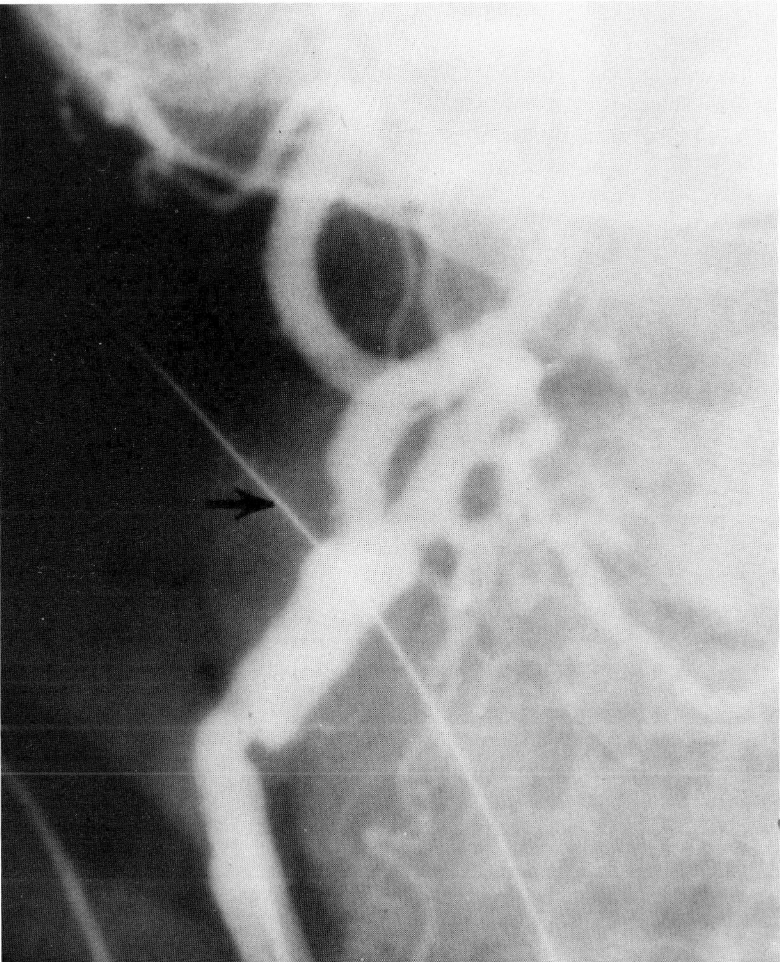

Figure 2 *Operative angiogram*: An excellent internal carotid pulse dictated the performance of this angiogram. The defect at the origin of the internal carotid artery proved to be gray shag (thrombus) at the suture line. (From Ref. 43, p. 491, used with permission.)

function with nonoperative supportive therapy. Patients with acute post-operative carotid thrombosis are most likely to recover function if successful thrombectomy is performed within 1 to 2 hours of the development of the neurologic deficit. Even with prompt intervention, only about 50% of these patients can be expected to demonstrate substantial recovery (7,9).

Other Acute Postoperative Complications

Hematoma

The incidence of significant neck hematomas after carotid endarterectomy is quite low. In a series of 1140 procedures, 0.7% required reoperation (15) Hematomas may develop due to several factors including inadequate hemostasis, excessive anticoagulation during endarterectomy, leakage from the suture line, and postoperative hypertension. Most hematomas remain small and do not require operative therapy. Rapidly expanding hematomas and those of substantial size may produce airway obstruction and require immediate management. Patients in respiratory distress should have sutures removed and the wound opened immediately. Only rarely, if ever, will emergent tracheostomy or cricothyroidotomy be required.

At reoperation, intubation may be difficult due to laryngeal edema. The arteriotomy is explored, and any suture line leaks appropriately repaired. Most patients bleed from miscellaneous bleeding points, which are controlled in the usual manner. Meticulous hemostasis should be obtained before closure in the usual fashion. The use of a drain is optional. Any drainage system should be removed within 24 hours. The long-term danger of postoperative neck hematoma is that of late wound infection with possible disruption of the arterial suture line, which while uncommon has disastrous results.

Frank arterial disruption after endarterectomy is an extremely rare occurrence that usually happens on the day of operation. The bleeding is controlled manually while the patient is returned to the operating room. The nervous surgeon should not blindly apply clamps in an attempt to obtain arterial control because damage to the cranial nerves is almost assured. With digital control of the bleeding, anesthesia is established, the wound opened, and arterial control obtained in the usual manner. Under most conditions, a simple suture or two will control whatever bleeding has occurred. If the arterial wall has broken loose because it was weakened, this diseased wall should be resected and a closure reperformed. Under these conditions, patch angioplasty is almost always required to restore a normal lumen.

Wound Infection

The incidence of wound infection in elective carotid arterial surgery is extremely low, and was .09% in the series of 1140 operations (15). Factors that predispose to wound complications include reexploration of the neck for bleeding and residual hematoma. If a prosthetic patch becomes infected, acute disruption of the suture line or false aneurysm may develop. Those patients should be given intravenous antibiotics, the patch removed, and the artery reconstructed with replacement autogenous tissue. The reconstruction should then be covered with adequate soft tissue, with the skin being left open to heal by secondary intention.

Recurrent Disease

The long-term durability of carotid endarterectomy has been well established by several reports (2,6,16,17) in the past two decades. With the increasing noninvasive diagnostic screening of postoperative carotid endarterectomy patients, a variable and often higher than expected percentage of recurrent stenosis has been identified (Table 1). The incidence of recurrent symptoms in these patients remains quite low. Therefore, a careful distinction must be made between noninvasively detected abnormalities and clinical symptoms when reviewing long-term results of this surgical procedure.

Transient Ischemic Attacks

Incidence and Etiology

The late occurrence of neurologic symptoms after carotid endarterectomy has been well documented by two recent reports. Owens and co-workers (18) evaluated the postoperative courses of patients with 121 carotid endarterectomies and found that 14 patients had TIAs in the distribution of the operated carotid artery (for an incidence of 12%). Ten of these 14 events occurred within the first postoperative week and four occurred between 4 and 18 months postoperatively. The late neurologic status of 325 operative survivors from 1 to 11 years postoperatively by Lees and Hertzer (16) demonstrated TIAs in the ipsilateral carotid distribution in 6.8% of patients. In those patients undergoing subsequent arteriography, recurrent disease manifested by restenosis and ulcerative plaques as well as an intimal injury thought to be due to shunt insertion were listed as potential etiologies for these neurologic deficits.

Table 1 Recurrent Carotid Stenosis Diagnosed by Noninvasive Examination

Author	Year	No.	Restenosis Rate	Diagnostic Methods
Kremen et al. (36)	1979	173	9.8%	OPG-G
Turnipseed et al. (37)	1980	80	8.8%	POD, SSA, Flowmap
Bodily et al. (23)	1980	69	17.7%	Duplex
Cantelmo et al. (38)	1981	199	12.1%	OPG-K, CPA, UA
Zierler et al. (24)	1982	89	19.0%	Duplex
Lynch et al. (39)	1983	54	5.6%	OPG-G, Duplex
Baker et al. (17)	1983	133	10.0%	OPG-K, CPA, POD, SSA
Salvian et al. (26)	1983	105	11.4%	OPG-G
Gonzalez et al. (40)	1984	265	2.6%	OPG-G, CPA, Duplex
Thomas et al. (29)	1984	257	15.0%	Duplex
Pierce et al. (41)	1984	75	6.7%	DSA
O'Donnell et al. (22)	1985	276	12.3%	B-mode ultrasound
Nicholls et al. (30)	1985	145	17.1%	Duplex
Keagy et al. (42)	1985	122	16.4%	OPG-G, Duplex
Das ct al. (31)	1985	1726	3.8%	CCT, POD, DSA

CCT = carotid compression tonography; CAPA = carotid phonoangiography; DSA = digital subtraction angiography; Duplex = combined B-mode and Doppler ultrasound with sound spectrum analysis; Flowmap = Doppler flow map imaging; OPG-G = ocular pneumoplethysmography – Gee; OPG-K = oculoplethysmography – Kartchner; POD = Periorbital Doppler examination; SSA = Sound spectrum analysis; UA = Ultrasonic arteriograph.

The preoperative preparation, operative technique, and postoperative care for patients requiring reoperation for late TIAs are essentially identical to that for restenosis.

Restenosis After Carotid Endarterectomy

Incidence

The true occurrence of hemodynamically significant restenosis of the carotid artery after endarterectomy has not been well defined. The two variables that most affect determination of this complication are the diagnostic technique used to evaluate the patients postoperatively and the intensity and duration of follow-up examinations. Consequently, a wide scatter of reported incidences of recurrent stenosis is found in the surgical literature. Those series (3,19-22) using clinical symptoms and signs to reevaluate patients have demonstrated restenosis rates ranging from 0.6 to 3.6%. Several reports using noninvasive diagnostic techniques including OPG-Kartchner, OPG-Gee, carotid phonoangiography, duplex Doppler scanning with spectral analysis, periorbital Doppler, and digital subtraction angiography have demonstrated restenosis rates from 2.6 to 19% (Table 1). An analysis of the criteria used for noninvasive identification of hemodynamically significant lesions affords some explanation for this discrepancy in incidence figures. Bodily and associates (23) using duplex Doppler examination, evaluated mean velocity ratio, maximum velocity in the internal carotid artery, and fractional broadening of the frequency spectrum. This technique demonstrated a 49% incidence of flow abnormalities consistent with a 50% or greater diameter stenosis. Interestingly, several lesions appeared to regress over time. In a similar study, Zierler and co-workers (24) reported an initial hemodynamically significant stenosis rate of 36%, but 41% of these patients subsequently exhibited regression of their lesion. Certainly, the evaluation of postoperative carotid endarterectomy patients with duplex Doppler scanning requires careful interpretation because it appears that either the initial stenotic lesions undergo a remodeling and regression or that the initial postoperative examination itself is affected by changes in arterial compliance, soft tissue edema, and so on.

Potential identification and interpretation errors are also present with other noninvasive diagnostic techniques. The surgeon must rely on the technique or techniques proven reliable in his or her vascular laboratory for postoperative assessment.

Etiology

Stoney and String (25) separated recurrent carotid lesions into two groups, the first being intimal fibrosis and the second being recurrent atherosclerosis. Fibrotic lesions appeared within 2 years of endarterectomy, while atherosclerotic lesions occurred later in the postoperative period. The pathogenesis of these lesions is not clearly separate and may very well represent a continuum.

Technical problems at the time of original endarterectomy may play a role in the development of later lesions, either through hemodynamic alterations or by serving as a nidus for thrombosis and platelet aggregation. Salvian and colleagues (26) reported a 75% incidence of problems with the end point of endarterecomy in those patients later developing restenosis based on noninvasive testing with an OPG-Gee. Specifically, the most common problem was the inability to obtain a feathering out of the plaque, requiring the use of tacking sutures distally. Even in routine operations, the segment of artery undergoing endarterectomy exposes collagen to the blood elements, resulting in some degree of platelet aggregation. Activation of these platelets may release a mitogenic factor that promotes proliferation of smooth muscle cells. Myointimal cell proliferation results and, in this group of patients, may be excessive, causing a dense, firm, rubbery lesion with a whitish, glistening luminal surface.

These findings of fibrous hyperplasia (or myointimal hyperplasia) are characteristic for lesions occurring within the first 2 years after carotid endarterecomy. Histologic characteristics of these lesions include stellate cells with exuberant growth and a paucity of lipid (19,25,27). The absence of neovascularization, hemosiderin, and fibrin deposition seems to exclude organizing mural thrombus as a cause of restenosis. Other factors that may be variably involved include hyperaggregable platelets, abnormalities in lipid metabolism, excessive smoking, and the female sex (22,28-31). The reasons for the increased incidence of restenosis in females may simply be due to the smaller size of the artery.

The pathologic lesion of late restenosis is quite different. These late lesions resemble atherosclerosis, with the familiar, irregular, and ulcerated plaque commonly found at initial endarterectomy (27). Abundant lipid deposition and lipid-laden cells are present immediately below the endothelium and at the intimal/medial interface. These plaques are also enveloped by fibrous caps and all have neovascularization in their periphery. There may also be a modest proliferation of myointimal cells. This lesion may only represent progression of fibrous hyperplasia in those patients more prone to aggressive arteriosclerosis.

Preoperative Management

The preoperative preparation of a patient with recurrent carotid stenosis differs little from that of a patient initially presenting with symptoms related to carotid arterial disease. After noninvasive examination, standard biplane carotid angiography should be obtained. These studies may also suggest the etiology of the recurrent stenosis. Myointimal hyperplasia is usually a smooth or regular lesion at the exact site of endarterectomy. The recurrent athero-sclerotic lesion tends to be irregular, ulcerated, and more prominent at one or both ends of the segment undergoing endarterectomy. In those centers with adequate experience with duplex Doppler scanning and digital subtraction angiography, standard intra-arterial arteriography may not be required pre-operatively. The clinical efficacy of perioperative antiplatelet agents, specifically aspirin and dipyridamole, has not been established, but certainly merits consideration since the pathogenesis of recurrent stenosis may involve abnormalities in platelet aggregation.

Technical Considerations

Although reoperative arterial surgery can be technically more demanding than virgin operations, the tenets of good carotid endarterectomy still follow (32). The operation needs to be performed as usual so that intraoperative embolization is avoided, a complete thromboendarterectomy is performed, non-obstructed flow to the internal and, if possible, the external carotid arteries results, and functional damage to the adjacent cranial nerves is avoided.

The first stage in reoperative carotid surgery is to obtain and read the initial operative note. Special attention should be paid to nuances in normal anatomy. Did the internal jugular vein appear to be displaced anteriorly? Were the cranial nerves in their usual position, or was the vagus nerve much more anterior than usual? Did the surgeon comment about difficulty of exposure at either end of the incision? Was there any problem in the performance of the endarterectomy? Was the end point well seen? Were tacking sutures used that might limit a reendarterectomy? Was there difficulty with the closure in any way? And, finally, was an operative arteriogram obtained? The answer to all of these questions can be obtained from a perusal of the original carotid endarterectomy dictation and will be helpful in planning any new operation.

Once the incision has been made, carotid endarterectomists are divided as to whether the scissors or the knife is the instrument of choice. All agree that the instrument used should sharply incise the tissues and avoid trauma to the carotid artery. In reoperative surgery, the use of scissors in general is not possible. Most of the loose areolar planes have been replaced with fibrous tissue that varies from being hard and firm to cementlike. In our experience, sharp dissection with the knife is far less traumatic and, in fact, creates less tissue damage than the use of a scissors. Using forceps and an experienced first assistant, proper tissue planes can be identified without undue injury to surrounding structures. Although occasionally the planes exist around the arteries, blunt dissection is to be discouraged.

The operation begins by reopening the original incision unless the previous operative note suggests that the original incision was inadequate. The anterior border of the sternocleidomastoid muscle is dissected, and the internal jugular vein is identified. Care should be taken during this dissection not to enter the internal jugular vein that may be densely adherent to the sternocleidomastoid muscle. If the operator finds himself at sea during this phase of the operation, he may extend the incision so that a more proximal dissection may be performed. Identification of the internal jugular vein and the common carotid artery low in the neck through previously undissected regions will allow him to approach the scarred segment of the neck with more confidence. The lymph nodes and fibrous tissue on top of the internal jugular vein are dissected off of the vein and reflected anteromedially. The ansa hypoglossal nerve lies within this mass of lymph nodes and scar and is, thus, preserved. The common carotid artery is identified and is sharply dissected in an immediately adjacent plane. The operator who dissects too far away from the common carotid artery increases the risk of injuring the vagus nerve. Once the common carotid artery has been identified, and it has been established that the vagus nerve is not still adherent to the common carotid artery, the dissection is carried immediately adjacent to the common carotid artery onto the internal carotid artery. Again, care must be taken not to traumatize the carotid artery lest an embolism occurs intraoperatively.

When the operator reaches the carotid bifurcation, the dissection is continued anteriorly. Staying close to the external carotid artery, the mass of tissue anteriorly is swept in an anterior and superior direction. This tissue will contain the hypoglossal nerve. If a proper periarterial plane is maintained, trauma to the nerve is unlikely. The dissection is carried anteriorly and posteriorly, but not necessarily circumferentially around the external carotid artery. The dissection is performed distally so that a vascular clamp can comfortably be applied to obtain external carotid control without compromising the proposed endarterectomy.

The internal carotid artery is sometimes rather difficult to dissect out because of scar and lack of exposure. Patients with high-lying bifurcations are especially troublesome. Often recurrent stenosis or new atherosclerosis grows at this distal endarterectomy site and, thus, control must be obtained some distance distally. Although tedious, this portion of the operation is essential.

Once satisfactory control has been obtained, heparin is given, arterial clamps applied, and the old arteriotomy reopened. Patients with recurrent atherosclerosis may have a surprisingly easily found cleavage plane between the atherosclerotic lesion and the wall of the artery. In these patients, the endarterecomy is reperformed. In other patients with myointimal hyperplasia, only an adherent, fibrotic, white-appearing smooth surface will be encountered. If this recurrent lesion is heaped up in one area, sharp knife dissection will be required to pare down this intraluminal obstruction. In other patients with a smooth circumferential lesion, an endarterectomy is not attempted, but the artery is enlarged during the closure with patch angioplasty or replaced with a suitably sized graft. After the intima of the artery has been manipulated, we irrigate with heparinized saline solution to ensure that all fronds of material have been completely removed. In secondary as well as primary operations, the distal end point is of paramount importance. If any doubt exists as to the adherence of the remaining intima, longitudinally oriented sutures of 7-0 polypropylene are used to tack down this remaining shelf of normal artery.

It is our practice to close all of these arteries with a patch angioplasty. In this clinic, saphenous vein or external jugular vein is used preferentially. In other clinics, polytetrafluoroethylene and Dacron are the materials of choice. Care must be taken to restore a normal-sized lumen to the internal carotid artery, but not to overcompensate and create an iatrogenic aneurysm (Fig. 3).

Some patients will present with a second recurrent stenosis or with unusable internal carotid arteries for other reasons. In these patients, the artery is replaced with an interposition graft of autogenous vein. Although every effort is made to preserve the external carotid artery, in some cases, this is technically deemed not feasible and this latter artery is merely suture ligated. Although the patients do well after ligation of the external carotid artery, the surgeon should realize that this makes any future ipsilateral extra-cranial-intracranial bypass impossible without additional external carotid artery revascularization.

The arguments for and against temporary indwelling carotid shunts are the same in reoperative as well as virgin carotid endarterectomies. Reoperations often require more time, and the surgeon feels more at ease with a shunt in place. Others note that if the patient could tolerate the original operation without a shunt and that the angiogram has not changed appreciably since that first operation, then the patient should survive well without a shunt the second time. The arguments for and against shunt usage are beyond the scope of this discussion, and the surgeon is urged to seek other information regarding this issue.

Reoperative surgery is often associated with more blood loss than usual. The planes are not fresh, and the scar tissue tends to ooze an inordinate amount. Most of these patients have been placed on aspirin or other anti-platelet agents further complicating this problem. If, indeed, after the liberal use of cautery, suture ligature, and application of pressure, oozing persists, a drain may be necessary. We have not used suction drains, but have relied on

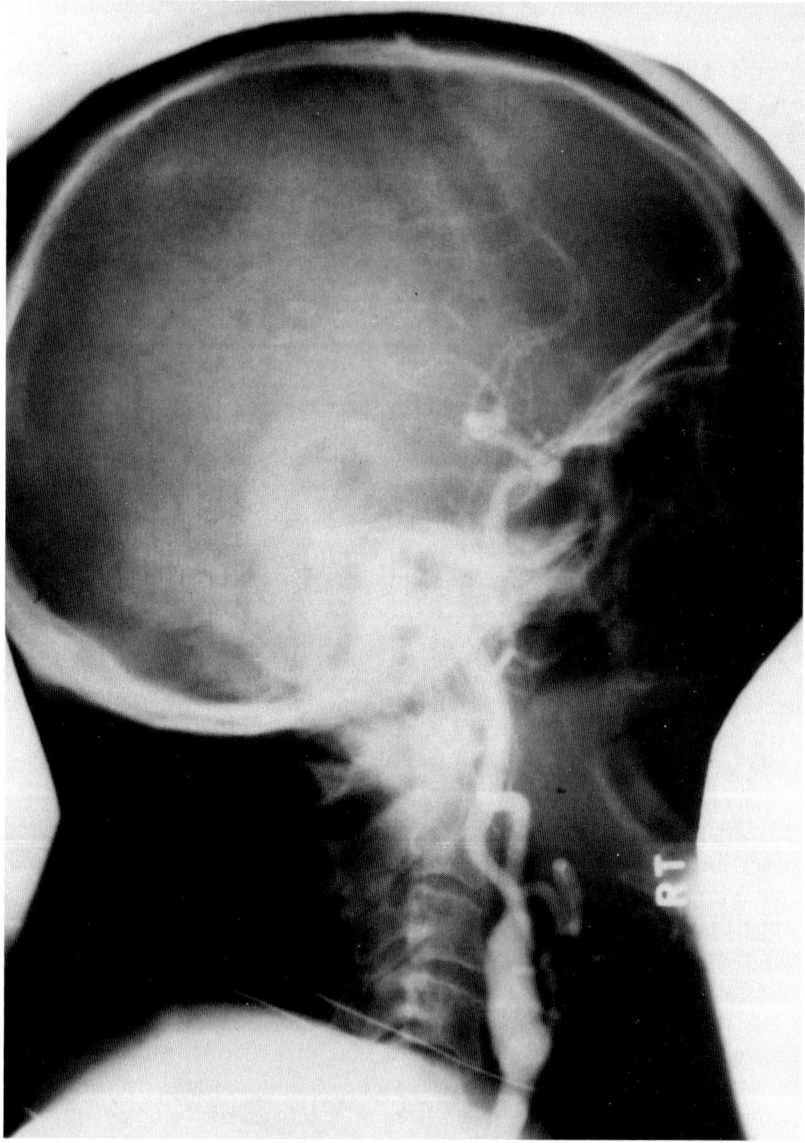

Figure 3   This patient returned with TIAs related to this "aneurysm" of the carotid. He had a carotid endarterectomy with Dacron patch angioplasty 16 months previously.

soft Penrose drains. Upon inspection of the neck that night, if the drain is not functioning and the neck is not enlarged, the drain is quickly removed. Surgeons should be aware that a drain is a two-way street, and that infection of a patch angioplasty closure may lead to either exsanguinating hemorrhage or false aneurysm formation.

Postoperative Management

The patient undergoing repeat carotid endarterectomy should be treated in essentially the same fashion as a patient undergoing initial endarterectomy. An additional consideration involves the use of postoperative antiplatelet agents, probably aspirin and dipyridamole, to prevent further platelet-mediated stenosis, but the efficacy of this treatment has not been established at this time. Because these patients may be subject to developing restenosis at a higher rate than the overall population of patients with carotid endarterectomy, careful follow-up at frequent intervals is a vital component of their postoperative care. An initial noninvasive assessment should be made before discharge and then at 3 month intervals for at least the first year after operation. Although several diagnostic techniques have been demonstrated to be effective either alone or in combination, we prefer the direct Doppler scan with spectral analysis, using the criteria of a peak systolic frequency of greater than 8000 Hz or a ratio of internal carotid artery to common carotid artery peak sysolic frequency greater than 3.5 as being suggestive of recurrent stenosis (33). Additionally, the B-mode scan has been useful in some cases to define anatomic characteristics of recurrent lesions (22).

Results

The long-term efficacy of repeat endarterectomy has not been well documented in the literature. A higher incidence of repeat stenosis may be suspected, but cannot be quantitated. Das and co-workers (31) from the Cleveland Clinic followed up 59 patients for a mean of 22 months and could identify only three subsequent neurologic events. With the performance of a technically perfect operation and use of antiplatelet agents, the durability of repeat endarterectomy should be quite good, although it may not achieve that for the population of patients undergoing initial carotid endarterectomy.

Restenosis has proven to be a problem in two of our patients who have had radiation therapy to the neck. In these patients, we recommend that at the original endarterectomy vein patch angioplasty be performed utilizing vein from a nonradiated area. In reoperations in these patients, the entire artery should be resected and replaced with a graft from an untreated area. Hopefully, these latter measures will reduce the incidence of a second recurrent stenosis.

Late Complications

False Aneurysm

The incidence of postendarterectomy false aneurysm formation is quite rare
(0.6% in a series (16) of over 900 patients). The instances may occur from 2
weeks to several years after operation (34,35). The causes most often
described in the literature involve dissolution of silk sutures used in Dacron
patch angioplasty at original operation and infection of either a prosthetic
patch angioplasty or the original suture line. The clinical presentation of such
patients is quite variable, including neurologic deficits, late wound infection,
and expanding neck masses. Preoperative assessment should include
angiography and B-mode scanning of the neck to identify aneurysm
formation. At surgery, early proximal and distal control are mandatory, with
resection of the false aneurysm. Depending on the clinical situation, appropriate treatment may consist of simple suture repair of the arterial defect,
trimming of the edges of the artery with subsequent patch angioplasty, or
resection of the segment of artery involved with interposition saphenous
vein or Dacron grafting. Patients in whom infection is suspected should have
only autologous tissue used for arterial reconstruction. For patch angioplasty,
saphenous vein is recommended by some surgeons over external jugular vein
because of a fear of late aneurysm formation. External jugular vein has been
used in this clinic because of its easy availability. We recently had one patient
treated elsewhere for an aneurysm at the site of the closure after external
jugular vein was used as angioplasty material (Fig. 4). The details of this
aneurysm formation are not known to us. Until other cases are reported, we
continue to recommend that either vein may be used as a patch material.

Late Infection

Late infection of the carotid artery is quite rare and occurs most often in
those patients undergoing prosthetic patch angioplasty or experiencing
complications at the time of original surgery, such as reoperation for hemorrhage or persistent wound hematoma. B-mode ultrasound as well as
angiography are useful to determine the extent of arterial involvement with
infection. Any cases involving prosthetic patch angioplasties require total
resection of the prosthetic material and replacement with autologous tissue.
Cases not involving prosthetic material require total excision of the infected
artery. If any infected prosthetic or nonprosthetic material is left behind,
recurrent problem is almost assured. In these patients, saphenous vein has
been used to replace the common carotid and internal carotid arteries, ligating

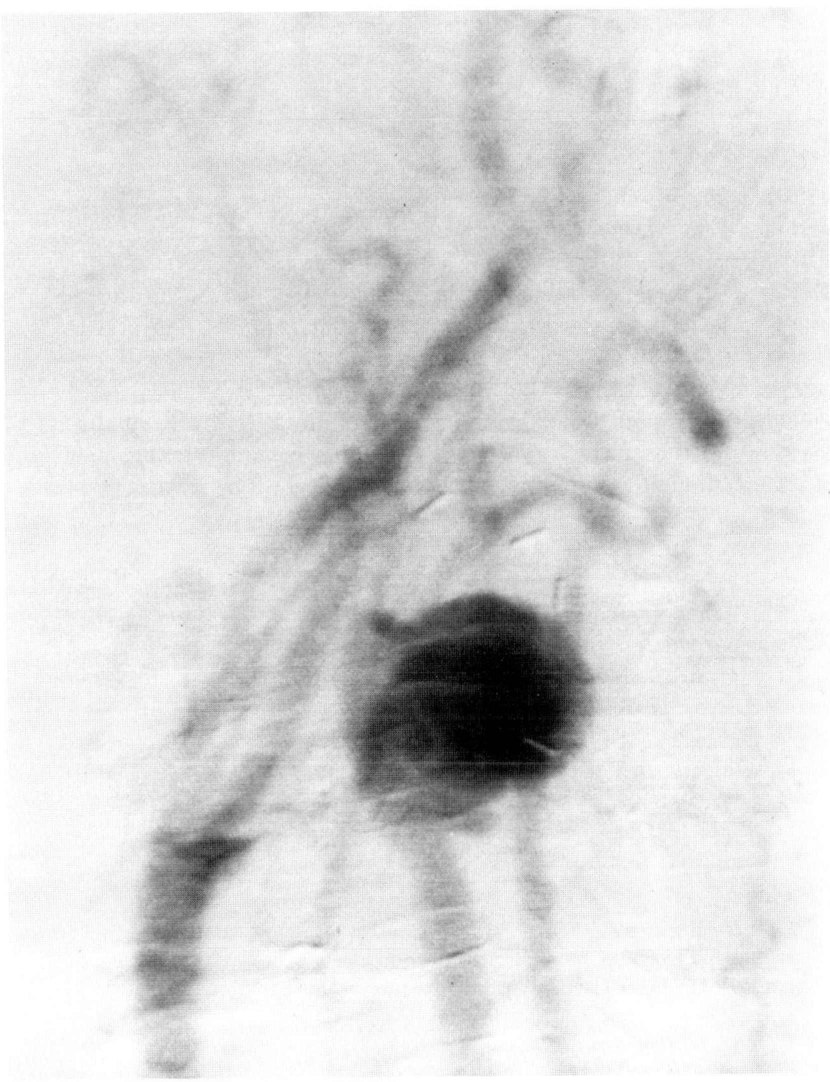

Figure 4   This false aneurysm developed 4 months after endarterectomy and patch angioplasty using autogenous external jugular vein. (From Ref. 44, used with permission.)

the external carotid artery. Soft tissue coverage of the infected site is required. The skin is usually left open and intravenous antibiotic therapy continued for 1 to 2 weeks. Although our experience is limited, results to date have been encouraging.

Rare Complications

True aneurysm formation in the segment of artery undergoing endarterectomy is rare. Duplex ultrasound and arteriography are both helpful in defining the anatomic extent of the lesion. Interposition grafting of either Dacron or saphenous vein is required to replace the resected aneurysmal artery. In some patients with aneurysms limited to the internal carotid artery, flow can be restored utilizing external carotid to internal carotid artery transpositions. In patients with far distal aneurysms, exposure may be obtained by anterior dislocation of the mandible or severance of the mandibular ramus. In very high aneurysms, it may be prudent to ligate the internal carotid artery after an extracranial-intracranial bypass has been extablished.

Conclusion

Restenosis of the carotid artery after endarterectomy occurs in approximately 10% of patients, but clinical manifestations of restenosis occur less frequently. Reoperations on the carotid artery are technically demanding and should be avoided by the inexperienced or occasional vascular surgeon. Despite the increased degree of technical difficulty, good results are anticipated.

References

1. Rutkow IM, Ernst CB: An analysis of vascular surgical manpower requirements and vascular surgical rates in the United States (abstract). Proceedings of The International Society for Cardiovascular Surgery, North American Chapter, Baltimore, Maryland, June 7, 1985, p. 54.
2. DeWeese JA, Rob CG, Satran R, Marsh DO, Joynt RJ, Summers D, Nichols C: Results of carotid endarterectomies for transient ischemic attacks-five years later. Ann Surg 178:258-264, 1973.
3. Thompson JE, and Talkington CM: Carotid endarterectomy. Ann Surg 184:1-15, 1976.
4. Imparato, AM, Ramirez A, Riles T, Mintzer R: Cerebral protection in carotid surgery. Arch Surg 117:1073-1078, 1982.

5. Baker WH, Littooy, FN, Hayes AC, Dorner DB, Stubbs D: Carotid endarterectomy without a shunt: the control series. J Vasc Surg, 1:50-56, 1984.
6. Thompson JE, Austin DJ, Patman RD: Carotid endarterectomy for cerebrovascular insufficiency: long-term results in 592 patients followed up to thirteen years. Ann Surg 172:663-679, 1970.
7. Treiman RL, Cossman DV, Cohen JL, Foran RF, Levin PM: Management of postoperative stroke after carotid endarterectomy. Am J Surg 142: 236-238, 1981.
8. Perdue GD: Management of postendarterectomy neurologic deficits. Arch Surg 117:1079-1081, 1982.
9. Rosenthal D, Zeichner WD, Lamis PA, Stanton PE, Jr: Neurologic deficit after carotid endarterectomy: pathogenesis and management. Surgery 94:776-780, 1983.
10. Blaisdell FW, Lim R Jr, Hall AD: Technical result of carotid endarterectomy. Arteriographic assessment. Am J Surg 114:239-246, 1967.
11. Alpert J, Brener BJ, Parsonnet V, Meisner K, Sadow S, Brief DK, Goldenkranz RJ: Carotid endarterectomy and completion contact arteriography. J Vasc Surg 1:548-554, 1984.
12. Zierler RE, Bandyk DF, Thiele BL: Intraoperative assessment of carotid endarterectomy. J Vasc Surg 1:73-83, 1984.
13. Kwaan JH, Connolly JE, Sharefkin JB: Successful management of early stroke after carotid endarterectomy. Ann Surg 190:676-678, 1979.
14. Novick WM, Millili JJ, Nemir P: Management of acute postoperative thrombosis following carotid endarterectomy. Arch Surg 120:922-925, 1985.
15. Thompson JE: Complications of carotid endarterectomy and their prevention. World J Surg 3:155-165, 1979.
16. Lees CD, Hertzer NR: Postoperative stroke and late neurologic complications after carotid endarterectomy. Arch Surg 116:1561-1568, 1981.
17. Baker WH, Hayes AC, Mahler D, Littooy FN: Durability of carotid endarterectomy. Surgery 94:112-115, 1983.
18. Owens ML, Atkinson JB, Wilson SE: Recurrent transient ischemic attacks after carotid endarterectomy. Arch Surg 115:482-486, 1980.
19. Cossman D, Callow AD, Stein A, Matsumoto G: Early restenosis after carotid endarterectomy. Arch Surg 113:275-278, 1978.
20. Hertzer NR, Martinez BD, Benjamin SP, Beven EG: Recurrent stenosis after carotid endarterectomy. Surg Gynecol Obstet 149:360-364, 1979.
21. Cossman, DV, Treiman RL, Foran RF, Levin PM, Cohen JL: Surgical approach to recurrent carotid stenosis. Am J Surg 140:209-211, 1980.
22. O'Donnell TF, Callow AD, Scott G, Shepard AD, Heggerick P, Mackey WC: Ultrasound characteristics of recurrent carotid disease: hypothesis explaining the low incidence of symptomatic recurrence. J Vasc Surg 2: 26-41, 1985.

23. Bodily KC, Zierler RE, Marinelli MR, Thiele BL, Greene FM Jr, Strandness DE: Flow disturbances following carotid endarterectomy. Surg Gynecol Obstet 151:77-80, 1980.
24. Zierler RE, Bandyk DF, Thiele BL, Strandness DE: Carotid artery stenosis following endarterectomy. Arch Surg 117:1408-1415, 1982.
25. Stoney RJ, String ST: Recurrent carotid stenosis. Surg 80:705-710, 1976.
26. Salvian A, Baker JD, Machleder HI, Busuttil RW, Barker WF, Moore WS: Cause and noninvasive detection of restenosis after carotid endarterectomy. Am J Surg 146:29-34, 1983.
27. Callow AD: Recurrent stenosis after carotid endarterectomy. Arch Surg 117:1082-1085, 1982.
28. Clagett GP, Rich NM, McDonald PT, Salander JM, Youkey JR, Olson DW, Hutton JE: Etiologic factors for recurrent carotid artery stenosis. Surgery 93:313-318, 1983.
29. Thomas M, Otis SM, Rush M, Zyroff J, Dilley RB, Bernstein EF: Recurrent carotid artery stenosis following endarterectomy. Ann Surg 200: 74-79, 1984.
30. Nicholls SC, Phillips DJ, Bergelin RO, Beach KW, Primozich JF, Strandness DE Jr: Carotid endarterectomy. Relationship of outcome to early restenosis. J Vasc Surg 2:375-381, 1985.
31. Das MB, Hertzer NR, Ratliff NB, O'Hara PJ, Beven EG: Recurrent carotid stenosis. A five-year series of 65 reoperations. Ann Surg 202:28-35, 1985.
32. Baker WH. (Ed.) Carotid endarterectomy. In: Diagnosis and Treatment of Carotid Artery Disease, 2nd Edition, Futura Publishing Company, Inc., Mount Kisco, New York 1985, pp. 181-212.
33. Michelini MA, Boynton AS, Mahler DK, Foldes MS, Hayes AC, Littooy FN, Baker WH: Combining carotid tests: if three is good, can two be better? Bruit IX:20-22, 1985.
34. Buscaglia LC, Moore WS, Hall AD: False aneurysm after carotid endarterectomy. JAMA 209:1529, 1969.
35. Ehrenfeld WK, Hays RJ: False aneurysm after carotid endarterectomy. Arch Surg 104:288-291, 1972.
36. Kremen JE, Gee W, Kaupp HA, McDonald KM: Restenosis or occlusion after carotid endarterectomy. Arch Surg 114:608-610, 1979.
37. Turnipseed WD, Berkoff HA, Crummy A: Postoperative occlusion after carotid endarterectomy. Arch Surg 115:573-574, 1980.
38. Cantelmo NL, Cutler BS, Wheeler HB, Herrmann JB, Cardullo PA: Noninvasive detection of carotid stenosis following endarterectomy. Arch Surg 116:1005-1008, 1981.
39. Lynch TG, Hobson RW, Berry SM: The role of real-time B-mode ultrasonography and ocular pneumoplethysmography following carotid endarterectomy. Am Surg 49:31-36, 1983.

40. Gonzalez LL, Partusch L, Wirth P: Noninvasive carotid artery evaluation following endarterectomy. J Vasc Surg 1:403-408, 1984.

41. Pierce GE, Iliopoulos JI, Holcomb MA, Rieder CF, Hermreck AS, Thomas JH: Incidence of recurrent stenosis after carotid endarterectomy determined by digital subtraction angiography. Am J Surg 148:848-854, 1984.

42. Keagy BA, Edrington RD, Poole MA, Johnson G: Incidence of recurrent or residual stenosis after carotid endarterectomy. Am J Surg 149:722-725, 1985.

43. Baker WH: Management of stroke during and after carotid surgery. In Bergan JJ, Yao JST (Eds): Cerebrovascular Insufficiency. New York, Grune & Stratton, 1983.

44. Baker WH, Stefani RH, Hayes AC: Recurrent transient ischemic symptoms. In Bergan JJ, Yao JST (Eds): Reoperative Arterial Surgery. Orlando, Grune & Stratton, 1985, p. 573.

8

Renovascular Reoperation After Prior Renal Artery Reconstructive Surgery

JAMES C. STANLEY
University of Michigan Medical School, Ann Arbor, Michigan

Arterial reconstructive surgery has proven to be a highly successful means of treating renovascular hypertension (1). Unfortunately, certain patients managed in this manner manifest persistent or recurrent hypertension that necessitates reoperation. Secondary surgical procedures are more technically demanding and carry a greater risk of nephrectomy than primary operations. Although complications associated with the surgical therapy of renovascular hypertension and their operative management have been alluded to in many surgical series, comprehensive reports on the subject are few in number (2-5).

The largest published experience (4) on reoperative renovascular surgery is from the University of Michigan, where 72 secondary procedures for complications of prior renal artery reconstructive surgery were undertaken in 58 patients from 1961 to 1983. This latter report evolved from the treatment of 373 patients who underwent 425 primary operations for renovascular hypertension. Secondary operations were performed 10 times in pediatric patients after 42 primary procedures (24%), 44 times in adult fibrodysplastic patients after 199 initial operations (22%), and 18 times in atherosclerotic patients after 184 primary operations (10%). Secondary procedures included nephrectomy (n=31), bypass grafts with vein (n=15) or prosthetic conduits (n=8), angioplasty or reimplantation (n=12), thrombectomy (4), and operative dilation (n=2). Benefits regarding hypertension control were afforded 91% of these patients. One death occurred among the 72 reoperations, representing a 1.4% operative mortality rate. This figure is more representative of contemporary practice than the 28% mortality accompanying reoperation reported in the Cooperative Study (6).

Reoperative renal artery procedures for complications of renal revascularization often present formidable technical problems. However, data from the literature on this topic should not be viewed as a worse case scenario to support nonsurgical management of renovascular hypertension, but instead should be viewed in the overall context of surgical therapy. For instance, in the most recent decade of the Michigan experience, the frequency of secondary operations was 9.7%, and only two patients classified as failures of surgical therapy during this period did not undergo reoperation (4). Thus, nearly 90% of all patients benefited from initial surgical treatment, being either cured or improved regarding their hypertension during a follow-up period extending considerably beyond that usually reported with nonsurgical forms of therapy. It is also noteworthy that of the 425 primary operations in this series, there were only nine nephrectomies performed when revascularization procedures proved technically impossible. Although primary surgical treatment of renovascular hypertension appears well established, reoperations remain a challenge for those performing renovascular surgery (7-15).

Reoperative renovascular procedures are complicated by two major factors. First, reoperation usually necessitates dissection in an operative field of fibrous scar tissue. That this represents a commonly encountered feature of these secondary operations is an understatement. In such cases, use of intraoperative Doppler ultrasonography to identify small vessels may be required to lessen the risk of irreparable vascular injury accompanying blind dissection. The second major complicating factor is that only a few millimeters of artery distal to the primary revascularization may be available as an entry point for the repeat revascularization. This is more likely to occur with reoperations for fibrodysplastic renovascular hypertension, the most frequent disease entity requiring secondary procedures (4,9,16).

Successful reoperation often depends on timely recognition of the failed primary procedure. In this regard, persistent or recurrent hypertension is the most common manifestation of a primary reconstructive failure and should lead to prompt diagnostic studies. Intravenous urography, isoptopic renograms, and renal scans have been advocated to document the existence of a functioning kidney when reconstructive failures are suspected in the immediate postoperative period. However, these studies are inconsistently helpful because most kidneys in such cases have extensive preformed collateral blood vessels that maintain renal function despite failed reconstructions. Conventional arteriographic examinations in these circumstances should be considered the most reliable and accurate means of detecting early or late reconstructive failures (17,18).

Because the risks of secondary operation are considerable, reoperative procedures should be contemplated only when persistent or recurrent post-reconstructive hypertension has been documented to be a consequence of an inadequate primary operative procedure (8). Specific complications leading to secondary operations as well as the various reoperative approaches warrant individual comment. Clearly, no single reoperative approach is applicable to all failures of prior renal artery reconstructive surgery.

Early Renal Artery Graft Thromboses

One of the most common complications of renovascular surgery is acute occlusion of an aortorenal, iliorenal, or other type of renal artery bypass. In the past, the frequency of this complication with vein graft reconstructions has been reported (17,18) to range as much as 8 to 14%, and may have been even more common with reconstructions using prosthetic grafts. The frequency of early vein graft occlusion in most contemporary practices is much less than that encountered during earlier years. For instance, acute thromboses occurred in only 2 of 100 recent consecutive aortorenal bypass grafts to the main renal artery at my institution (4). Infrequent early occlusions as noted in the Michigan experience have also been reported by others (19). Perioperative graft thromboses are usually related to technical complications such as intimal flaps or anastomotic constrictions.

Operative intervention for acute thromboses involving renal artery reconstructions should be undertaken promptly if the risk of irreparable kidney ischemia is to be lessened. Reoperation performed during the first 72 to 96 hours after the primary revascularization, before dense fibrous scar tissue forms, usually requires little additional dissection beyond that of the initial procedure. An exception relates to acute occlusions associated with distal anastomotic narrowings. Secondary procedures in these cases may require isolation of the renal vessels as they enter the kidney parenchyma. Control of renal artery backbleeding in this situation may be best achieved by cautious insertion of intraluminal dilators, rather than using microvascular clamps or traction loops on the smaller segmental arteries. Intraluminal balloon catheters may also be used to achieve control of backbleeding in such cases, but these devices can cause vascular injury if overinflated, and their use should be undertaken with great caution.

Early reoperations for anastomotic thromboses usually include complete replacement of the previously inserted graft or angioplastic repair of the obstructed anastomosis. In the latter case, generous patches should be used so that late strictures will not develop (Fig. 1). In addition to intimal flaps and distal anastomotic narrowings, acute thromboses may also result from graft kinking or graft narrowing at the aortic anastomosis. These faults are relatively easy to identify during reoperation. They may be managed by either local revision and repositioning of the initially placed graft or, as is usually the case, by replacement of the proximal conduit with a more properly positioned aortic anastomosis.

Kidney viability may be difficult to assess during exploration for acute thromboses, and often may not be ascertained until after the repeat revascularization. Documentation of cortical blood flow by Doppler ultrasonography or intraoperative arteriography has proven useful in establishing the adequacy of difficult reoperative procedures in such cases. In this regard, it is important to recognize that the renal circulation is very vasoreactive, and that intraoperative arteriograms often document narrowing of parenchymal arteries due to spasm rather than thrombus. Such phenomena often make interpretation of operative arteriograms difficult.

Renal Artery Occlusion After Resection and Reanastomosis or Aortic Reimplantation

Resection of renal artery stenosis with primary reanastomosis of the vessel or aortic reimplantation of the distal renal artery may lead to early thromboses. This is especially true if accompanied by inadequate anastomotic spatulation or undue anastomotic tension. The Michigan experience with this type of primary renal revascularization, because of these complications, has been poor in contrast with acceptable results reported by others (9,20).

Reoperation for acute occlusions after reimplantation or reanastomosis usually entails performance of a conventional bypass originating from the aorta or iliac arteries to the distal renal artery, rather than revising the failed primary vascular reconstruction. Local angioplasty may be technically more difficult and hazardous in this setting.

Arterial Thromboses After Operative Dilation

Advancement of rigid dilators through select renal artery stenoses is an invaluable adjunct in treating certain cases of renovascular hypertension. How-

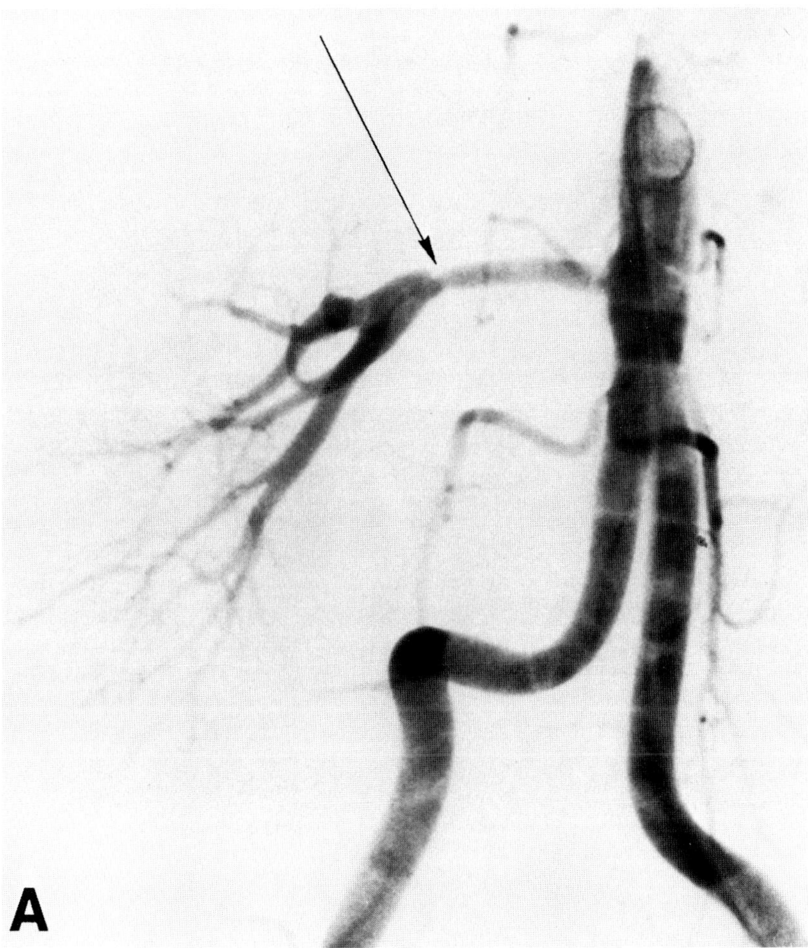

Figure 1 *A*: Early postoperative arteriogram documenting distal anastomotic stricture (*arrow*) in a patient with fibrodysplastic renal artery disease who underwent aortorenal bypass with reversed autogenous saphenous vein. *B*: Arteriographic study 1 week after reoperation with vein patch angioplasty repair of anastomotic stricture. Note the generous character of the patch graft (*arrow*). *C*: Arteriographic study at 12 months, documenting normal appearance of reconstruction. (From Ref. 4, used with permission.)

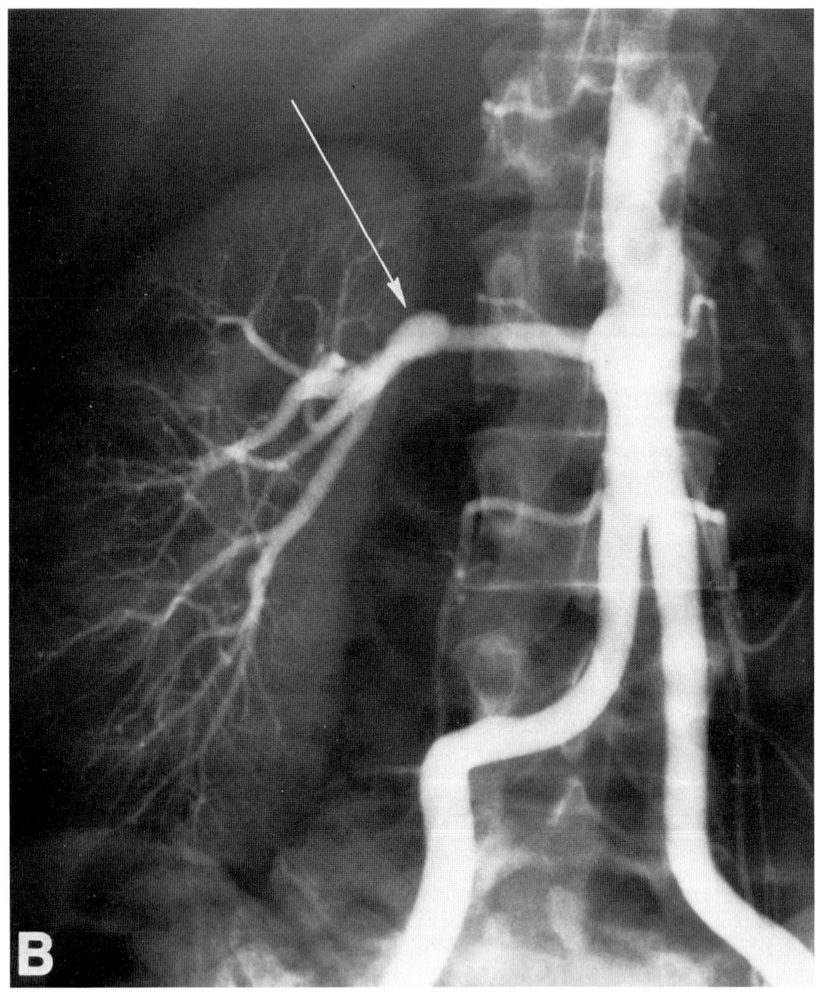

Figure 1   (Continued)

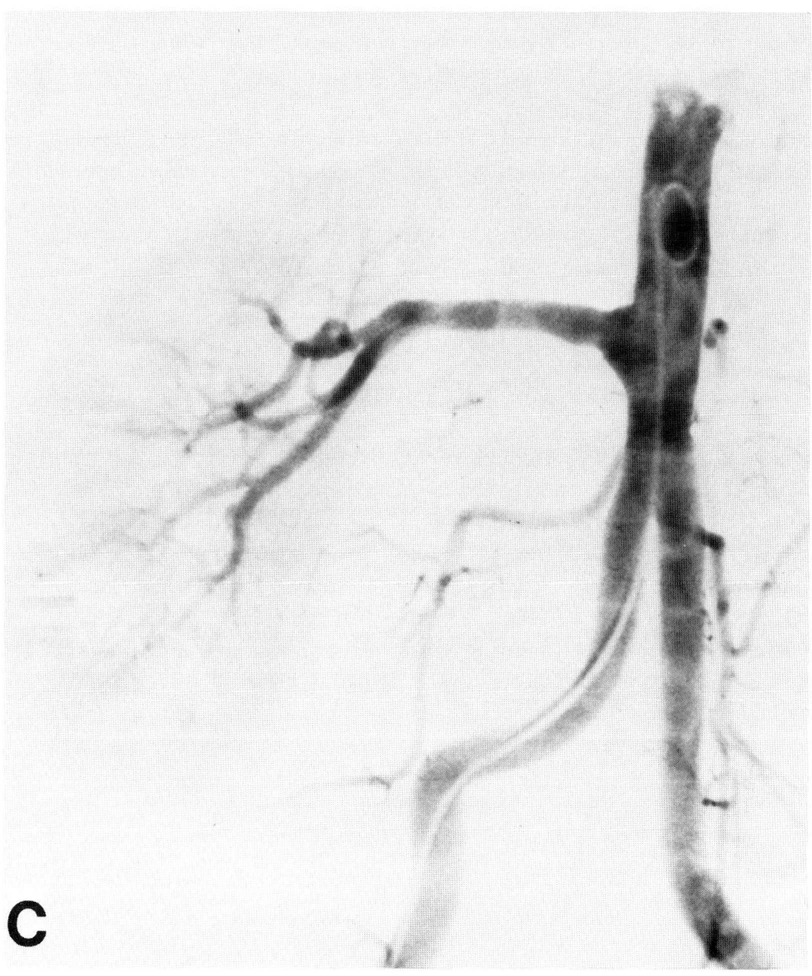

Figure 1   (Continued)

ever, overzealous dilation can cause intimal disruption and acute thromboses. Such a complication most often results in nephrectomy. Because of the distal location of many lesions treated by operative dilation, ex vivo reoperation may be necessary if the jeopardized kidney is to be salvaged after failure of primary therapy. Standard ex vivo reconstructive techniques should be pursued in these circumstances, adhering to careful microvascular reconstructive technique (21). If partial nephrectomy is required, it should probably be performed early after the thrombosis, rather than late when fibrous scar may make identification of uninvolved renal vessels difficult.

Postendarterectomy Thromboses

Renal artery occlusions after endarterectomy for atherosclerotic lesions occurred in 9% of the Michigan series. This incidence, although similar to that reported by others (22), is much greater than that observed at institutions where this operation is performed on a more frequent basis (23,24). Acute thromboses, when they do occur, are more likely to accompany endarterectomies performed through limited renal arteriotomies than with transaortic endarterectomies.

Conventional bypass procedures are usually undertaken in managing acute postendarterectomy thromboses. Lesser procedures may be successful if a well localized cause for the occlusion, such as an intimal flap, is identified and appears correctable without undue technical difficulty. The most common of the later reoperations involves creation of a long renal arteriotomy beyond the area of occlusion, and closure with a patch graft. Late stenoses or thromboses after endarterectomy are uncommon (20,24,38). Similarly, aneurysmal dilation at the site of an endarterectomy is an infrequently recognized complication (20).

Late Stenoses and Occlusions of Renal Artery Bypass Grafts

Late compromise of renal artery bypass grafts is most often the result of: (a) anastomotic stricture due to faulty operative technique; (b) accumulation of dysplastic fibrous tissue at an anastomosis; (c) graft trauma due to application of vascular clamps causing progressive mural fibrosis; (d) intraluminal trauma, especially in small renal arteries during passage of dilators when calibrating or attempting to increase the diameter of these vessels during primary operation; or (e) construction of a conduit by an organized perigraft hematoma. The majority of graft occlusions recognized in the late postoperative period have probably evolved from events occurring in the early perioperative period (17,18,25,26).

Stenoses of autogenous saphenous veins used in renal revascularizations have been documented in as many as 41% of patients (20). Stenoses specifically involving the anastomoses have been recognized in 17% of vein grafts (17). Many of the former stenoses were considered functionally inconsequential and, as such, were not demanding of reoperation. In contradistinction to these benign lesions, late stenoses of hemodynamic and functional importance have been observed in approximately 8% of vein grafts used in renal artery reconstructions (17). Similar stenoses or thromboses of explanted arterial autografts are uncommon (27-30), but have been noted with higher than expected frequencies in some reports (22,31). In a related matter, direct splenorenal arterial anastomoses are an appropriate means of renal revascularization in select adult cases, but carry an unacceptably high incidence of stenoses and thromboses in pediatric cases (32).

Two reoperative approaches to late failures of renal artery reconstruction exist, namely: (a) repeat renal revascularization, and (b) nephrectomy. The later is acceptable therapy only when diseased renal vessels are unreconstructable or irreparable parenchymal injury has occurred. Details of these two treatment modalities deserve discussion.

Reoperative renal artery reconstructions for late occlusions usually encompass standard in situ surgical procedures. Exposure is critical to the performance of successful surgery in these instances. In this regard, a supraumbilical transverse abdominal incision is recommended, being extended from the opposite midclavicular line to the midaxillary line on the side of the affected kidney. This particular incision provides a technical advantage in the handling of instruments perpendicular to the longitudinal axis of the body, which during more complex procedures, greatly facilitates the ease of reconstruction. Midline vertical abdominal incisions can also be used for renal revascularization, but provide a somewhat less generous exposure.

The right kidney vessels as well as the inferior vena cava and aorta are exposed by first incising the lateral parietes along the ascending colon and reflecting it, the duodenum, as well as pancreas medially in an extended Kocher-like maneuver. Dissection of the renal artery or the previously placed graft usually begins just lateral to the vena cava. If one dissects the more distal renal vessels first, troublesome injuries to small arterial and venous branches are more likely. Alternatively, when treating proximal stenoses, the inferior vena cava may be retracted laterally and the first portion of the renal artery or graft near its aortic origin may be exposed.

Periarterial fibrosis is common after prior revascularization procedures, and identification of vascular structures within the region of the initial operative field may be exceedingly difficult. Accurate localization of segmental renal arteries is often facilitated by intraoperative Doppler ultrasonography (33). Circumferential dissection of distal renal arteries in these circumstances is hazardous. Rather than dissect the distal native renal artery when it is embedded in dense fibrous scar tissue, it is often best to open the graft or vessel and control backbleeding with the careful placement of rigid olive-tipped intraluminal dilators. The renal artery or graft beyond the occlusion may then be opened over the metal dilator, and patch graft repair or anastomosis of a replacement interposition graft can be accomplished with this device remaining inserted until the last few sutures are placed. As in the case of acute occlusions, use of intraluminal balloon catheters in this setting may injure delicate segmental arteries.

The left kidney vessels and the aorta are exposed in a retroperitoneal manner similar to that described for right-sided operations, with reflection of the viscera, including the descending colon, medially. This retroperitoneal approach offers better visualization of the left renal pelvis than does an anterior approach through the central mesocolon and root of the small bowel mesentery. Exposure of the left renal artery may be extended with mobilization of the renal vein, including ligation and transection of its gonadal and adrenal branches.

Autologous saphenous vein grafts are preferred for replacing stenotic renal bypass grafts in adults, and autologous hypogastric artery grafts are favored in pediatric-aged patients. Local procedures such as patch graft angioplasty of a stenotic anastomosis may be more practical than replacing an entire bypass conduit in some instances. Veins for aortorenal bypass or patch grafting should be carefully procured, gently handled, and cautiously irrigated with cold heparinized blood prior to implantation. Infiltration of papaverine along the course of the vein before its excision or addition of this drug to irrigation media may lessen venospasm and the early loss of endothelium from these conduits. Procurement of the hypogastric artery for use as an ex vivo or in situ interposition graft should proceed in a similar manner. Dacron or expanded polytetrafluoroethylene (PTFE) grafts may also be utilized for certain reoperative procedures. These synthetic prostheses, especially the newer thin-walled expanded PTFE grafts, should be used in preference to fibrotic or small caliber veins. It is important to remember that synthetic conduits are technically more difficult to use when revascularizing small arteries or treating extensive distal graft stenoses affecting segmental vessels.

Systemic anticoagulation during reoperations is best accomplished by intravenous administration of sodium heparin, 150 units/kg intravenously, before clamping the aorta or renal artery. Regional heparinization may not provide consistent anticoagulation and is not recommended in these cases. When undertaking reoperative renal artery bypasses, the infrarenal aorta is dissected about its circumference for approximately 5 cm above the inferior mesenteric artery. Other sites of origin for renal grafts may be preferable when extensive aortic disease or dense periaortic fibrosis from earlier operations make dissection or clamping of this vessel hazardous. The common iliac and hepatic arteries are the most frequent nonaortic donor vessels used in such circumstances (Fig. 2). The proximal anastomosis is almost always constructed first in the case of aortorenal bypasses, with a side-biting vascular clamp used to partially occlude the aorta. An aortotomy is made with its length approximately two to three times the diameter of the graft. In cases of severe calcific aortic atherosclerosis, an ellipse of aorta may be excised. The graft is then beveled or spatulated and the aortic anastomosis is performed using continuous 4-0 or 5-0 monofilament suture.

The most direct route for right-sided aortorenal grafts is beneath the inferior vena cava, taking origin from a lateral aortotomy. However, in many reoperations, the retrocaval region is densely fibrotic as a consequence of the primary procedure. In these situations, it may be better if replacement grafts are taken from an anteriorly placed aortotomy and carried in front of the inferior vena cava to the renal vessels. Grafts used for left-sided reoperations are usually positioned beneath the renal vein unless this vessel is markedly adherent to the underlying artery as a consequence of an earlier operation. The aortic clamp should remain in place during completion of the renal anastomosis because to remove it and place a vascular clamp on a saphenous vein or hypogastric artery graft might injure the latter conduits.

Performance of the distal anastomosis is then undertaken. The renal artery or graft is transected, and in most instances an end-to-end, new graft-to-renal artery or new graft-to-old graft, anastomosis is completed. In the former reconstruction, this is facilitated by spatulation of the graft posteriorly and of the distal renal artery anteriorly. In adults, these anastomoses are fashioned with a continuous 5-0 or 6-0 monofilament suture. In pediatric-aged patients, three or four sutures are placed in a discontinuous manner to allow subsequent vessel growth. In the case of arteries smaller than 2 mm diameter, these anastomoses are best completed with individual interrupted sutures about the entire circumference. After establishment of antegrade renal blood flow, the anticoagulant effects of heparin are reversed with intravenous

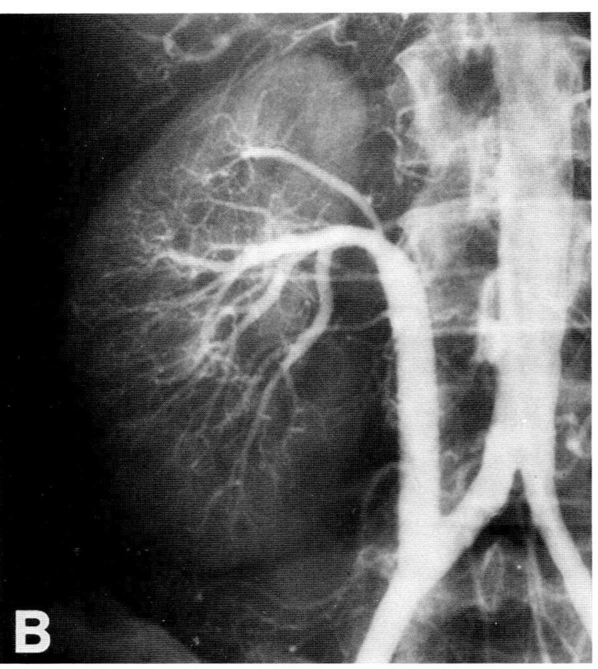
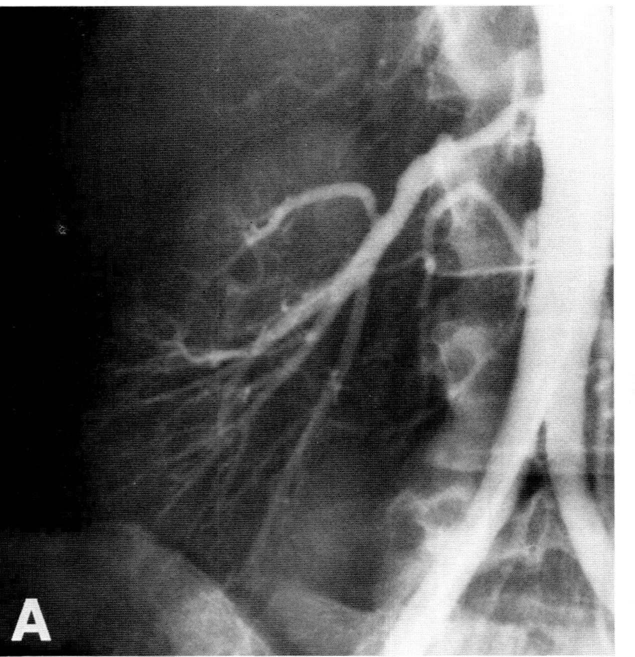

Figure 2 *A*: Segmental stenosis of an aortorenal autogenous saphenous vein bypass 8 months postoperatively. *B*: Iliorenal prosthetic bypass performed at reoperation, with satisfactory appearance at 12 months. (From Ref. 5, used with permission.)

administration of 1.2 mg of protamine sulfate for each 100 units of heparin given previously. Intraoperative arteriography is performed only if Doppler assessment suggests inadequate repair or in any situation where technical faults are suspected. In all cases, postoperative arteriography should be undertaken before discharge to define the anatomic status of the reoperative procedure and provide a baseline for continued follow-up (Fig. 3).

Extirpative procedures may become necessary treatment in cases of unreconstructable vessels or renal infarction. A few caveats regarding total or partial nephrectomy in these instances deserve mention. First and foremost is that intracapsular nephrectomy is much simpler than removing the kidney with its perinephric fat and adnexa in an extracapsular fashion. Bleeding from preformed collateral vessels occurring with advanced renal artery occlusive disease may be considerable in these cases. When performing an intracapsular nephrectomy, an incision is made through Gerota's fascia and the anterior kidney capsule with a cautery knife blade. Once a plane between the renal parenchyma and capsule is established, the kidney can easily be freed using blunt digital dissection about its entire circumference. Vessels within the renal pelvis should be independently dissected, allowing the artery and vein to be individually ligated with nonabsorbable sutures and transected. The ureter is similarly ligated and divided. The kidney is then removed, its capsule being left intact within the retroperitoneum. Pre-existing collateral vessels traversing the capsule may be easily identified from within and ligated or cauterized.

Partial nephrectomy for renovascular hypertension after a failed primary operation poses certain unique problems. The most disconcerting of these is differentiation of the kidney's normal from abnormal circulation. In most instances, the anatomic area requiring resection is adequately delineated by preoperative arteriographic studies. In other cases, use of fluorescent or vital dyes may be necessary to distinguish the ischemic from nonischemic tissue. Careful attention to transection of the renal parenchyma is essential to avoid leaving marginally perfused tissue behind. Parenchymal vessel ligation and repair of the collecting system when it has been opened are done in a conventional manner using absorbable stutures. Closure of the capsule over the exposed renal parenchyma must be performed without tension, to avoid construction of the underlying cortex and development of a "Page-kidney" form of secondary hypertension.

Aortorenal Graft Dilation

A relatively common phenomenon in renal reconstructive surgery using autogenous vein has been the late increase in vein graft lengths and diameters (25).

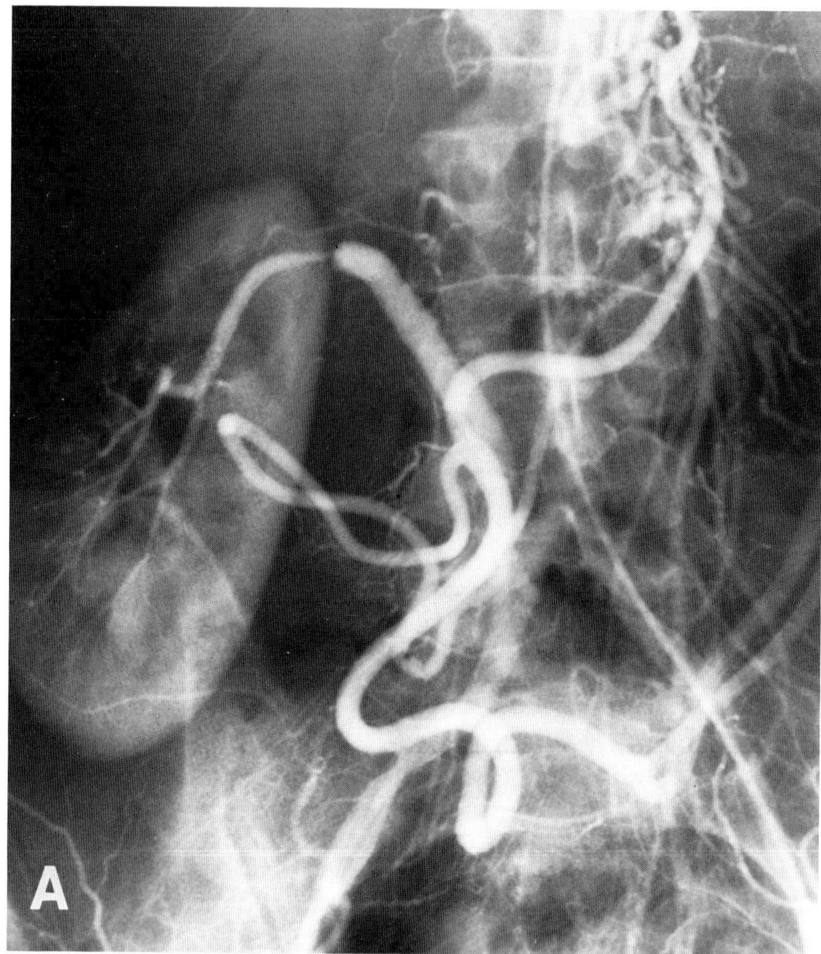

Figure 3 *A*: Postoperative appearance at 124 months of iliorenal auto-genous saphenous vein bypass to segmental renal artery demonstrating high grade distal anastomotic stricture. A large collateral artery within the mesenteric circulation is also apparent. *B*: Digital subtraction arteriogram revealing satisfactory vein patch angioplasty of the distal stricture 1 week postoperatively. (From Ref. 4, used with permission.)

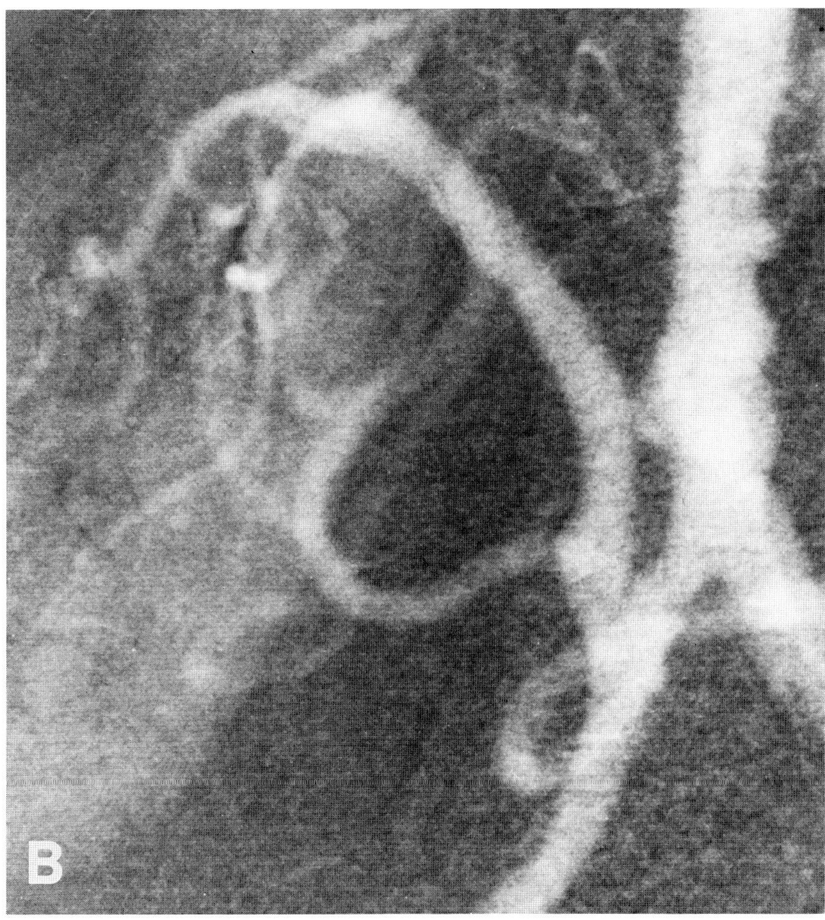

Figure 3 (Continued)

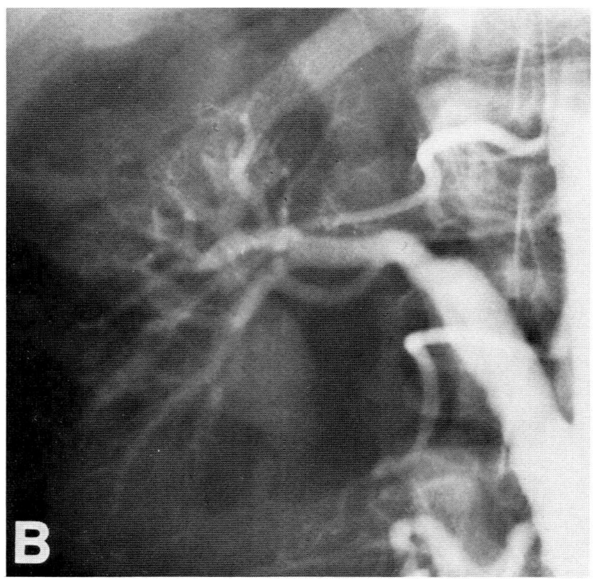

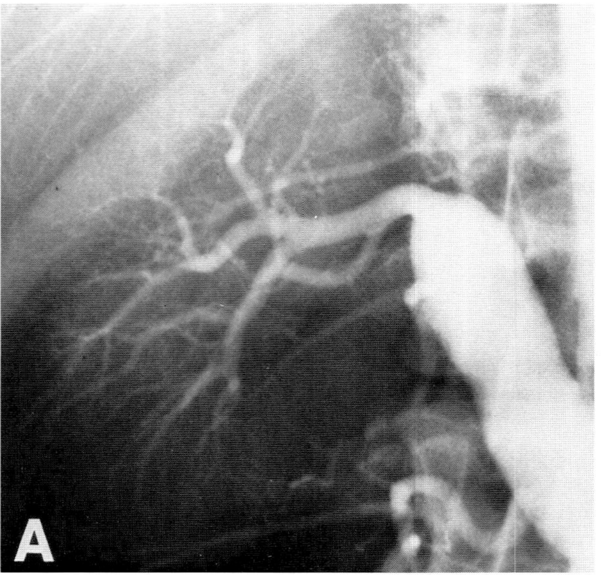

Figure 4 *A*: Aneurysmal aortorenal autogenous saphenous vein bypass 16 months postimplantation. *B*: Reduced vein graft diameter at 18 months after operative plication of the dilated conduit. (From Ref. 5, used with permission.)

Limited graft expansion has been reported to affect 20 to 40% of such conduits (17,18). Greater expansion in the form of actual aneurysms has been documented in 6% of implanted autogenous saphenous veins (18) and as many as 20% of those placed in pediatric-aged patients (34). In only a small number of cases do vein graft aneurysms appear to be poststenotic in etiology (7,18). Mural ischemia and cellular injury in veins transplanted into the renal arterial circulation are the most likely events leading to aneurysmal dilation. Perhaps the precarious intrinsic blood supply of veins in children accounts for a greater degree of mural ischemia occurring in transplanted veins of younger patients compared with adults. Autogenous arterial grafts are not immune to aneurysmal change, but this complication appears to be much less prevalent with this type of conduit (17,28).

Aneurysmal dilation of vein conduits may result in stagnant luminal blood flow and surface thrombus formation, with distal embolization of mural thrombotic debris causing renal infarction. It is this complication, not the potential for rupture, that makes it appropriate to treat progressive aneurysmal changes in vein grafts operatively. In reoperation for advanced aneurysmal vein grafts, a new conduit, usually a synthetic graft, should be used to replace the deteriorated vein. As an alternative therapy, plication of an aneurysmal graft has been advocated as a means of reducing lateral wall pressure. This has been undertaken twice in the Michigan series, and appears to limit further aneurysmal dilation, although the long-term durability of this procedure has yet to be established (Fig. 4).

Synthetic Aortorenal Graft Infection and Enteric Fistulas

Synthetic grafts were among the first conduits utilized in the reconstruction of diseased renal arteries. Prophylactic administration of perioperative antibiotics may lessen the incidence of synthetic graft infection, yet this complication is always a risk when using this type graft. When infection occurs, the prosthesis must be removed. This is usually accompanied by nephrectomy, although in cases of a solitary kidney, extra-anatomic renal revascularization using an autologous conduit is certainly appropriate. Incomplete synthetic graft removal in the presence of infection is unacceptable. Exsanguination due to aortoduodenal fistulas associated with graft remnants not removed in the presence of infection has been documented by others (4,35,36). Similarly, enteric erosions associated with infected prosthetic grafts used in renal revascularizations are often catastrophic, with reported survivals being few in number (37-40).

Reoperation for failures of primary renovascular reconstructive surgery represents a serious therapeutic undertaking. A major detriment to successful reoperation appears to be a delay in recognizing the underlying complication. This prevents the performance of an *early* reoperation, when the involved vessels may be dissected and repaired more easily with less hazard than during *late* reoperation. Prompt arteriographic studies in patients with persistent or recurrent hypertension combined with an appropriately executed reoperation will provide better results in treating this subgroup of patients with renovascular hypertension.

References

1. Stanley JC, Ernst CB, Fry WJ: Surgical treatment of renovascular hypertension: results in specific patient subgroups. In Stanley JC, Ernst, CB, Fry WJ (Eds): Renovascular Hypertension. Philadelphia, W. B. Saunders, 1984, pp. 363-371.
2. Dean RH: Complications of renal revascularization. In Bernhard VM, Towne JB, (Eds): Complications in Vascular Surgery, 2nd Edition. New York, Grune & Stratton, 1985, pp. 229-246.
3. Kaufmann JJ: Complications of renovascular surgery, In Smith RB, Skinner DG (Eds): Complications of Urologic Surgery. Philadelphia, W.B. Saunders, 1976, pp. 113-128.
4. Stanley JC, Whitehouse WM Jr, Zelenock GB, Graham LM, Cronenwett JL, Lindenauer SM: Reoperation for complications of renal artery reconstructive surgery undertaken for treatment of renovascular hypertension. J Vasc Surg 2:133-143, 1985.
5. Stanley JC, Whitehouse WM Jr, Graham LM: Complications of renal rerevascularization. In Bernhard VM, Towne JB (Eds): Complications in Vascular Surgery. New York, Grune & Stratton, 1980, pp. 189-210.
6. Franklin SS, Young JD Jr, Maxwell MH, Foster JH, Palmer JM, Cerny J, Varady PD: Operative morbidity and mortality in renovascular disease. JAMA 231:1148-1153, 1975.
7. Bergentz SE, Ericsson BF, Husberg B: Technique and complications in the surgical treatment of renovascular hypertension. Acta Chir Scand 145:143-148, 1979.
8. Ekestrom S, Liljeqvist L, Nordhus O, Tidgren B: Persisting hypertension after renal artery reconstruction. A follow-up study. Scand J Urol Nephrol 13:83-88, 1979.
9. Eigler FW, Dostal G, Montag H, Jakubowski HD: Results of a ten-year period of reconstructive surgery for renovascular disease. Thorac Cardiovasc Surg 31:45-48, 1983.

10. Jakubowski HD, Eigler FW, Montag H: Results of surgery in fibrodysplastic renal artery stenosis. World J Surg 5:859-861, 1981.
11. Lankford NS, Donohue JP, Grim CE, Weinberger MH: Results of surgical treatment of renovascular hypertension. J Urol 122:439-441, 1979.
12. Lawrie GM, Morris GC Jr, Soussou, ID, Starr DS, Silvers A, Glaeser DH, DeBakey ME: Late results of reconstructive surgery for renovascular disease. Ann Surg 191:528-533, 1980.
13. Morris GC Jr, DeBakey ME, Crawford ES, Cooley DA, Zanger LCC: Late results of surgical treatment for renovascular hypertension. Surg Gynecol Obstet 122:1255-1261, 1966.
14. Stefanini P, Benedetti-Valentini F Jr, Fiorani P: Selection for surgery and long-term results in renovascular hypertension. Int Surg 63:73-81, 1978.
15. Straffon R, Siegel DF: Saphenous vein bypass graft in the treatment of renovascular hypertension. Urol Clin North Am 2:337-350, 1975.
16. Foster JH, Maxwell MH, Franklin SS, Bleifer KH, Trippel OH, Julian OC, DeCamp PT, Varady PT: Renovascular occlusive disease. Results of operative treatment. JAMA 231:1043-1048, 1975.
17. Dean RH, Wilson JP, Burko H, Foster JH: Saphenous vein aortorenal bypass grafts: serial arteriographic study. Ann Surg 180:469-478, 1974.
18. Stanley JC, Ernst CB, Fry WJ: Fate of 100 aortorenal vein grafts: characteristics of late graft expansion, aneurysmal dilatation, and stenosis. Surgery 74:931-944, 1973.
19. Dean RH: Indications for operative management of renovascular hypertension. JSC Med Assoc 73:523-525, 1977.
20. Ekelund L, Gerlock J Jr, Goncharenko V, Foster J: Angiographic findings following surgical treatment for renovascular hypertension. Radiology 126:345-349, 1978.
21. Stoney RJ, Silane MF: Surgical treatment of renovascular hypertension: ex vivo reconstruction. In Stanley JC, Ernst CB, Fry WJ (Eds): Renovascular Hypertension. Philadelphia, W.B. Saunders, 1984, pp. 320-326.
22. Pechan BW, Novick AC, Stewart BH, Straffon RA: Endarterectomy and patchgraft angioplasty in treatment of atherosclerotic renovascular hypertension. Urology 14:487-490, 1979.
23. Thevenet A, Mary H, Boennec M: Results following surgical correction of renovascular hypertension. J Cardiovasc Surg 21:517-528, 1980.
24. Wylie EJ: Endarterectomy and autogenous arterial grafts in the surgical treatment of stenosing lesions of the renal artery. Urol Clin North Am 2:351-363, 1975.
25. Ernst CB, Stanley JC, Marshall FF, Fry WJ: Autogenous saphenous vein aortorenal grafts. A ten-year experience. Arch Surg 105:855-864, 1972.
26. Foster JH, Dean RH, Pinkerton JA, Rhamy RK: Ten years experience with the surgical management of renovascular hypertension. Ann Surg 177:755-766, 1973.

27. Kaufman JJ: Renovascular hypertension: the UCLA experience. J Urol
    121:139-144, 1979.
28. Lye CR, String ST, Wylie EJ, Stoney RJ: Aortorenal arterial autografts.
    Late observations. Arch Surg 110:1321-1326, 1975.
29. Novick AC, Stewart BH, Straffon RA: Autogenous arterial grafts in the
    treatment of renal artery stenosis. J Urol 118:919-922, 1977.
30. Stoney RJ, De Luccia N, Ehrenfeld WK, Wylie EJ: Aortorenal arterial
    autografts. Long-term assessment. Arch Surg 116:1416-1422, 1981.
31. Stanley P, Gyepes MT, Olson DL, Gates GF: Renovascular hypertension
    in children and adolescents. Radiology 129:123-131, 1978.
32. Novick AC, Straffon RA, Stewart BH, Benjamin S: Surgical treatment of
    renovascular hypertension in the pediatric patient. J Urol 119:794-805,
    1978.
33. Thuroff JW, Frohneberg D, Riedmiller R, Alken P, Hutschenreiter G,
    Thuroff S, Hohenfellner R: Localization of segmental arteries in renal
    surgery by Doppler sonography. J Urol 127:863-866, 1982.
34. Stanley JC, Fry WJ: Pediatric renal artery occlusive disease and reno-
    vascular hypertension. Etiology, diagnosis, and operative treatment. Arch
    Surg 116:669-676, 1981.
35. Keeffe EB, Krippaehne WW, Rosch J, Melynk CS: Aorto-duodenal
    fistula: complication of renal artery bypass graft. Gastroenterology 67:
    1240-1245, 1974.
36. Shaigany A, Gillespie L, Mock JP, Vasarhelyi L, Donovitch SH: Aorto-
    enteric fistula. A complication of renal artery bypass graft. Arch Int Med
    136:930-932, 1976.
37. Campbell HC Jr, Ernst CB: Aortoenteric fistula following renal revascu-
    larization. Am Surg 44:155-158, 1978.
38. Cerny JC, Fry WJ, Gambee J, Koyangyi T: Aortoduodenal fistula. J
    Urol 107:12-13, 1972.
39. Kaufman JJ: Dacron grafts and splenorenal bypass in the surgical treat-
    ment of stenosing lesions of the renal artery. Urol Clin North Am 2:365-
    380, 1975.
40. Howard RJ, Leonard JJ, Howard BD: Renal artery-cholecystoduodenal
    fistula. A late complication of Dacron patch angioplasty for renal artery
    stenosis. Arch Surg 113:888-890, 1978.

9

Vascular Techniques in Kidney Retransplantation

FUAD JOSEPH DAGHER
University of Maryland School of Medicine and Hospital,
Baltimore, Maryland

SAID A. KARMI
George Washington University Medical Center,
Washington, D.C.

"...the only way to transplant more patients successfully is to perform more transplants."

Kountz and Belzer

After failure of a transplanted kidney, regardless of cause, the choice for further treatment is either retransplantation or chronic hemodialysis.

Before the introduction of cyclosporine A, the recent and most promising immunosuppressive agent to date, and as reported by the Standards Committee of the American Society of Transplant Surgeons (2) approximately 30 to 40% of patients who receive a cadaver kidney transplant will lose their grafts within 1 year from irreversible rejection. The results of the Southeast Organ Procurement Foundation (SEOPF) study (3), which reported the experience of 39 SEOPF institutions during a 58 month period, revealed a cadaver graft survival rate of 52% percent at 1 year and 45% and 36% at 2 and 3 years, respectively. Thus, by the third year, over 30% of cadaveric kidney transplant patients could lose their grafts. A few other cadaveric kidney recipients as well as living, related transplant patients may ultimately lose their kidneys from chronic rejection. These patients, too, become potential candidates for retransplantation.

Whether or not second, third, fourth, or even fifth kidney transplants do well has been the subject of numerous reports (4,5). Also, the selective and therapeutic factors affecting the success and outcome of multiple kidney transplants have been addressed by a number of centers in a number of reports. The Minnesota Group (6) for example, reported the overall patient survival rate in the retransplant population to be 10% less than in the dialysis population. They also reported that the best results of graft function and patient survival were noted in younger patients who were nondiabetic patients who received two sequential, living, related transplants and in those patients whose first graft was lost to chronic rejection (i.e., rejection occurring at 6 months or longer after transplantation). The worst and poorest results were observed in patients with acute rejection occurring during the initial posttransplant periods, older patients who are older than 40 years of age, and diabetics. Although the SEOPF patient survival rates for secondary grafts showed no increased patient mortality, and unlike the Minnesota study, they did not show reduced secondary graft survival rates in patients older than 45 years old. The SEOPF data confirm the observation of the studies by Gifford and co-workers (7) and Oplez and associates (8) that prolonged function of the primary graft for more than 1 year was associated with improved second graft outcome. Furthermore, the results of Schulack and co-workers (5) from the University of Iowa on the feasibility and success of a third kidney transplant are also of interest. These authors reported three successful third transplantations with graft survival of 6, 3, and 1 year respectively, in recipients whose initial kidney transplant survivals were also more than 1 year. Thus, a large population of first kidney transplants along with a few second and third kidney transplant patients who had lost their kidneys to rejection or to some other causes remain candidates for re-transplantation.

Presently, with the availability of cyclosporine A and with future, more potent, immunosuppressive medications, a larger number of patients may undergo successful retransplant operations regardless of the cause of loss of previous transplanted kidneys and regardless of the length of time the original transplanted kidneys have stayed in the patient. A patient of one of the authors (F.J.D.) received his fourth kidney transplant after losing the first three from acute rejection in periods ranging between 3 to 7 months. He has now kept his fourth transplanted kidney with excellent function for more than 2 years. He had been treated initially with cyclosporine A and prednisone for the first 6 months after his fourth transplantation, at which time he was converted to conventional immunotherapy of Imuran and prednisone therapy.

Although factors influencing the outcome of multiple kidney transplants have been repeatedly addressed, little attention has been given to the technical aspects of retransplantation. More specifically, the operative techniques of reestablishing the vascular continuity in kidney re-transplantation are lacking. It is the purpose of this chapter to address the technical alternatives available for vascular anastomoses in patients considered for secondary renal transplantation.

The Location of the Transplant

When the decision to retransplant a patient has been made, the location of the new transplant depends on the number and anatomic sites of previous transplants, the size disparity between the kidney and the host, the length of ureter on the available kidney, and the number of renal arteries. The external iliac vein on the side where a previous, acutely rejected kidney had been removed may be thrombosed and, therefore, unusable. Also, the area may be difficult to dissect out and better avoided because of adhesions resulting from previous operations, previous inflammatory processes, and possible previous infection.

In a second transplant in the adult patient, the donor kidney is best placed in the recipient's contralateral iliac extraperitoneal space. Although a number of techniques are used to get access to this area (9), the technique we have used in over 400 kidney transplants avoids cutting any muscles. As shown in Figure 1, the incision extends along a line drawn from the pubis to just above the anterior superior iliac spine, approximately two finger widths above and parallel to the inguinal ligament through skin and subcutaneous tissues. The external oblique aponeurosis is then divided along its fibers throughout the length of the incision. Proximally, if the incision is rather long, this aponeurosis begins to merge with the external oblique and internal oblique muscles. Next, the anterior rectus sheath is opened longitudinally along the lateral border of the rectus muscle, also extending throughout the length of the incision (Fig. 2). The posterior rectus sheath along with the transversus abdominis are next opened to expose the preperitoneal fat. Here, with the help of a sponge stick, the intact peritoneum is gently retracted medially; the inferior epigastric vessels are identified and divided between ligatures (Fig. 3). When the dissection is complete and the intact peritoneum and its contents are retracted medially, the iliac arteries and veins are well in view (Fig. 4). While carrying the dissection to isolate the external iliac vein and the hypogastric artery, care should be taken to ligate or coagulate the lymphatic channels, which may be numerous at times, to avoid future excessive lymphatic leakage. The renal vein of the donor kidney is anastomosed end-to-side to the external iliac vein. The renal artery, if single and without a Carrel patch, is spatulated and sutured end-to-side to the external or com-

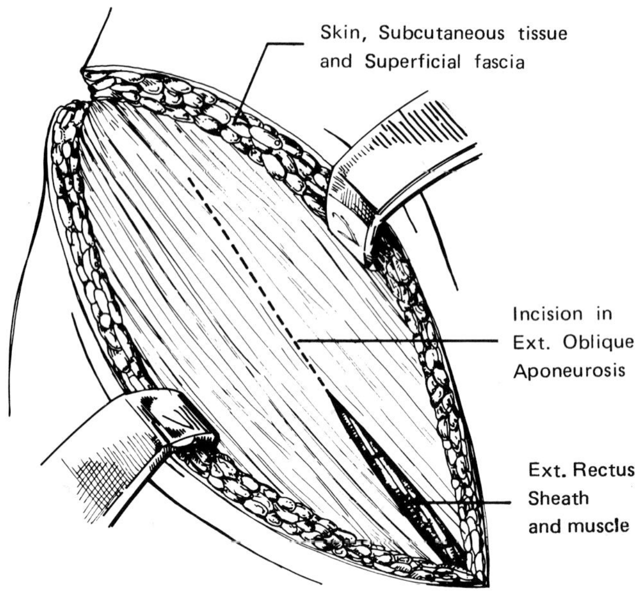

Figure 1   The incision through skin and subcutaneous tissue, revealing the external oblique aponeurosis.

mon iliac artery using double-arm 5-0 prolene sutures. Presently, however, because most renal arteries of cadaveric kidneys are removed en bloc with a segment of aorta at harvest time, a Carrel patch is easily fashioned at the end of the renal artery. This patch makes the end-to-side suture of the renal artery to the external or common iliac artery relatively easy. At the end of the procedure, the incision is then closed in two layers of continuous sutures of O vicryl.

The end-to-end anastomosis of the artery of the second renal transplant to the internal or hypogastric iliac artery on the contralateral iliac fossa should be avoided in the presence of an already ligated hypogastric artery on the opposite side. Ligating both hypogastric arteries may ominously alter the

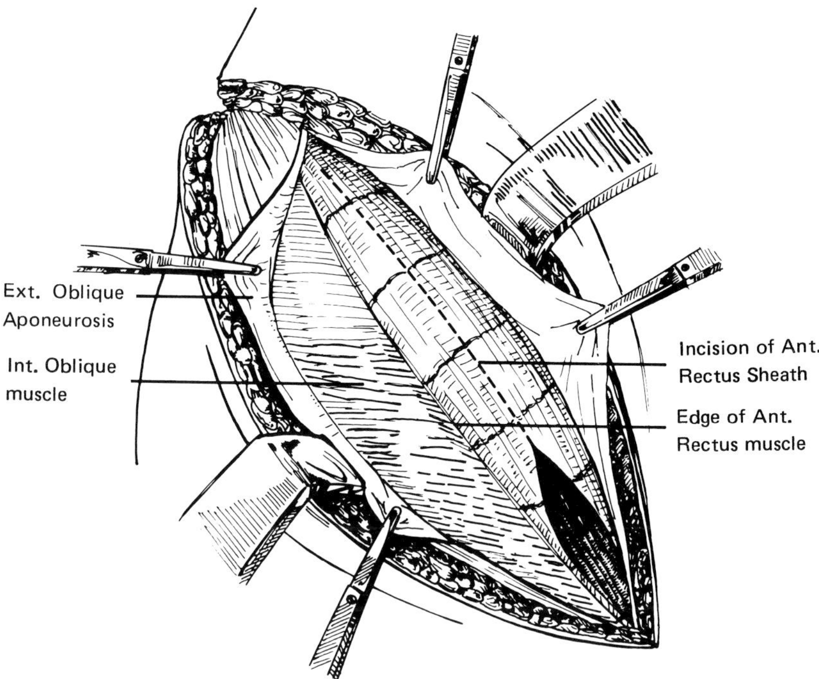

Figure 2 The external oblique aponeurosis is opened along its fibers, revealing the anterior rectus sheath and muscle.

normal pelvic arterial flow hemodynamics and possibly reduce arterial blood flow to the phallus, resulting in vasculogenic impotence (10-11).

In the case of a third, fourth, or even fifth transplant, while placing the kidney in either iliac retroperitoneal space can be achieved, it may be rather difficult or, at times, impossible. The iliac fossa where the kidney is to be placed may be limited by extensive adhesions and fibrosis, and the external iliac veins may be thrombosed or cordlike. The renal vein of the new kidney may then be anastomosed end-to-side to either the common iliac vein or to the inferior vena cava, while the renal artery with its Carrel patch is usually anastomosed end-to-side to either the common iliac artery or the lower aorta.

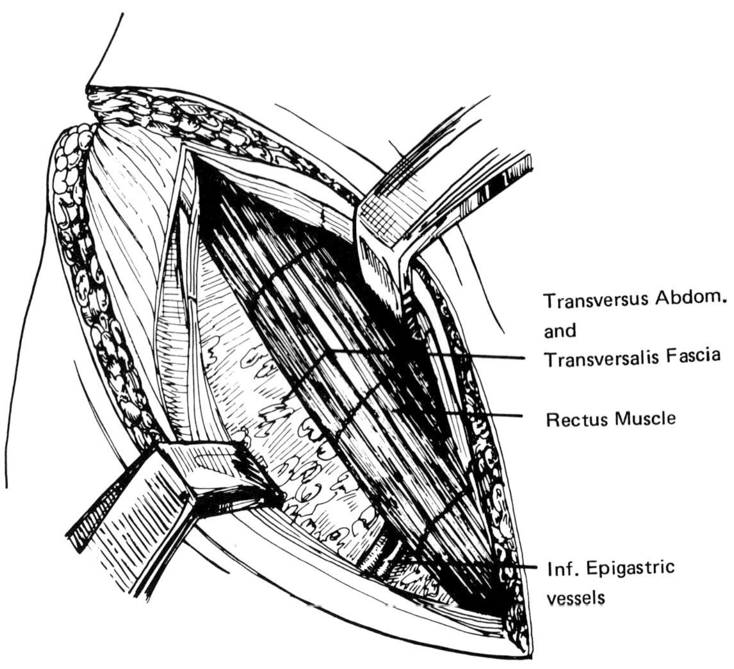

Figure 3 The anterior rectus sheath is opened throughout the length of the incision, revealing the posterior rectus sheath, transversus abdominis muscle, and transversalis fascia.

As an alternative method, either iliac fossa may also be approached through a midline abdominal incision in the adult patient undergoing third, fourth, or fifth transplants or in children undergoing first adult renal homografts. This technique was initially reported by Starzl and his co-workers (12) in 1964. In this technique, after entering the abdomen, an incision is made in the posterior peritoneum either to the right of the ascending or to the left of the sigmoid colon, depending on which fossa is chosen to place the kidney in. The periotoneum is then reflected medially, creating a proper fossa for the transplanted kidney to lay in. The terminal end of the inferior vena cava is freed and used for the end-to-side hookup of the renal vein if the kidney is

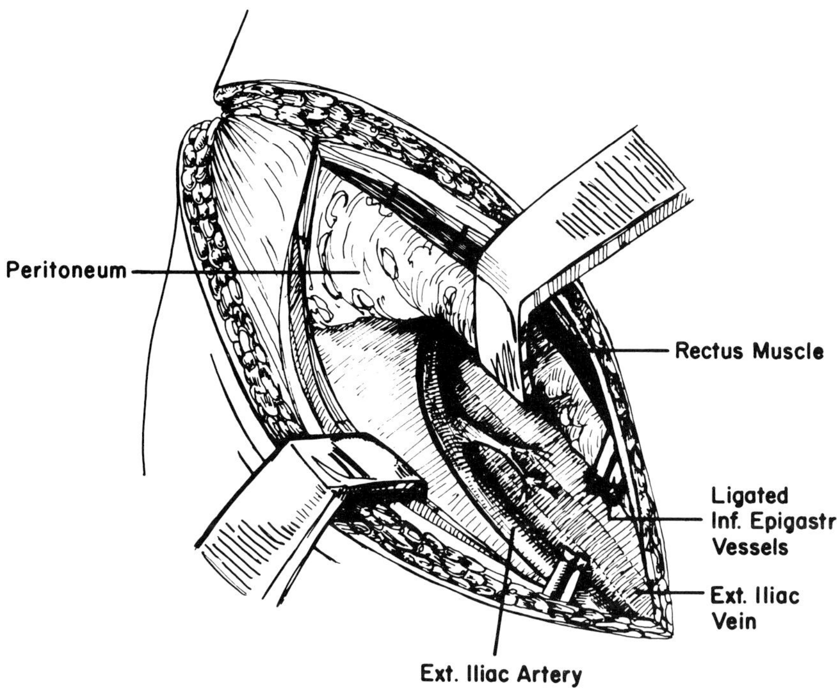

Figure 4 The retracted intact peritoneum and the ligated inferior epigastric vessels, exposing the iliac arteries and veins.

placed on the right side, and to the left common iliac vein when the kidney is placed on the left side. The renal artery with its Carrel patch can be sutured end-to-side to either the right or left common iliac artery. It may be sutured to the lower aorta if necessary (Fig. 5).

Technical Alternative for Multiple Renal Arteries

In the early days of organ retrieval, when cadaveric kidneys were harvested separately and individually, a number of kidneys with multiple or polar arteries were available. To use these otherwise normal kidneys, a number of

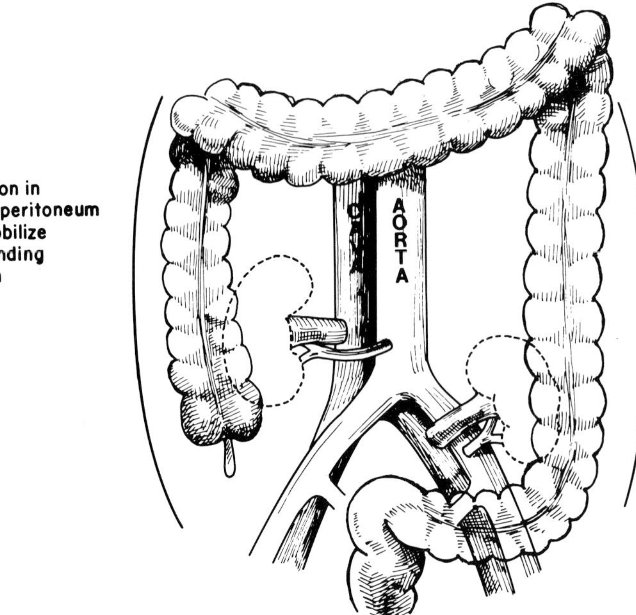

Figure 5 Kidney in third, fourth, or fifth transplants may be placed through an abdominal approach, either behind the ascending colon on the right or behind the descending colon or sigmoid on the left. The renal artery is sutured either to the aorta directly on the right or to the left common iliac artery on the left, while the renal veins may be sutured either to the vena cava on the right or to the common iliac vein on the left.

techniques addressing these multiple vessels were reported. In the case of the kidney with a sizeable polar artery, the need to preserve accessory lower polar renal arteries because of their frequent contribution to the ureteral vasculature is well recognized. Vineyard and Tilney (13) recommend anastomosing the spatulated end of the polar branch end-to-side to the main renal artery at a convenient and easily accessible site. Other alternatives include anastomosing the polar artery to the inferior epigastric artery of the recipient patient or creating a common trunk or channel between the end of the polar artery and the main renal artery, with subsequent direct anastomosis with the recipient hypogastric artery. However, if the segment of the aorta sur-

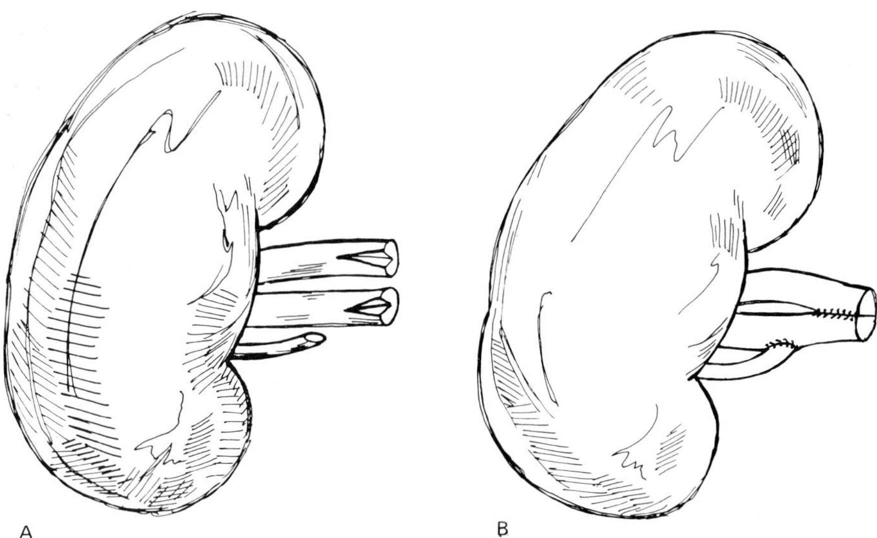

Figure 6 *A, B*   A common trunk is created between two separate renal arteries. Then the spatulated end of a third artery is anastomosed to the side of one of the arteries.

rounding the polar artery is available, a Carrel patch can be fashioned and used. When three separate hilar arteries of moderate size are present on a cadaver kidney, Dagher and colleagues suggest a technique of creating a common trunk or channel between the ends of at least two of the arteries, then anastomosing the spatulated end of the third artery to the side of one of the arteries, with subsequent direct anastomosis of the common channel with a recipient hypogastric artery in an end-to-end fashion (Figs. 6A and B). Other surgeons (15) recommend additional various alternatives to this problem. As seen in Figures 7A, B and C, in the case of two separate hilar arteries, one branch can be sutured end-to-end to the hypogastric artery, while the second artery sutured end-to-side to the common iliac artery (Fig. 7A). The two renal arteries can also be sutured end-to-end to the end branches of the hypogastric artery (Fig. 7B). Also, both ends of the two separate renal arteries may be each individually sutured end-to-side to the common or external iliac artery (Fig. 7C).

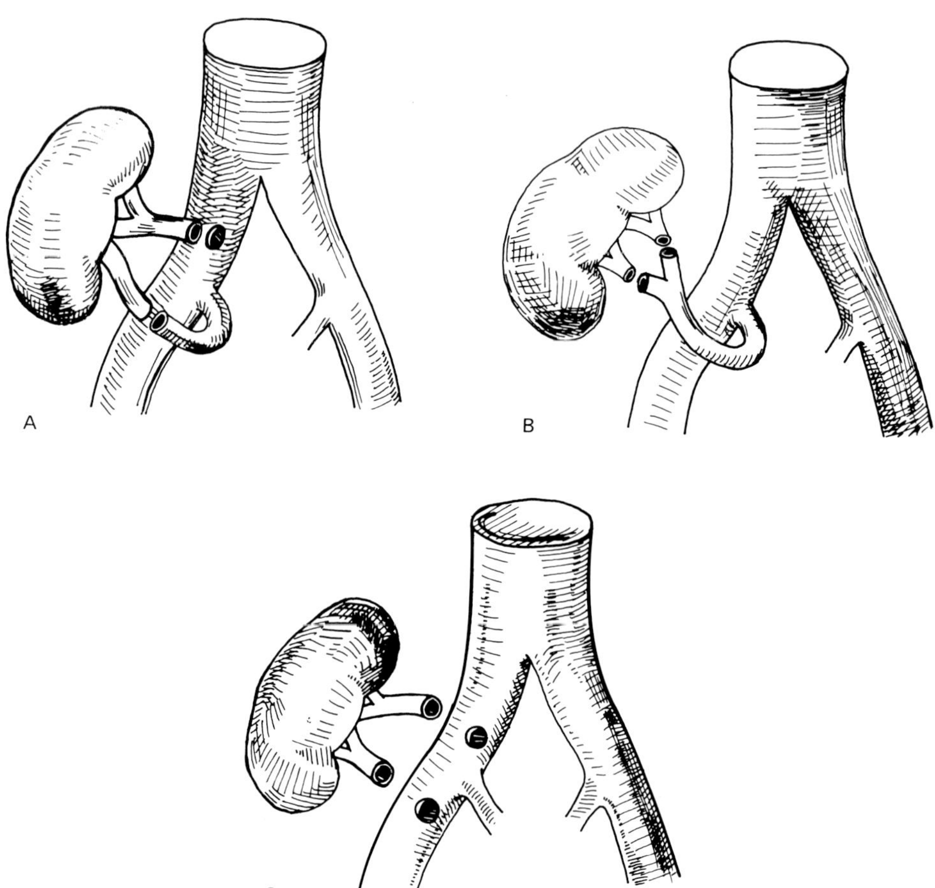

Figure 7 *A*: With two separate arteries, one branch can be sutured end-to-end to the hypogastric artery, while the second artery is sutured end-to-side to the common iliac artery. *B*: The two renal arteries can be sutured end-to-end to the end branches of the hypogastric artery. *C*: The ends of both separate renal arteries may be individually sutured end-to-side to the common or external iliac artery.

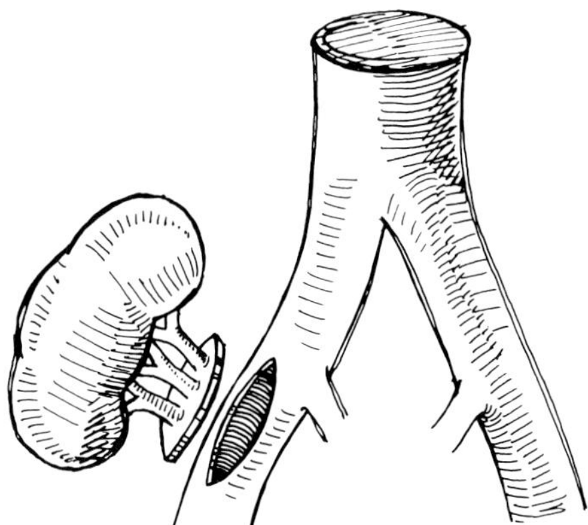

Figure 8 A Carrel patch with multiple renal arteries is fashioned and sutured to the side of the external or common iliac artery.

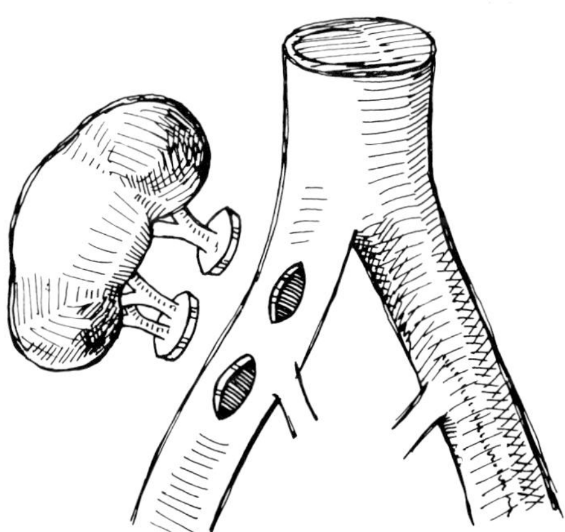

Figure 9 When hilar arteries are widely separated on the aorta, multiple Carrel patches with one or more arteries can be sutured end-to-side to the common or external iliac arteries.

Presently, however, with most cadaver kidneys harvested en bloc, the renal arteries regardless of their number are usually removed with a segment of the aorta. A Carrel patch with multiple arteries can be fashioned and sutured to the side of the external or the common iliac arteries (Fig. 8), as reported by Novick and co-workers (16). If the hilar arteries are multiple or if they are widely separated on the aorta, multiple Carrel patches with one or more arteries can be sutured end-to-side to the common or external iliac arteries (Fig. 9).

Further, in the presence of anomalous vessels, such as agenesis of the inferior vena cava and thrombosis of the external and common iliac veins, alternative locations and different arterial anastomoses may be sought. Talbot-Wright and co-workers (17) from Spain reported a case where in the presence of these venous anomalies, the kidney was placed orthotopically on the left side, anastomosing the renal vein end-to-side to the patient's own renal vein and the renal artery end-to-end to the patient's own splenic artery with successful outcome.

Cadaver kidneys from pediatric donors can be transplanted and do function well, even in adult recipients. If such kidneys are too small, en bloc transplantation of the double cadaveric kidneys can be performed and has been successfully reported (18). Here, with both kidneys removed en bloc in continuity with the aorta and vena cava, one end each of the aorta and vena cava is closed with a running vascular suture. The other end of the vena cava is sutured end-to-side to the external iliac vein, while the opposite end of the aorta is sutured either end-to-end to the hypogastric artery if no size discrepancy exists or end-to-side to the common or external iliac artery. The two small kidneys are usually placed in the iliac retroperitoneal space on one side or the other, as in the adult situation.

Technical Alternatives for Venous Anastomoses

The standard procedure with a single end-to-side renal vein to the external iliac vein anastomosis can be used most of the time. In patients undergoing second transplants on the contralateral iliac fossa, the external iliac vein should be freely mobilized and all of its tributaries suture ligated and divided to give it maximum mobility. Thus, the end-to-side anastomosis of the renal vein to the iliac vein can be done without tension, even though the renal vein in question may be short or even cut off flush with the hilum of the kidney. However, in the presence of a short vein or a vein cut off flush with the hilum of the kidney, a segment of free saphenous vein can be used to

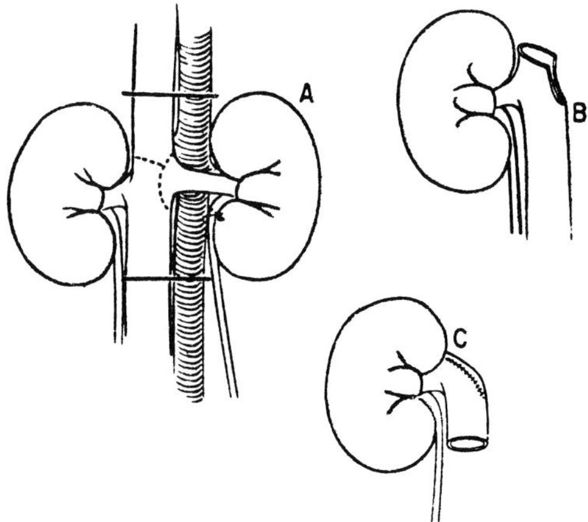

Figure 10 *A*: Technique of lengthening the right renal vein during harvesting of cadaveric kidneys. *B*: The venotomy in the vena cava is extended to open it above the right renal vein. *C*: The venotomy is then closed longitudinally with a running vascular suture. (From Ref. 19, used with permission.)

lengthen the renal vein. With the kidney in a basin filled with ice cold saline slush, one end of the free saphenous vein can then be sutured to the end of the short or hilar vein to prolong it. Subsequently, the other end of the saphenous vein can be sutured end-to-side to the iliac vein. While harvesting cadaveric kidneys and to avoid the problem of a short right renal vein, Corry and Kelly (19) devised a technique of lengthening the right renal vein at the time of en bloc harvesting of the kidneys. As seen in Figure 10, the left kidney is removed with a single cuff of the vena cava. The venotomy in the cava is next extended to open the vena cava just above the right renal vein. While the kidney is immersed in cold saline slush, the venotomy is closed longitudinally with a running vascular suture. The excess length of the vena cava is removed before suturing its end to the common iliac vein. In kidneys with normal-sized veins and several other smaller veins, the smaller veins can be suture ligated or tied. Occasionally, when two separate large renal veins are present, it is preferable not to form a common channel between the ends, but instead anastomose each end separately, end-to-side to the iliac vein. If each of the veins end separately in the vena cava of the donor, the patch of vena cava with these veins can be sutured directly to the iliac vein as a patch, with the two venous ostia coming out through it.

Arterial and Venous Complications

There remain the problems of acute arterial or venous thrombosis after retransplantation and how to deal with it successfully. A number of reports addressing this issue have been published. The diagnosis of arterial thrombosis is usually established by angiography, while blood flow technetium scanning of the kidney may also be extremely helpful. If recognized in the immediate posttransplant period, acute occlusion or thrombosis of the renal artery should be promptly explored surgically. Whether or not kidney function in the transplanted kidney can be restored depends to a large extent on the warm ischemic time that the kidney had been through and the extent of intrarenal thrombosis that may have occurred during the period of ischemia. The maximum warm ischemic tolerance of transplanted kidneys is not fully determined. However, the effects of varying periods of renal warm ischemia in both human and animal studies (21) show that up to 2 hours of warm time is consistent with the return of renal function after revascularization. In 1982, Melzer and co-workers (22) reported a patient in whom the artery of a renal allograft was kinked in the immediate postoperative period, obstructing the flow to the transplanted kidney, which on exploration was flaccid and cyanosed. After 3 hours of acute warm ischemic time, the patient was successfully treated by emergency exploration and reimplantation of the renal artery end-to-side to the common iliac artery. Others (23) reported two cases of renal artery thrombosis managed by immediate reexploration and restoration of blood flow to the transplanted kidney, with return of function after 2 and 5.5 hours of occlusion, respectively. From these reports, it seems reasonable to seriously consider surgical repair of acute arterial thrombosis provided that it can be accomplished within a reasonable time.

In reexploring a transplanted kidney for renal artery stenosis, the recommended approach is through the peritoneum. By this technique, the surgeon avoids the difficult dissection of the adherent peritoneum to the capsule of the kidney and, therefore, injury to the kidney. The posterior peritoneum over the stenosed suture line is opened and the vessels identified. With sharp dissection, the artery and vein are dissected and vessel loops are placed around them. The proximal end of the artery is clamped, the stenosis or thrombosed area is excised, and, with the use of a graduated plastic catheter,

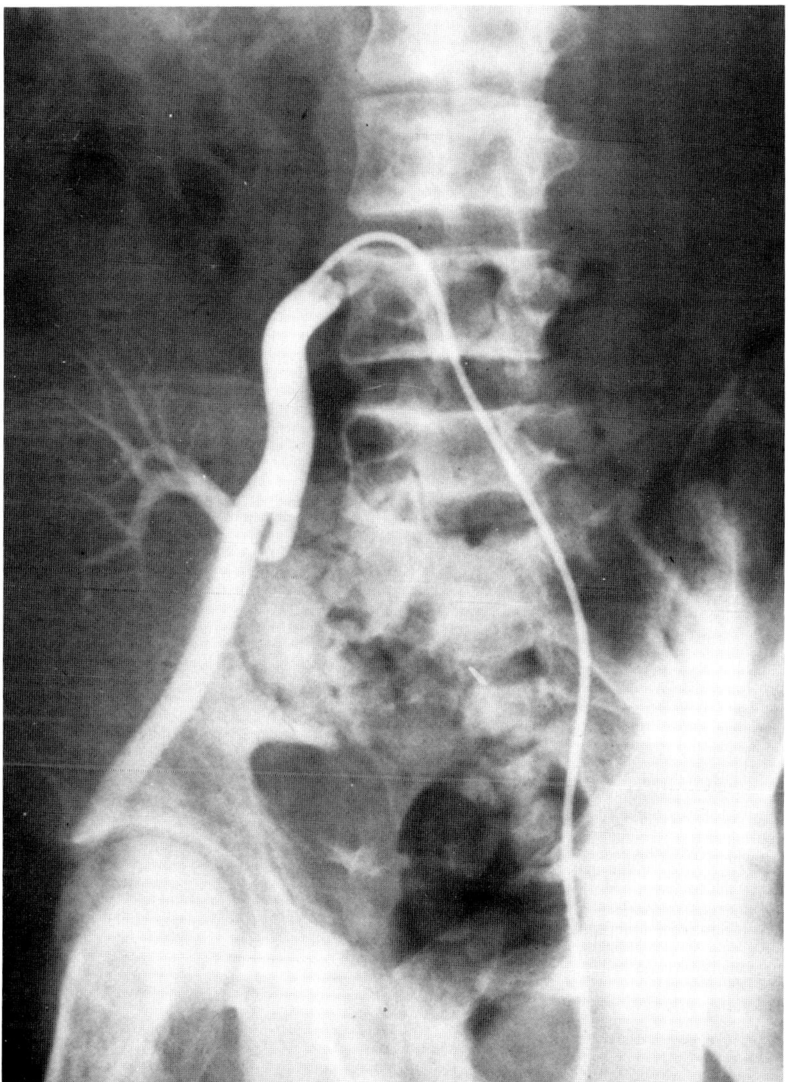

Figure 11 Severe renal artery stenosis at the site of end-to-end anastomosis, resulting in severe diastolic hypertension.

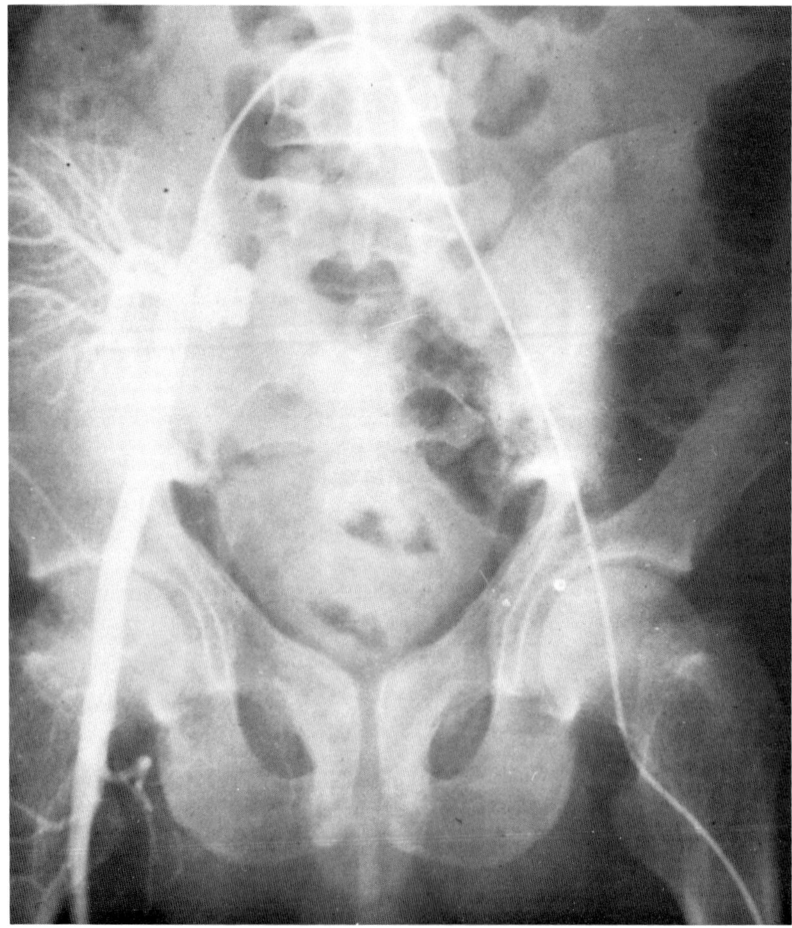

Figure 12   Pseudocyst appearing 6 months after repair of stenosis in the patient illustrated in Figure 11. This lesion was excised and successfully repaired using the peritoneal approach.

the distal renal artery is perfused with about 200 cc of heparinized cold Ringer's lactate solution. Reanastomosis is usually performed with double-arm 6.0 prolene sutures continuous on each side. The incision is then closed in the usual manner. We operated on a patient twice with this technique within a period of 6 months. Initially, as shown in Figure 11, for severe stenosis causing hypertension, the stenotic segment was resected with end-to-end anastomosis. Six months later, hypertension recurred and repeat angiography revealed a pseudoaneurysm of the renal artery (Fig. 12). Reexploration and excision of the aneurysm resulted in a normal blood pressure and continued good kidney function.

The outcome of acute renal vein thrombosis, however, is somewhat more dismal. Acute renal vein thrombosis in the immediate posttransplant patient, while rare, carries a much higher incidence of kidney loss. If and when suspected, the accepted approach is immediate exploration and thrombectomy. Such early diagnosis and prompt thrombectomy have occasionally resulted in graft salvage. More commonly, however, prolonged venostasis leads to a nonviable graft as often seen at the time of surgical exploration. Renal vein thrombosis occurring more than 1 month after transplantation is probably best treated with anticoagulation; by that time, established collateral venous channels are adequate enough to prevent loss of graft.

References

1. Kountz SL, Belzer FO: The fate of patients after renal transplantation, graft rejection and re-transplantation. Ann Surg 176:509, 1972.
2. Standard Committee of the American Society of Transplant Surgeons. Current results and expectation of renal transplantation. JAMA 246: 1330, 1981.
3. Spees EK, Vaughn WK, McDonald JC, Bollinger RR, Williams GM, Sanfilippo FP, Adams P, Mendez-Picone GG, Niblack G: Why do secondary transplants succeed? Results of the Southeast Organ Procurement Foundation Prospective Study, 1977-1982. J Urol 129:484, 1983.
4. Walter WC, Zincke H, Sterioff S, Offord KP, Frohnert PP: Renal transplantation after failure of first kidney graft. Surg Gynecol Obstet 152: 476, 1981.
5. Schulack JA, Nghiem DD, Ercolani L, Corry RL: The third kidney transplant. Am J Surg 147:269, 1984.
6. Ascher NL, Ahrenholz, DH, Simmons RLV, Najarian JS: 100 second renal allografts from a single transplantation institution. Transplantation 27:30, 1979.
7. Gifford RR Sr, Sutherland DE, Fryd DS, Simmons RL, Najarian JS: Duration of first renal allograft survival as an indicator of second allo-

graft outcome. Surgery 88:611, 1980.

8. Opelz G, Iwaki Y, Terasaki PI: Effect of HLA matching and pretransplant blood transfusion on survival of cadaver kidney transplants. In Cascianni CV, Adorno D (Eds): Tissue Typing and Renal Transplantation. Padua, Italy, Piccin Medical Books, 1978, p. 7.

9. Starzl TE, Marchioro TL, Dickinson TC, Rifkind D, Stonington OG, Waddell WR: Technique of renal homotransplantation. Arch Surg 89:87, 1964.

10. Billet A, Dather FJ, Queral LA: Surgical correction of vasculogenic impotence in a patient after bilateral renal transplantation. Surgery 91:108, 1982.

11. Billet A, Davis A, Linhardt GE, Queral LA, Dagher FJ: The effects of bilateral renal transplantation on plevic hemodynamics and sexual function. Surgery 95:415, 1984.

12. Starzl TE, Marchioro TL, Morgan WW, Waddel WR: A technique for use in adult renal homografts in children. Surg Gynecol Obstet 1066, 1964.

13. Vineyard G, Tilney N. An effective technique for management of transplant kidneys with polar branches. Arch Surg 111:407, 1976.

14. Dagher FJ, Ollodart RM, Ayella JJ, Mason GR: Kidney transplantation using cadaveric kidneys having three separate renal arteries. Am Surg 42:85, 1976.

15. Rijksen FF, Kookan WB, Walaszewki W, et al. Vascular complications in 400 consecutive renal allografts. J Cardiovasc Surg 23:91, 1982.

16. Novick AC, Magnusson M, Braun WE: Multiple artery renal transplantation: emphasis on extracorporeal methods of donar arterial reconstruction. J Urol 122:731, 1979.

17. Talbot-Wright R, Figuls J, Gelabert A, Carretero P, Solanas G, Gil-Vernet J: Alternative surgery in renal transplantation: spleno-renal anastomosis. Eur Urol 8:127, 1982.

18. Dreikorn L, Rohl L, Horsch R: The use of double renal transplant from pediatric cadaver donors. Bri J Urol 49:361, 1977.

19. Corry RJ, Kelly SE: Technique for lengthening the right vein of cadaver donor kidneys. Am J Surg 135:867, 1978.

20. Palleschi J, Novick AC, Braun WE, Magnusson MO: Vascular complications of renal transplantation. Urology 16:61, 1980.

21. Bidle J, Dahlager JI, Asnaess A, Jaglicic D: The influence of warm ischemia on renal function and pathology. Scand J Urol Nephrol 11:156, 1977.

22. Melzer JS, Sicard GA, Etheredge EE, Anderson CB: Successful revascularization of early post-transplant renal arterial occlusion. Surgery 91:168, 1982.

23. Gerard DF, Devin J, Halaz NA, Collins G: Transplant renal artery thrombosis. Arch Surg 117:361, 1982.

10

Reoperations After Femoropopliteal Bypass

JOSEPH M. GIORDANO
George Washington University Medical Center, Washington, D.C.

Femoropopliteal bypass plays a pivotal role in the management of lower extremity ischemia. Despite enormous experience with this procedure and improvements in the operative approach, the 5 year patency for femoropopliteal bypass remains at 50 to 70% (1-5). Although these results are considered acceptable, we must recognize that this means a failure rate of 30 to 50% for these operations. This far exceeds the late failure rate reported for other vascular procedures such as carotid artery endarterectomy, aortofemoral bypass, and abdominal aortic aneurysm resection. The vascular surgeon then must frequently treat patients with failed femoropopliteal bypasses whose original symptoms of ischemia and disabling claudication have returned or worsened. If other indications such as infection and false aneurysm formation are considered, it becomes clear that reoperative surgery after femoropopliteal bypass is common. As described in a chapter on general considerations of reoperative surgery (6), 46.3% of 2682 patients who underwent infrainguinal vascular reconstruction needed reoperation within 5 years of their original vascular procedure according to data from the Cleveland Vascular Registry.

Occlusion of femoropopliteal bypass grafts occurs at any time after the operative procedure. Two distinct groups are defined. Early occlusion occurs within 30 days of operation and late occlusion occurs after this. This time distinction has important clinical implications. The etiology, prevention, diagnosis, initial management, operative approach, and results significantly differ between early and late occlusion and, therefore, will be discussed separately.

Incidence and Etiology of Early Graft Occlusion

Early graft occlusion occurs in 10 to 25% of all femoropopliteal bypass procedures (7,8). This incidence is probably higher than generally realized because lifetable projections of graft patency usually exclude those occlusions successfully reopened within 48 hours of the original operation. The etiology of early bypass failure is due to inappropriate planning of the operation, technical problems associated with performance of the operative procedure, and adverse factors that occur in the immediate postoperative period. Failure to appreciate poor arterial inflow from disease in the aortoiliac system and inadequate delineation of popliteal artery outflow are important causes of failure (9). Proximal or distal anastomotic intimal flaps, stenoses of the distal anastomoses, improper graft tunneling causing twists or kinks, a structurally inadequate vein graft, and atheromatous embolic debris from the proximal arterial lesions are common causes of technical failure. Adverse systemic factors in the immediate postoperative period include hypotension and the hypercoagulable state, both of which exhibit undefined and possibly significant influences on the early outcome of femoropopliteal bypass grafts (10, 11).

Prevention of early graft failure depends on eliminating all of these potential pitfalls. Preoperative arteriography helps to determine the adequacy of arterial inflow and the appropriate site for the distal anastomosis. Any question of a stenotic lesion in the aorta or iliac artery is investigated at the time of arteriogram, with direct measurement of arterial pressure above and below the questionable area. A 15% reduction in systolic arterial pressure distal to the stenosis is significant and should be corrected if possible by percutaneous transluminal angioplasty. The arteriogram should clearly demonstrate the site on the popliteal artery for the distal arterial anastomosis. This area should be open and relatively free of atherosclerotic disease. Although bypass to an isolated popliteal artery segment is at times appropriate, it is better if the popliteal artery has runoff to at least one of the three trifurcation arteries. If stenotic lesions exist in the outflow vessels, it is more appropriate to place the anastomosis distal to these stenoses. If preoperative arteriography does not clearly define the optimal site for the distal anastomosis, then an operative arteriogram by direct puncture of the exposed popliteal artery is performed.

Meticulous attention to detail avoids other technical problems. A saphenous vein used in the reversed technique must be 4 mm in diameter and free of structural defects such as a thick wall from a previous episode of superficial phlebitis. The distal anastomosis is performed at a site in the popliteal artery free of calcific atherosclerotic disease. To avoid damage to arterial outflow, the popliteal artery is controlled with vessel loops, internal balloon catheters, or atraumatic clamps placed in the soft part of the popliteal artery, with minimum tension needed to prevent backbleeding. Just before completion of the anastomosis, I dilate with a balloon catheter, coronary artery dilator, or a small hemostat the distal popliteal artery at the site of the occluding clamp. At this time, if there is a question about the adequacy of the distal anastomosis, an operative arteriogram is performed through the graft prior to its tunneling. It is far easier to correct a technical problem at this point in the operative procedure than after the completion of the proximal anastomosis. The graft is tunneled under the sartorious muscle, carefully avoiding twists or kinks. Stripping a reversed saphenous vein with a marking pen before tunneling is helpful. Other authors (12) recommend placing a long black silk suture through the most superficial adventitia, picking up bites at 10 cm intervals. Polytetrafluoroethylene (PTFE) grafts will usually not kink, but the modified human umbilical vein graft will catch and twist as it is pulled under the sartorious muscle. This graft must always be inserted through a tunneller.

The proximal anastomosis is done in a soft part of the femoral artery. Anastomosis of the reversed saphenous vein to a thick-walled femoral artery is a common and poorly emphasized technical problem that causes stenosis of the proximal anastomosis. To avoid this, a patch graft angioplasty with vein or PTFE can be performed first, facilitating the proximal vein graft anastomosis. After completion of both anastomoses, an operative arteriogram should be obtained to rule out any of the technical problems mentioned.

Systemic problems in the immediate postoperative period affect graft patency. Both biologic and synthetic grafts are thrombogenic, particularly in the immediate postoperative period. If intravascular volume is not maintained, hypotension or low cardiac output may predispose the graft to thrombose. Adequate hydration monitored by urine output and central venous pressure is essential. The recently reported (13) improved early patency of femoropopliteal grafts noted with the intravenous administration

of low molecular weight Dextran in the immediate postoperative period may
be related to the effect of that drug on increasing intravascular volume.

Diagnosis: Early Occlusion

The diagnosis of failed femoropopliteal bypass grafts depends on frequent
evaluations of the peripheral pulses by experienced personnel. If the patient's
runoff included either an anterior or posterior tibial artery, ankle pulses are
usually palpable or at least easily audible by Doppler examination. If runoff
included only a blind popliteal segment or the peroneal artery, ankle pulses
may not be palpable, but a marked improvement of the ankle-arm arterial
pressure index should be present. Absence of these findings in the immediate
postoperative period indicates early failure of a femoropopliteal bypass graft.

Technical Management: Early Occlusion

The management of these patients is immediate operative reexploration.
Since technical errors are most likely responsible for early graft failure, every
effort is made to identify and correct these. A repeat preoperative arteriogram is not necessary. Intravenous heparin and antibiotics are given as soon as
the diagnosis of failed femoropopliteal graft is made. The initial operative approach is the same for vein, PTFE, or human umbilical vein grafts. The distal
anastomosis is explored first. A longitudinal incision is made in the graft up
to but not through the suture line. The thrombus is gently removed, the
anastomosis inspected, and obvious defects corrected. A balloon embolectomy catheter is passed proximally to reestablish arterial inflow. If the greater
saphenous vein was used for a bypass, valves may prevent proximal passage
of the catheter. The proximal anastomosis is explored, the vein graft opened,
and an irrigating catheter passed through the vein graft and out the opening in
the distal anastomosis. The balloon catheter is attached to the irrigating
catheter and pulled through to the proximal anastomosis. The balloon is
inflated and thrombus then removed. If arterial inflow to the graft is not adequate, then the proximal anastomosis is opened to correct any technical
problems. If there is a question of adequacy of graft inflow, arterial pressure
is measured directly and compared with the brachial arterial pressure. There
should be no significant difference. After completion of the thrombectomy
and correction of any technical problems, an operative arteriogram is always
performed.

Postoperative Management and Results: Early Occlusion

Although scientific proof of its efficacy is not established, I fully anti-coagulate the patient in the postoperative period with intravenous heparin and maintain this until discharge. The patient is closely monitored by examination and with Duppler ultrasound. Antibiotics are continued. The results of reexploration depend on the type of graft originally used. The patency of reexplored vein grafts, even when technical problems are identified and corrected, is considerably less than the expected patency for femoropopliteal vein grafts that do not initially fail. Craver and co-workers (8) reported on eight reexplored vein grafts that were treated by thrombectomy alone. By 3 months, all eight grafts had reoccluded. Because the viability of vein intima and part of the media depend on luminal diffusion of oxygen and nutrients, it is possible that during the period of occlusion, significant ischemic changes in the vein graft occur, accounting for the poor results of reexplored vein grafts. Reexplored PTFE and umbilical vein grafts give better results. Veith and associates (14) reported that PTFE grafts that were reexplored had patency rates similar to the grafts that did not need reexploration. They reported that nine PTFE grafts treated by thrombectomy alone or thrombectomy with graft extension remained patent. Hafner and Cranley (15) reported that 6 of 9 umbilical vein grafts originally placed in patients with claudication and 11 of 12 umbilical vein grafts placed in patients for limb salvage that underwent thrombectomy alone for early failure remain patent. These results, particularly with occluded PTFE and umbilical vein grafts, justify an aggressive approach in patients with early occlusions.

Incidence and Etiology of Late Graft Occlusion

Late failure of femoropopliteal bypass grafts is defined as graft occlusion more than 30 days after the operative procedure. Up to 65% of these occlusions occur within the first year, after which there is a slow loss of patency (16). Intimal hyperplasia, structural changes in the vein grafts, and progression of atherosclerotic occlusive disease are the major causes of late graft failure.

Neointimal hyperplasia generally occurs 3 to 18 months postoperatively. Smooth muscle cells and collagen-producing fibroblasts build up usually at the distal anastomosis, narrowing the lumen and eventually occluding the graft. This process more commonly affects synthetic grafts. Its etiology is unclear, but it may be due to arterial injury, either from the surgical procedure or from graft-host compliance mismatch. Some believe that platelets migrate to the site of the endothelial injury and release mitogenic growth factors, stimulating the proliferation of smooth muscle cells that are the hallmark of neointima. The etiology of this lesion, however, may not be that simple.

Structural changes in vein grafts also occur 12 to 48 months after the original operative procedure. Szilagyi and co-workers (17) documented eight different abnormalities affecting 33% of the grafts studied. Progressive lesions that ultimately affect the graft itself include diffuse intimal thickening, atherosclerotic changes in the vein graft, valve fibrosis, localized fibrotic stenosis, aneurysmal degeneration, and suture stenosis. Progression of atherosclerotic occlusive disease in the proximal arterial inflow and the distal arterial outflow occurs in the period 2 to 5 years after graft implantation. The lesions are more frequently distal popliteal artery stenoses and significant lesions of the tibial vessels. Lesions of proximal inflow, such as stenoses of the iliac and proximal common femoral artery, are less common than distal lesions. Stenosis of the arterial inflow or outflow and structural lesions in the body of the graft develop slowly after a successful bypass procedure.

Diagnosis: Late Occlusion

Before these lesions progress to complete graft occlusion, patients frequently complain of new symptoms that are usually not as severe as their original complaint (Fig. 1). Vascular laboratory examination will document a decrease in the ankle-arm index, indicating the development of a hemodynamically significant arterial stenosis (18). Even before new symptoms develop, routine evaluation of the ankle-arm index at 6 month intervals after bypass surgery will often detect develping stenosis. These patients are immediately investigated with arteriography to determine the location of the stenosis. Correction by operative exploration with patch angioplasty or percutaneous transluminal angiography is then performed. The importance of detecting a hemodynamically significant stenosis before vein graft occlusion occurs is emphasized in a study by Whittemore and colleagues (19) who reported that 85% of stenotic vein grafts treated with patch angioplasty remained patent, while only 19% of occluded vein grafts treated by thrombectomy and surgical revision remained patent.

Diagnosis of an occluded femoropopliteal graft is usually obvious. Most patients present with a recurrence of their original symptoms. Brewster and associates (16) reported that 67% of patients with failed grafts previously

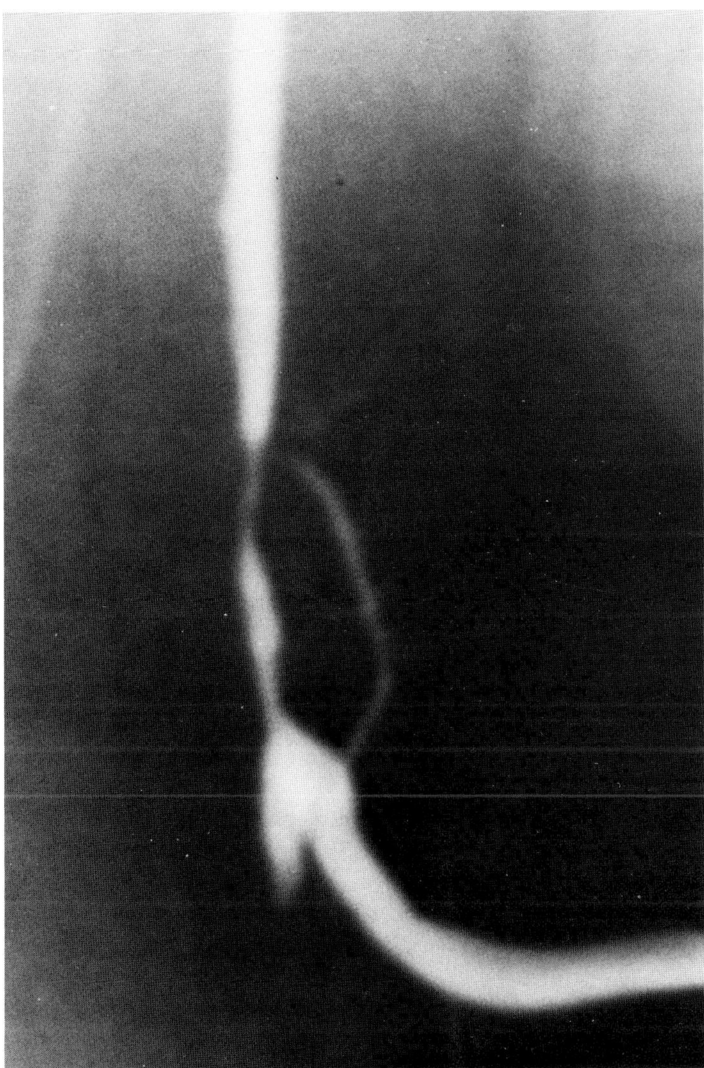

Figure 1 Proximal anastomosis of a previously performed femoropopliteal vein graft. The patient presented with recurrent symptoms and a significant reduction in the ankle-arm index. The arteriogram showed this stenotic lesion proximal to the anastomosis, which was treated successfully with patch angioplasty before graft occlusion occurred.

placed for claudication returned to their preoperative status, while 24%
became worse; only 9% were improved from their preoperative condition.
Similarly, 79% of patients with failed grafts previously placed for limb salvage
were again threatened with limb loss, while 21% were no longer at risk of
limb loss. This study indicates that a careful history alone can diagnose the
majority of occluded femoropopliteal grafts. When history is combined with
physical findings of an absent distal pulse, marked reduction in the ankle-arm
index, and the presence of ischemic changes, the diagnosis of an occluded
femoropopliteal graft becomes apparent.

Management of late failure of a femoropopliteal graft depends on a mature
judgment as to the current status and needs of the patient. A failed graft does
not always threaten the patient with limb loss, even if the original operation
was done for limb salvage. Certain patients can be best managed non-
operatively. However, if the patient is again threatened with limb loss, the
surgeon must decide between a new attempt at revascularization or a primary
amputation. Previous arteriograms, especially those obtained at the last
operation, are often of great assistance in making this determination. If the
runoff was marginal and no autogenous vein is available, a new attempt at revascularization is often inappropriate. Also, if the patient's medical condition
has deteriorated, the mortality of reoperation might be excessive. Some
authors (20,21) have suggested that a new attempt at revascularization of an
ischemic limb, if unsuccessful, raises the level of amputation, but others
(15,19,22) have found this not to be true. After careful consideration of
these points, an aggressive approach is usually indicated for patients threatened
with limb loss from a failed femoropopliteal grafts.

If a failed femoropopliteal graft was originally done for claudication, the
patient's current needs should be assessed. Perhaps the patient's life style
has changed so that the symptoms of claudication are no longer disabling or
sufficiently limiting to justify reoperation. As will be discussed, reoperation
on occluded femoropopliteal bypasses yields acceptable results, but not as
good as those reported for primary femoropopliteal bypass. This should limit
the enthusiasm for reoperative surgery in patients not threatened with limb
loss.

Technical Considerations: Late Occlusion

If reoperation is contemplated, arteriography is mandatory to determine the
feasibility of a secondary reoperation. The procedure is done from the opposite groin with the intention of documenting the adequacy of proximal

arterial inflow and the anatomy of the distal arterial runoff, including the presence of an intact pedal arch. If the distal circulation is not adequately visualized, then an operative arteriogram through either the common femoral artery, the popliteal artery, or one of the trifurcation vessels is necessary. The angiographer should be skilled in the technique of percutaneous transluminal angioplasty to dilate stenotic lesions of the proximal arterial system if this is appropriate.

Definitive operative treatment depends on the type of graft originally used. Occluded vein grafts may be treated with thrombectomy and correction of underlying stenotic lesions, but the results in this approach have been quite discouraging. Whittemore and colleagues (19) reported a 19% patency at 5 years in 18 patients who were treated with thrombectomy and correction of underlying stenotic lesions. A better approach for patients with occluded vein grafts is to place a new vein graft using either the greater saphenous vein from the opposite leg, the lesser saphenous vein, or arm veins. Whittemore and colleagues (19) reported a 37% 5 year patency with revascularization of an occluded vein graft with a new saphenous vein bypass graft. In the same series, prosthetic grafts used to bypass an occluded vein graft did not do well: all grafts placed failed at 5 years. Brewster and associates (16) reported a 63% 5 year patency rate for new vein grafts used in secondary femoropopliteal reconstructions.

Thrombectomy and surgical revision as outlined by Veith and co-workers (14) is the approach for late occlusion of PTFE grafts. The surgeon explores the distal anastomosis, makes a longitudinal incision up to the suture line, and removes clot at the site of the anastomosis. A thrombectomy of the proximal graft and the distal popliteal artery is then performed. This step usually restores adequate arterial inflow, but when unsuccessful, the proximal anastomosis must also be explored and appropriately revised. Once arterial inflow is reestablished, attention is directed toward the arterial outflow problems. The distal anastomosis is directly inspected. If intimal hyperplasia is present, the arteriotomy is extended through the suture line into the popliteal artery. A patch angioplasty with PTFE is performed. One technical problem needs clarification. An incision through the anastomosis divides the old suture line that may then unravel, forming a false aneurysm. Several techniques are available to avoid this potential problem. Interrupted sutures can be placed at the toe of the anastomosis during the primary procedure. If reexploration becomes necessary, incision through the anastomosis does not interrupt the continuity of the suture line. If a running suture was used for the entire anastomosis, the ends of the old suture can be tied to a new suture and fixed in place. Another approach is to place interrupted mattress sutures between the graft and artery on each edge of the incised anastomosis to ensnare the suture used originally.

If intimal hyperplasia is not identified, the longitudinal arteriotomy is closed and an operative arteriogram is performed. A distal stenotic lesion is treated with a jump bypass, preferably with autogenous vein from the distal PTFE graft to a point distal to the stenotic lesion. At times, no specific lesion in the anastomosis or distal arterial system is identified. If proximal inflow is adequate, a thrombectomy alone is satisfactory treatment. Finally, when managing failed PTFE grafts, the surgeon should always be prepared to perform a new bypass with autogenous vein graft, if available.

The management of occluded umbilical vein grafts may, on occasion, be similar to that described with PTFE grafts. One major difference in this circumstance is the dense connective tissue that incorporates the biograft, making dissection of the proximal and distal anastomoses difficult. Often it is easier to perform a new bypass graft with either the greater saphenous vein or another umbilical vein graft. However, if dissection of the graft is successful, thrombectomy and graft revision can be performed. This must be done with great care since the luminal surface of the umbilical vein graft can easily be damaged by balloon catheter thrombectomy.

Postoperative Management and Results: Late Occlusion

Anticoagulation is usually not indicated in the initial management of patients with failed femoropopliteal grafts, regardless of whether a reoperation is contemplated. After reoperation, if the runoff is marginal, I will frequently prescribe warfarin and attempt to keep the patient's prothrombin time at about 1½ times the control value. The results of reoperation for occluded PTFE grafts have been good and far superior to those reported for vein grafts that underwent reoperation. Veith and associates (14) reported 22 late PTFE occlusions, with 18 requiring reexploration. Fourteen of these remained patent 2 to 27 months after reoperation. Baker and co-workers (23) reported thrombectomy and graft revision in 12 patients with seven grafts remaining patent. O'Donnell and colleagues (24), however, reported that only two of six occluded PTFE grafts remained patent after thrombectomy and graft revision.

The results of reoperative surgery for occluded umbilical vein grafts have been good. Hafter and Cranley (15) reported that six of eight occluded umbilical vein grafts treated by thrombectomy alone remained patent.

Boontje (25) reported on 49 of 57 occluded umbilical vein grafts that underwent reoperations. Thirty-eight (77%) of the 49 reoperations, consisting of thrombectomy and surgical revision, were initially successful. Dardik (26) recently reported that five of nine umbilical vein grafts that occluded more than 6 months after the original operation were reopened.

Thrombolytic Therapy: An Alternative

Thrombolytic drugs are an alternative to thrombectomy and surgical revision (27-33). These agents have been available for at least 20 years and, although initially plagued with problems of standardization and allergic reaction, they are currently available in reliable commercial preparations. Streptokinase and urokinase are most frequently used; the former has been preferred in the past because it is less expensive, although allergic reactions are common. Other potent fibrinolytic agents with few side effects are soon likely to be commercially available at reasonable cost.

These drugs work by converting fibrinogen to fibrin, a powerful thrombolytic agent. If high doses are given intravenously, the sytemic fibrinolytic system is activated, lysing clots anywhere in the body with potential serious hemorrhagic complications. A preferred method for treating occluded grafts is to administer low doses of the drug directly into the graft. This local infusion technique lyses the thrombus without fully activating the systemic fibrinolytic system so that hemorrhagic complications are reduced. The common femoral artery on the side of the occluded graft is punctured, cannulated, and a catheter is directed under fluoroscopy into the occluded graft. Streptokinase (5000 units/hour) or urokinase (4400 units/kg per hour) is infused directly in the clot. Every 12 hours, radiopaque contrast is injected through the catheter to document clot resolution and advance the catheter further into the clotted graft. If within 24 hours no progress occurs, the procedure is terminated. If there is evidence of thrombolysis, the procedure should be continued for up to 72 hours or until the graft is completely open to the distal popliteal artery. If the arteriogram shows a significant stenosis in the vein graft, distal anastomosis or popliteal artery transluminal angioplasty can then be performed. If this is unsuccessful, operative correction of the stenosis is mandatory.

Hemorrhage is the major complication of fibrinolytic drugs. Although the advantage of the local infusion technique is that low doses of the drug are used, sometimes sufficient quantities of the drug are administered to cause changes in the coagulation profile. Bleeding may occur at the site of a previously performed arteriogram. To reduce this occurrence, arteriography in patients who are potential candidates for thrombolytic therapy should be done from the contralateral groin so that the thrombolytic drugs can be administered with a direct puncture of the femoral artery on the side of the occluded graft away from the puncture wound performed for arteriography.

It is often stated that thrombolytic therapy is most effective on thrombi less then 2 weeks old. These clots are soft, less organized, and, therefore, more amenable to lytic therapy. Success, however, has been reported in grafts occluded for up to 2 months (28). The therapy usually is contraindicated if the graft has occluded within two weeks of implantation because local infusion therapy will lyse clots at the site of the anastomoses and cause bleeding.

Low dose fibrinolytic therapy has achieved encouraging successes. Katzen and co-workers (29) reported 7 of 10 occluded grafts were opened. Eight of these 10 patients had femoropopliteal bypasses. Hargrove and colleagues (30) were able to reestablish and maintain patency in four of six vein grafts occluded from 5 to 6 weeks. Transluminal angioplasty was used to dilate underlying stenoses. These two reports were particularly encouraging since patency of vein grafts treated by thrombectomy is unsatisfactory. Dardik and co-workers (33) reported that 8 of 16 occluded grafts were successfully opened with lytic therapy. Therapy was unsuccessful in all 10 grafts occluded for more than 7 days. These studies all suggest that low dose intra-arterial lytic therapy is often initially successful to restore patency in occluded grafts. Treatment of the underlying causes of occlusion yielded acceptable long-term results.

An aggressive approach to late occlusion of femoropopliteal bypass grafts is warranted. Each case must be considered individually, and reoperations should always be planned taking into consideration the current medical status and present needs of the patient. If the viability of the limb is threatened, the surgeon has a choice among lytic therapy, reoperation, or primary amputation. Flinn and associates (34) reported on 52 patients who underwent repetitive distal revascularization. Twenty-seven patients underwent secondary femorodistal bypass, 14 patients had a third bypass, 20 had a fourth attempt, and 1 patient underwent a fifth reoperation. The overall limb salvage rate was 61% after 18 months of follow-up. The operative mortality was 3.8%. If one compares these results with the functional disability and mortality of an amputation, a well planned reoperation in many patients is advisable.

Anastomotic False Aneurysms: Incidence and Etiology

Anastomotic false aneurysm is an uncommon but serious complication of arterial bypass procedures. In 1975, Szilagyi and associates (35) reported an incidence of false aneurysms of 1.7% of all anastomoses performed for peripheral arterial vascular disease. Most occur in the femoral anastomosis of an aortobifemoral bypass graft. Anastomotic aneurysms in femoropopliteal bypasses account for a small percentage of all anastomotic aneurysms. Hollier and co-workers (36) reported that only 2 of 87 femoral anastomotic aneurysms came from femoropopliteal bypasses. Szilagyi and associates (35) reported 9 of 163 anastomotic aneurysms developed in the popliteal artery. Chavez (37) reported 8 of 34 false aneurysms occurred in femoropopliteal bypasses, 7 in the proximal suture line and 1 in a distal suture line.

Multiple factors are responsible for the development of anastomotic aneurysms (38-43). Most false aneurysms develop because sutures pull out of the arterial wall. This occurs if arterial sutures were not placed deep enough in the arterial wall, hematoma formation prevented the incorporation of the graft by surrounding tissue, or the arterial wall was weakened by infection, extensive atherosclerosis, or previously performed endarterectomy. Compliance mismatch between the prosthetic graft and the artery is an additional factor in the development of anastomotic false aneurysms (40). Prosthetic grafts lose compliance and become stiff after implantation. The arterial wall maintains its compliance so that with each arterial pulsation, the arterial wall expands but the prosthetic wall does not. This places tension on the arterial suture line and causes anastomotic disruption and false aneurysm formation. The importance of compliance mismatch is supported by the low incidence of an anastomotic false aneurysm in vein grafts that retain most of their compliance after implantation. Breakdown of suture material, particularly silk, and the structural defects of prosthetic grafts have also been implicated as the cause of anastomotic false aneurysms (39).

False Aneurysms: Preoperative Management

The patient presents with a pulsatile mass in the groin, a large painful hematoma, or lower extremity ischemia due to graft thrombosis or distal emboli. Anastomotic false aneurysms can still occur in the groin even if the femoropopliteal bypass has been occluded. I have personally treated four false aneurysms of clotted bovine heterografts (Fig. 2). Although sonography and computerized tomography scans have been advocated, arteriography is presently the most appropriate method for definitive diagnosis because it will

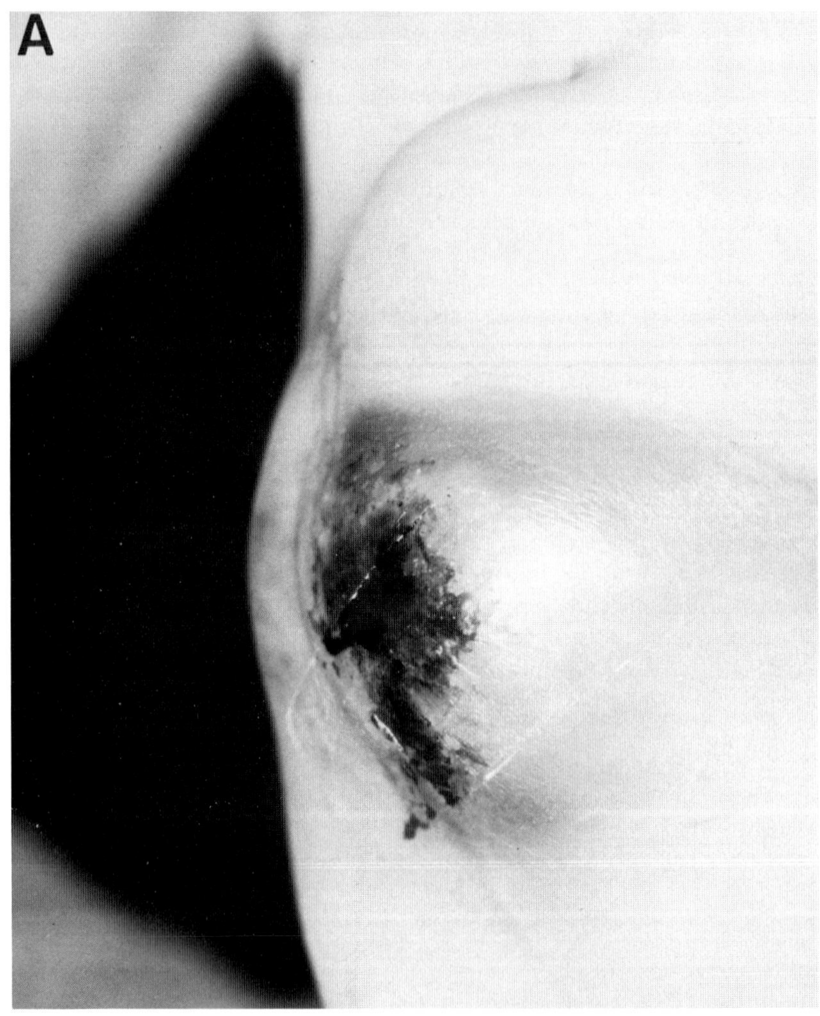

Figure 2

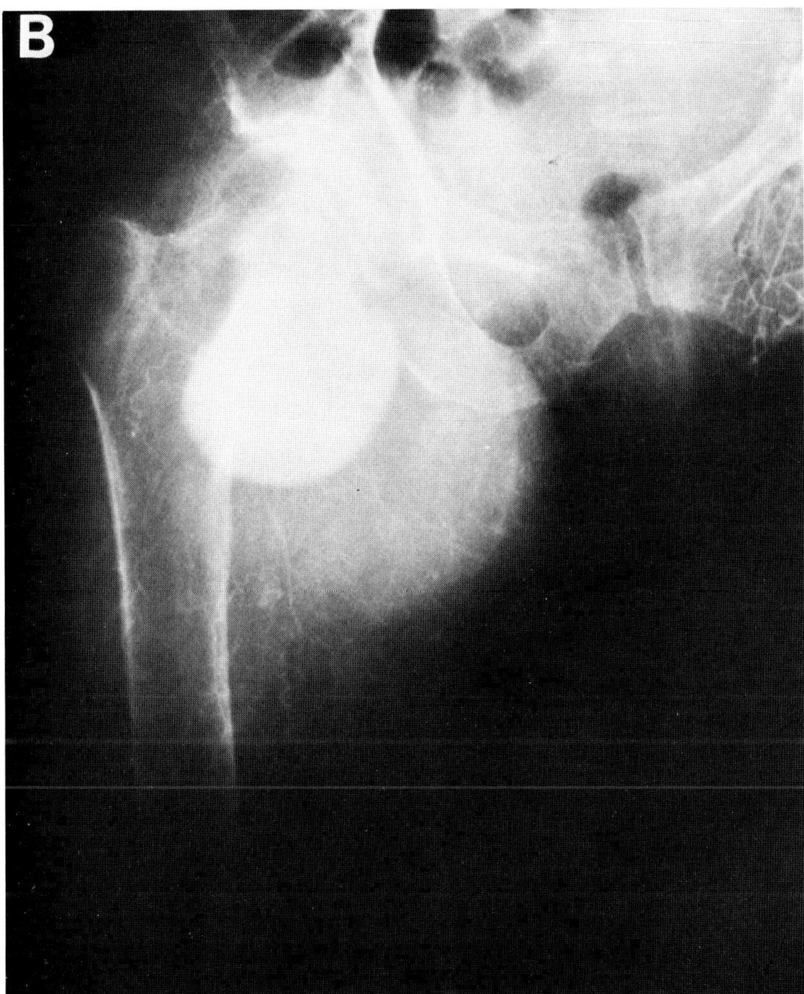

Figure 2 *A*: The patient presented with a ruptured false aneurysm of the groin. *B*: The arteriogram demonstrating false aneurysm. The false aneurysm occurred in a previously clotted bovine xenograft used for femorpopliteal bypass performed 10 years previously.

usually demonstrate the false aneurysms as well as outline the status of the autogenous vessels and the bypass conduit.

False aneurysms involving femoropopliteal bypass grafts require repair. A nonoperative approach or delay until the aneurysm reaches a certain size may be dangerous. If the graft is patent and treatment is delayed, the patient may present with an acutely ischemic limb after graft occlusion or distal peripheral emboli. Even in previously occluded grafts, the aneurysms may rupture, necessitating emergency operations. These situations are far more difficult to manage than elective repair of anastomotic false aneurysms.

Technical Considerations

The operative approach in the groin is first to dissect and control both the common femoral artery proximal to the graft and the graft distal to the aneurysm. The superficial femoral artery and the profunda artery are not exposed. The false aneurysm is opened and thrombus removed. Backbleeding from the profunda femoris artery is controlled internally with an occlusion balloon catheter. The anastomosis is carefully inspected to determine the cause of the false aneurysm. The prosthesis still attached to the arterial wall is removed, and a specimen is sent for culture. The arterial wall is dissected from surrounding tissue, debrided, and prepared for anastomosis. If the femoropopliteal graft is open, a small segment of prosthetic graft is sutured end-to-side to the prepared artery and end-to-end to the old graft. If the graft had previously occluded, a synthetic patch graft is placed on the common femoral artery at the site from which the occluded graft had been removed.

When false aneurysms involve the distal anastomosis of a femoropopliteal graft, the graft is always patent. The graft and the popliteal artery distal to the false aneurysm are first explored and controlled. The aneurysm is then excised, and the popliteal artery at the site of the aneurysm is ligated. A new graft is sutured end-to-end to the old graft and end-to-side to the popliteal artery distal to the site of the old anastomosis.

Postoperative Management and Results

An important aspect of postoperative management involves antibiotic treatment and close observation if infection was a possible factor in aneurysm formation. Intraoperative cultures should be obtained for this purpose. Few studies in the literature report the results of operation for false aneurysm of femoropopliteal bypass grafts. Most papers that discuss false aneurysm in the groin do not distinguish the results from repair of false aneurysms that occur after aortobifemoral bypass grafts from repair of false aneurysms from femoropopliteal bypass grafts. I have successfully treated four false aneurysms of clotted bovine heterografts placed in the late 1960s. Szilagyi and associates (35) reported nine false aneurysms of the popliteal artery, with seven treated successfully. One patient underwent amputation and one patient died. Elective operations for false aneurysms involving femoropopliteal bypass yield reasonably good results.

References

1. Cranley JJ, Hafner CD: Revascularization of the femoropopliteal arteries using saphenous vein, polytetrafluoroethylene, and umbilical vein grafts. Arch Surg 117:1543, 1982.
2. Harmon M, Giron F, Jacobson JH: The expanded polytetrafluoroethylene graft. Three year experience with 362 grafts. Arch Surg 114: 673, 1979.
3. Dardik H, Ibrahim IM, Jarich M: Three year experience with glutaraldehyde stabilized umbilical vein for limb salvage. Br J Surg 67:229, 1980.
4. Szilagyi DE, Hageman JH, Smith RF, Elliott JP, Brown F, Dietz P: Autogenous vein grafting in femoropopliteal atherosclerosis: the limits of its effectiveness. Surgery 86:836, 1979.
5. Veith FJ, Gupta SK, Samson RH, Scher LA, Fell SC, Weiss P, Janko, G, Flores SW, Rifkin H, Bernstein G, Haimovici H, Gliedman ML, Sprayregen S: Progress in limb salvage by reconstructive arterial surgery combined with new or improved adjunctive procedures. Ann Surg 194:386, 1981.
6. DePalma RG and Trout HH III: Reoperative surgery: general considerations. In Reoperative Vascular Surgery. New York, Marcel Dekker, 1986.
7. LiCalzi LK, Stansel HC Jr: Failure of autogenous reversed saphenous vein femoropopliteal grafting: pathophysiology and prevention. Surgery 91:352, 1982.
8. Craver JM, Ottinger LW, Darling RC, Austen WG, Linton RR: Hemorrhage and thrombosis as early complications of femoropopoliteal bypass grafts: causes, treatment, and prognostic implications. Surgery 74:839, 1973.
9. Blackshear WF Jr, Thiele BL, Strandness DE: Natural history of above- and below-knee femoropopliteal grafts. Am J Surg 140:234, 1980.

10. Collins GJ Jr, Heymann RL, Zajtchuk R: Hypercoagulability in patients with peripheral vascular disease. Am J Surg 130:2, 1975.
11. Towne JB, Bernhard VM, Hussy C, Garancis JC: Antithrombin deficiency — cause of unexplained thrombosis in vascular surgery. Surgery 89: 735, 1981.
12. Cambria RP, Abbott WM: The autogenous vein as an arterial graft. In Rutherford RB (Ed): Vascular Surgery. Philadelphia, WB Saunders Company, 1984, p. 376.
13. Rutherford RB, Jones DN, Bergentz S, Bergqvist D, Karmody AM, Dardik H, Moore WS, Goldstone J, Flinn WR, Comerota AJ, Fry WJ, Shah DM: The efficacy of dextran 40 in preventing early postoperative thrombosis following difficult lower extremity bypass. J Vasc Surg 1: 765, 1984.
14. Veith FJ, Gupta S, Daly V: Management of early and late thrombosis of expanded polytetrafluoroethylene (PTFE) femoropopliteal bypass grafts: favorable prognosis with appropriate reoperation. Surgery 87: 581, 1980.
15. Hafner CD, Cranley JJ: Problems encountered in the use of umbilical vein grafts. In Bernhard VM, Towne JB (Eds): Complications in Vascular Surgery. Orlando, Florida, Grune & Stratton, 1985, pp. 619-638.
16. Brewster DC, LaSalle AJ, Robison JG, Strayhorn EC, Darling C: Femoropopliteal graft failures. Clinical consequences and success of secondary reconstruction. Arch Surg 118:1043, 1983.
17. Szilagyi DE, Elliott JP, Hageman JH, Smith RF, Dallolmo CA: Biologic fate of autogenous vein implants as arterial substitutes. Ann Surg 178: 232, 1973.
18. O'Mara CS, Flinn WR, Johnson ND, Bergan JJ, Yao JS: Recognition and surgical management of patent but hemodynamically failed arterial grafts. Ann Surg 193:467, 1981.
19. Whittemore AD, Clowes AW, Couch NP, Mannick JA: Secondary femoropopliteal reconstruction. Ann Surg 193:35, 1981.
20. Kazmers M, Satiani B, Evans WE: Amputation level following unsuccessful distal limb. Salvage operations. Surgery 87:683, 1980.
21. Schlenker JD, Wolkoff JS: Major amputations after femoropopliteal bypass procedures. Am J Surg 129:495, 1975.
22. Maini BS, Mannick JA: Effects of arterial reconstructions on limb salvage. Arch Surg 113:1297, 1978.
23. Baker WH, Hadcock MM, Littooy FN: Management of polytetrafluoroethylene graft occlusions. Arch Surg 115:508, 1980.
24. O'Donnell TF Jr, Mackey W, McCullough JL Jr, Maxwell SL Jr, Farber SP, Deterling RA, Callow AD: Correlation of operative findings with

angiographic and noninvasive hemodynamic factors associated with failure of polytetrafluoroethylene grafts. J Vasc Surg 1:136, 1984.

25. Boontje AH: Occlusion of femoropopliteal bypass (biografts). J Cardiovasc Surg 38:385, 1984.

26. Dardik H: Reoperative surgery for complications following femorodistal bypass with umbilical vein grafts. In Bergan JJ, Yao JST (Eds): Reoperative Arterial Surgery. Orlando, Florida, Grune & Stratton, 1986, pp. 331-342.

27. Bell WR, Meek AG: Guidelines for the use of thrombolytic agents. N Engl J Med 301:1266, 1979.

28. Breda AV, Robison JC, Feldman L, Waltman AC, Brewster DC, Abbott WM, Athanasoulis CA: Local thrombolysis in the treatment of arterial graft occlusions. J Vasc Surg 1:103, 1984.

29. Katzen BT, Edwards KC, Albert AS, Breda AV: Low dose direct fibrinolysis in peripheral vascular disease. J Vasc Surg 1:718, 1984.

30. Hargrove WC, Berkowitz HD, Freiman DV, McLean G, Ring EJ, Roberts B: Recanalization of totally occluded femoropopliteal vein grafts with low-dose streptokinase infusion. Surgery 92:890, 1982.

31. Hargrove WC, Barker CF, Berkowitz HD, Perloff LJ, McLean G, Freiman D, Ring EJ, Roberts B: Treatment of acute peripheral arterial and graft thromboses with low-dose streptokinase. Surgery 92:981, 1982.

32. Wolfson RH, Kumpe DA, Rutherford RB: Role of intraarterial streptokinase in treatment of arterial thromboembolism. Arch Surg 119: 697, 1984.

33. Dardik H, Sussman BC, Kahm M, Greweldinger J, Adker J, Mendes D, Svoboda J, Ibrahim I: Lysis of arterial clot by intravenous or intraarterial administration of streptokinase. Surg Gynecol Obstet 158:137, 1984.

34. Flinn WF, Harris JP, Rudo ND, Bergan JJ, Yao JST: Results of repetitive distal revascularization. Surgery 91:566, 1982.

35. Szilagyi DE, Smith RF, Elliott JP, Hageman JH, Dall'olmo CA: Anastomotic aneurysms after vascular reconstruction: problems of incidence, etiology, and treatment. Surgery 78:800, 1975.

36. Hollier LH, Batson RC, Cohn I Jr: Femoral anastomotic aneurysms. Ann Surg 191:715, 1980.

37. Chavez CM: False aneurysms of the femoral artery: a challenge in management. Ann Surg 183:695, 1976.

38. Satiani B, Kazmers M, Evans WE: Anastomotic arterial aneurysms. Ann Surg 192:674, 1980.

39. Starr DS, Weatherford SC, Lawrie GM, Morris GC Jr: Suture material as a factor in the occurrence of anastomotic false aneurysms. Arch Surg 114:412, 1979.

40. Mehigan DG, Fitzpatrick B, Browne HI, Bouchier-Hayes DJ: Is compliance mismatch the major cause of anastomotic arterial aneurysms? J Cardiovasc Surg 26:147, 1985.
41. Richardson JV, McDowell HA: Anastomotic aneurysms following arterial grafting: a 10-year experience. Ann Surg 184:179, 1976.
42. Nichols WK, Stanton M, Silver D, Deitzer WF: Anastomotic aneurysms following lower extremity revascularization. Surgery 88:366, 1980.
43. Knox WG: Peripheral vascular anastomotic aneurysms: a fifteen-year experience. Ann Surg 191:715, 1980.

11

Reoperation After Infrapopliteal In Situ Saphenous Vein Bypass

ROBERT P. LEATHER and DHIRAJ M. SHAH
Albany Medical Center, Albany, New York

Until recently, reversed autogenous saphenous vein has been considered the conduit of choice for infrainguinal arterial bypass. The saphenous vein is histologically similar to an artery and is usually available, accessible, expendable, and generally of adequate length and diameter. Its superior performance as compared with prosthetic grafts was responsible for this acceptance; thus, the reversed saphenous vein became the standard by which all other grafts were compared. Nonetheless, despite some opinions that autogenous vein used as a free graft is still the optimum arterial substitute, there has been a growing awareness of the development of degenerative and proliferative changes in the vein wall that may ultimately lead to graft failure. In addition, as arterial bypasses were carried to the crural vessels, it became apparent that these long bypasses with low flow often exceed the physiologic limits of reversed vein graft performance as indicated by a 30 day failure rate of 15 to 30%.

This failure rate led to development of criteria of operability in an attempt to define factors responsible for success. Synthetic grafts and reversed saphenous bypasses would presumably be used only when there was a reasonable expectation of success. For reversed saphenous grafts, criteria include a normal thin-walled vein of at least 4 mm in diameter (available in no greater than 66% of patients requiring infrapopliteal bypass) and a distal perfusion bed with the minimum angiographic characteristics of a patent tibial vessel in continuity with an intact pedal arch (available in less than 60% of threatened limbs). These constraints, therefore, limited the number of legs threatened by ischemia that could be salvaged to fewer than 50% of those requiring tibial bypass for limb preservation.

As a result, interest and experience with the saphenous vein used in situ as an arterial bypass have been revived. The existence of a viable, physiologically active, and hence antithrombogenic endothelial flow surface within the in situ bypass is a unique and important attribute of this conduit. In addition, the gradual distal taper of the in situ bypass and the size match of the bypass to the inflow and outflow arteries result in more optimal flow characteristics than those associated with reversed vein grafts (1). Although first suggested and subsequently reported by Hall (2) more than 25 years ago, the in situ bypass was not adopted widely because of its operative complexities and, until recently, because of lack of evidence of its superiority over the simplicity of reversed vein grafts (3-8).

The essential requirement of in situ vein bypasses and, in fact, the only reason for vein excision and reversal, is removal of the valvular obstructions to distal flow. Among the various techniques to produce valvular incompetence, division of the valve leaflets has proved to be expeditious, effective, and minimally traumatic, and can be used successfully in veins as small as 2.5 mm in diameter. Use of the saphenous vein in situ, however, begets new problems. These problems occur intraoperatively, in the immediate perioperative period within 30 days, and in the remote postoperative period.

Incidence and Etiology

Early Postoperative Bleeding

Return to the operating room for bleeding has almost universally been due to inadequate ligature of the divided branches of the arterialized saphenous vein. Metal clips singly applied to such branches have been particularly prone to become dislodged by arterial pressure. As a result, we recommend that the most clearly satisfactory method of branch control is an appropriately sized and applied suture ligature.

The vein preparation, the subsequent arterialization of the saphenous vein, and the construction of the distal anastomosis require only minimal systemic heparinization (i.e., less than 50 mg/kg or 2000 to 3000 units intravenously);

thus, bleeding caused by excessive heparin (5000 to 10,000 units) is avoided. In addition, the necessity for reversal by the administration of protamine, which in itself may be productive of significant complications, is unnecessary.

Residual Fistulae

In the early perioperative period after the construction of an in situ bypass, particularly when exposure of the entire length of the vein was not carried out, edema will commonly develop along the thigh portion. In approximately 33% of these, discrete areas of induration and erythema with pain and tenderness will also occur. These are manifestations of superficial arteriovenous (A-V) communications undergoing the spontaneous thrombosis that most often occurs. This inflammatory process, which consists of superficial endophlebitis, is sterile and self-limiting. These require only symptomatic treatment. Central skin necrosis, although sporadically reported (9), has occurred only twice in more than 800 cases, and in both instances was complicated by additional factors (i.e., one patient on chronic total steroid replacement, the other superimposed on a hematoma). Both healed spontaneously.

On rare occasions (13 of 845 cases), fistulous flow will progressively enlarge in the early perioperative period. These were readily recognized by a decrease in the distal pulses when palpable. Decreased segmental Doppler pressure and pulse volume recording amplitude with concomitant dampening of the pulse wave contour confirm the diagnosis. In such patients in the early postoperative period, it is best to carry out repeat angiography. More than half have exhibited flow diversion from more than one fistula. More recently, complementary duplex ultrasound scanning has been used, not only for identification and location of fistulae, but more specifically for quantification of the magnitude of their individual flow rates.

After discharge from the hospital, persistent or worsening edema in those patients with clear evidence of a fistula required subsequent ligation in an additional 27 limbs. These late fistulae are usually readily localized by Doppler ultrasound, and are treated by ligation under local anesthesia on an outpatient basis. In only three instances has angiography been necessary either because of multiplicity of fistulae or because of a fistula coursing parallel to the bypass, rendering its precise origin difficult to determine.

Wound Infection

Postoperative wound infection has been an infrequent occurrence (less than 2%) in spite of the fact that more than 50% of the patient population in the series are insulin-dependent diabetics. Careful and precise sharp dissection technique, minimal exposure, and scrupulous avoidance of lymph node-bearing areas in the femoral region have contributed to this low incidence. In contrast, bypasses in immunosuppressed patients have demonstrated a much higher wound complication rate (i.e., greater than 30%), and almost half of these resulted in life-threatening hemorrhage. Therefore, these patients require very careful care and attention to assure graft coverage and healing of the skin envelope.

Postoperative Stenoses

The most important and only late bypass-threatening lesion intrinsic to the in situ conduit is the development of a stenotic lesion. Such lesions have also been observed in excised vein grafts, both in the coronary and peripheral positions, in up to 25% of such bypasses meticulously followed by serial angiography (10-12). Vein graft stenoses are, therefore, not unique to the in situ bypass. In excised veins, stenotic lesions have been described as being invariably caused by endothelial hyperplasia, and are usually located at valve sites. A similar phenomenon also has been found to be true in the in situ bypass.

Among 845 in situ conduits constructed, 50 stenotic lesions have developed in 43 patients. The majority of these have occurred within the first 12 months (35 of 50), and most frequently occurred in the distal mobilized segment (22 of 50). Seventeen were present in the proximal mobilized segment, and 11 in the midportion of the bypass conduit. They also tended to occur with increased frequency in smaller veins (i.e. 29 [9%] occurring in 326 veins of 3.0 mm or less as compared with 20 [4%] in 483 veins of 3.5 mm or larger). All of these stenoses were treated operatively by vein patch angioplasty, and all but one remained patient beyond 30 days.

Preoperative Management in Reoperative Procedures

Early detection of stenoses and correction of defects of in situ conduits before occlusion occurs can be achieved by a comprehensive follow-up program (13). Our patients are seen and examined every 6 to 8 weeks for the first 6 months, every 8 to 10 weeks up to the first year, and every 6 months thereafter. Each examination includes pulse volume recordings and segmental pressures, audible Doppler assessment along the course of the bypass, and, more recently, direct visualization of the conduit and estimates of volume flow at serial levels by duplex ultrasound scanning.

The most sensitive indicator of developing stenosis has been a decreasing slope of the dP/dt segment of the pulse wave contour, usually accompanied by decreased amplitude of the pulse wave and lowered segmental pressure distally. When possible, postexercise treadmill examination will further increase the sensitivity of these observations and earlier detection of these lesions. Such findings are indications for immediate angiographic and operative correction.

Technical Considerations

Complications requiring operative revision are frequently related to the unusual problems in the preparation of in situ saphenous vein conduits. These include recognition of reductions in pulse pressure and/or flow that can be caused early by fistulae, competent valve leaflets, spasm, or platelet aggregates on areas of endothelial injury. Later complications include fistulae and stenotic lesions. Because these complications account for nearly all of the reoperative procedures, this discussion of reoperative surgery of the in situ bypass will begin with a description of intraoperative techniques required to ensure in situ bypass patency.

Platelet Aggregation

In the prepartion of in situ conduits, the constant exposure of its inner surface to blood for periods of time during which there is little or no flow is a novel and unavoidable departure from the preparation of most vascular conduits. However, stagnant blood in the vein left in situ is well tolerated because of the presence of an intact endothelium. When the integrity of the endothelial surface is disrupted, the result is platelet deposition. In the absence of boundary layer flow or high shear velocity, the accumulation of platelet aggregates continues unopposed. Platelet aggregates may result in high grade, significant stenoses or, ultimately, in complete obstruction. Conditions for maximum potential platelet aggregation end with the institution of arterial flow through the bypass. Doppler ultrasound and performance of a completion angiogram are used to detect platelet accumulations. Angiographically, these are characterized by interruption of the normally clear and distinctly smooth outline of the bypass conduit by an irregular and foamy mass.

Platelet accumulations are densely adherent to the area of injury. Although tempting, the worst possible solution for this problem is an attempt to remove the platelet mass by balloon embolectomy catheter. Not only is it impossible to completely dislodge the adherent platelet plug, but the balloon itself may produce further endothelial injury and compound the problem. Therefore, direct removal with a longitudinal venotomy extending over the entire involved segment and repair by patch angioplasty are required (Fig. 1) (14). When pulsatile flow is restored, platelet thrombosis usually does not recur unless the endothelial injury is circumferential and extends over a considerable length of vein. Rarely, complete replacement of the injured vein segment may be required. This injured segment is excised and replaced with a portion of vein segment from the ipsilateral lesser saphenous system, the lateral accessory vein, or, when available, a more distal portion of the greater saphenous. With improvements in technique and instrumentation (15), the frequency of such platelet lesions has progressively declinded to an incidence of less than 1%.

Residual Valve Leaflets

To comprehend the problems encountered with valve lysis, it is important to have a clear concept of venous valve function. The normal closing mechanism of the symmetrical venous valve is initiated by expansion of the valve sinus in response to increased intraluminal pressure. This creates tension along the leading edge of the valve, which brings the cusps toward the center of the lumen. Reverse flow then forces the cusps into a closed and competent position. In a segment of vein where a valve has been mechanically opened from below by passage of an instrument in the proximal direction (e.g., valvulotome or balloon catheter), a valve leaflet may remain temporarily adherent to the wall of the valve sinus in the open position. This phenomenon is most likely to occur in asymmetrical valves because the normal closing mechanism may not be operative. Subsequent closure of such an artifically opened valve leaflet will result in partial or complete obstruction to prograde arterial flow. In these circumstances, an incompletely lysed leaflet can close during extraluminal manipulation of the vein (e.g., during attempts to palpate the presence of a pulse). Therefore, before the operation is completed, deliberate attempts are made to precipitate closure of any incompletely lysed valves by the following maneuver: with the distal vein open and free flow observed, a sponge is rolled along the in situ conduit from top to bottom. It is desirable to detect this problem before construction of the distal anastomosis. The most reliable test of the absence of a flow-limiting stenosis in the bypass conduit before construction of the distal anastomosis is to observe free flow through the distal divided end of the arterialized in situ vein. Strong, persistent, pulsatile flow is absolute evidence that no proximal,

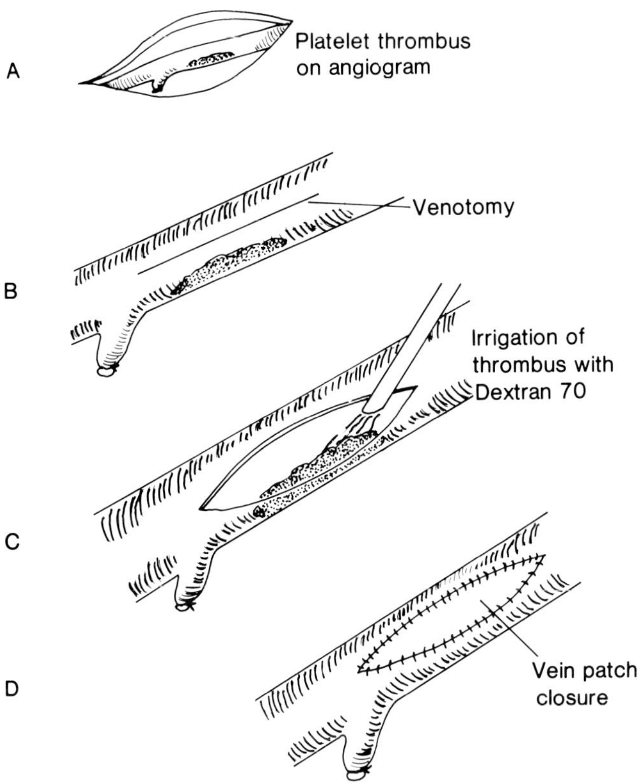

Figure 1 *A*: Platelet thrombus located on postoperative angiogram, and site exposed. *B*: Venotomy of conduit. Note that the incision extends beyond the limits of the platelet thrombus. *C*: Irrigation of platelet aggregate with Dextran-70 to free it from conduit wall. *D*: Closure with vein patch.

hemodynamically significant, stenotic lesion exists after the previously described maneuver has been performed.

The second intraoperative step specific to the *in situ* conduit is a completion angiogram that is required for the identification of A-V fistulae. In general, only fistulae that carry enough radiocontrast material to visualize the deep venous system require interruption. If a recognizable pulse amplitude deficit persists after ligation of such fistulae and, in the absence of an identifiable stenosis either due to spasm or platelet deposition, the most likely cause is the presence of a residual valve leaflet. Unfortunately, such leaflets are usually not visible on a properly timed completion angiogram. Partially occlusive intact leaflets may only show on an unusually late film after the radiopaque material has been washed out. The appearance is that of a pocket of contrast between the valve sinus and retained valve cusp. The symmetrical curvilinear defect frequently seen on venograms and occasionally on completion angiograms in the region of a valve sinus does not represent a valve leaflet, but is in reality the insertion ridge of the valve cusps that is projecting from the endothelial surface into the lumen.

The valves most likely to be missed are those at the ends of the proximal and distal mobilized segments and those located between the below-knee incision and the distal most point of passage of the intraluminal valve cutter. These areas of the conduit, therefore, merit specific attention during the procedure.

The Use of Intraoperative Audible Doppler Ultrasound

The use of intraoperative Doppler ultrasound is very helpful in identifying the previously described, hemodynamically significant, stenotic lesions by the generation of a localized continuous high-pitched (high velocity) signal (16, 17). Both fistulae and stenoses will produce a similar continuous high-pitched flow signal. Differentiation between a fistula and a stenosis can be made by digital compression of the bypass immediately distal to the site of the high velocity signal. If the continuous high-pitched signal persists, a fistula is present (Fig. 2A). If the high-pitched signal disappears with digital compression of the conduit (Fig. 2B) and persists when the digital pressure is released (Fig. 2C), this is diagnostic of intraluminal stenosis. In the absence of arteriographically visible platelet aggregates or spasm producing such a flow disturbance, this site should be checked with a retrograde valvulotome for the presence of an undivided valve leaflet. In addition, when digital palpation of the pulse or Doppler examination fails to locate the stenosis, retrograde passage of a pressure catheter will objectively confirm not only the presence but the precise location of a pressure gradient requiring correction.

There have been 28 residual valve leaflets (3.3%) overall, 10 intra-operatively (i.e., detected and corrected by valve incision before wound closure) and 18 postoperatively, 7 of which were completely occlusive within 24 hours after operation. Hence, frequent monitoring of pulse volume and Doppler flow in the bypass is required during this period. It is preferable to detect flow abnormalities before complete occlusion of the in situ conduit occurs. Revision of these cases by valve incision or excision with patch angioplasty resulted in continued patency in 15 of 18 instances.

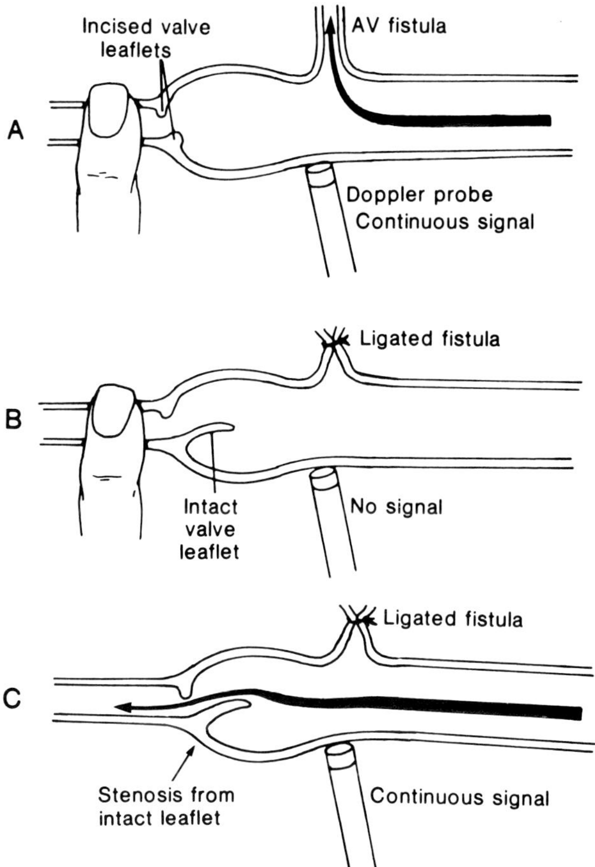

Figure 2 *A*: Continuous Doppler signal produced by flow through residual A-V fistula. *B*: Doppler signal abolished by distal compression, indicating no undetected A-V fistula. *C*: Persistent high-pitched Doppler signal produced by flow past a stenosis caused by residual valve leaflet.

Venous Spasm

In the process of preparation of either in situ or excised saphenous vein for bypass, surgical manipulation usually induces marked venous spasm. In the excised vein, this problem is immediately and permanently solved by hydrostatic dilation irrespective of the temperature and nature of fluid medium that is used. When the vein is left in situ, however, the problem of venous spasm assumes a new dimension. Not only is spasm initiated by the neuromuscular responses in the vein wall during its exposure, but it may recur because the smooth muscle wall retains the ability to contract.

The best means of treating venous spasm is by prevention. Minimal exposure of the vein should be the invariable rule to achieve this end. Most particularly, circumferential dissection of the vein should be avoided where possible. The work of LoGerfo and co-workers (18) has led us to use pre-incision perivenous papaverine infiltration 10 to 15 minutes before exposure. The earliest possible arterialization is the most physiological method to prevent or reverse spasm utilizing oxygenated blood under arterial pressure. Only rarely will arterialization fail to reverse the venous spasm and maintain the normal caliber of the vein.

Although venous spasm occurs to some extent in every vein, it is more prevalent and vexing in small caliber veins less than 3.5 mm in diameter. Reflex spasm occurring in protracted form in the midportion of the bypass can create a significant obstruction to flow; this problem can be very difficult to manage because further physical manipulation often increases its severity and persistence. The best treatment is the use of perivenous and topical (sponge-saturated) 1% papaverine solution (1 mg/ml); the gentle but inexorable relaxation produced by intraluminal arterial pressure will then invariably occur. When treating venous spasm, patience is a virtue that ultimately ensures success.

If an artificial form of hydrostatic dilation is used, the intraluminal pressure exerted should not exceed 300 mmHg. Pressure should be applied steadily to the vein and allowed to work slowly. An excellent way to accomplish this is to keep the fluid medium in a plastic container to which a pneumatic transfusion cuff is externally applied and controlled at no greater than 300 mmHg. When this pressure system is applied intraluminally, venous spasm can be reversed without digital pulsing. Powerful pulses with a small caliber syringe can cause pressure peaks up to 1000 mmHg (19). This maneuver may produce visible longitudinal fractures throughout the entire vein wall; as a consequence, the temptation to use this expedient should be avoided.

There is also a substantial risk of serious endothelial damage when intraluminal instrumentation is attempted within or through spastic vein segments. When such instrumentation is necessary, it is essential that spasm be completely relieved before instruments are passed through the vein lumen. Failure to achieve relief of spasm potentiates frictional shear of the instruments against the endothelial surface and causes further injury.

Intraoperative A-V Fistulae

When the saphenous vein is left in situ perforating branches may divert the flow of arterialized blood away from the patent distal arterial perfusion bed. Branches with the most important diversionary capability are the perforating veins that run directly between the saphenous vein and the deep venous system. Not only are these perforating veins short, but their valves open away from the saphenous vein, allowing flow to take place without obstruction. The arterial flow rapidly empties into the high capacity, low pressure, deep venous system with little outflow resistance. The amount of flow that can be diverted through these perforators can be considerable. In contrast, a superficial fistula, formed by a vein that is a tributary from the skin or subcutaneous tissue, is much less threatening. The hemodynamic effect of these superficial fistulae is considerably smaller than that from those involving the perforating branches.

The reduction in the palpable pulse pressure in the distal conduit may be related to the magnitude of flow diversion by the fistulae. If the diversion is substantial, the surgeon may be misled into believing that the reduced pulse is secondary to an obstructing lesion such as a proximal competent valve or an area of endothelial damage with fibrinoplatelet or thrombus deposition. It is important to be aware that alterations in palpable pulse pressure in the bypass can occur solely because of fistula diversion, either proximal or *distal* to the point of palpation. With a large fistula proximal to the point of palpation, the diversion of flow is so considerable that there is a reduction in both the flow and arterial pressure transmitted distally. With fistulae distal to the point of palpation, the actual flow rate through the vein is high, but the runoff into the deep venous system is so profound that the systolic arterial pressure in the vein is reduced substantially. This then also results in a reduced palpable pulse pressure. These high flow patterns are readily detected by Doppler examination. Correction of such high flow fistulae will correct the low pressure at the distal end of the in situ conduit.

Apart from confusing the surgeon, the presence of functioning fistulae has little physiological effect until the distal anastomosis has been performed. In fact, it is quite beneficial to allow them to function up to this time since they provide an outflow tract for the arterialized vein. They must, however, be controlled by interruption in continuity to allow maximum flow into the arterial outflow tract. The completion angiogram, with a needle-marked grid, will identify A-V fistulae. In general, *only* those fistulae that carry sufficient radiocontrast material to visualize the deep venous system require interruption.

Varices of the Saphenous Vein

It is safe to use the saphenous vein in presence of varices. In fact, most varices occur in communicating venous branches, and it is surprising how infrequently the main trunk of the greater saphenous vein itself is involved. When a varix is identified on the preoperative venogram or ultrasound image and is part of the saphenous vein, however, it must be surgically exposed and repaired. Interrupted suture of the defect by gathering the excess dilated vein wall in continuity with a transverse orientation of the closure is usually adequate (Fig. 3). Variceal excision with patch closure of the defect by angioplasty is only rarely required. Failure to identify and repair large and thin-walled varices may result in rupture and acute hemorrhage. Thirteen in situ bypasses with 19 varices have been used, and the only instance of rupture has occurred when a known varix was not exposed and repaired. Subsequent repair of the ruptured varix with patch angioplasty has not affected its continued patency.

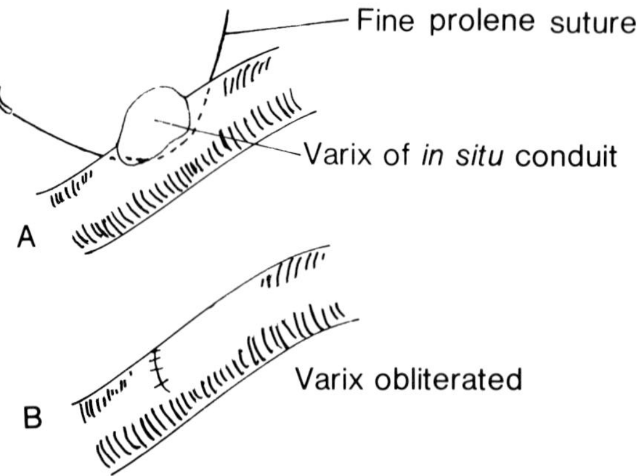

Figure 3 *A* and *B*: Repair of varix of in situ vein conduit with interrupted sutures.

Extrinsic Compression

Bypasses to the distal anterior tibial artery, particularly at or below the malleolar level, are vulnerable to extrinsic compression by the skin envelope sufficient to reduce flow. Such external compression can be caused by the closure of the parallel incisions, one of which is required to mobilize the distal saphenous vein and the other to expose the anterior tibial or dorsalis pedis artery. Occasionally, it has been necessary to leave one or even both incisions open, achieving closure of the wound with meshed split-thickness skin grafts. In addition, to ensure coverage with native skin and subcutaneous tissue of the bypass at its distal anastomosis, it is advisable to make the incision for exposure of the artery lateral to its axis (Fig. 4).

Postoperative Management

An in situ bypass should be considered completed only after obtaining defect-free completion angiography and Doppler assessment, with particular attention to the flow patterns. Normal postoperative Doppler flow patterns are characterized by continuous velocity signals extending through diastole over the distal conduit (6). When both these examinations are satisfactory, it is unusual to encounter perioperative occlusion or deterioration of flow requiring revision. The program of postoperative management to detect stenoses or other problems before occlusion occurs is similarly employed after redo operations, and has been previously described (13).

Results

Among 845 operations, there were 59 perioperative occlusion or deterioration of graft flow, 53 of which were revised as indicated in Table 1. Twenty-three of these revisions remained patent beyond 30 days; their subsequent performance has not been significantly different from those bypasses that did not require revision. The incidence of perioperative occlusion has decreased steadily in frequency as greater care and control have been exercised to prevent endothelial injury, particularly in the distal mobilized vein segment. There is ample experimental evidence that the preservation of endothelial integrity is best achieved by avoidance of the summation of a variety of injuries (i.e., spasm, the subsequent truama of hydraulic dilation required for its relief particularly if a pressure exceeding 300 mmHg is used, exposure to nonhemic solutions, warm ischemic time exceeding 30 minutes, and the more obvious mechanical trauma of dissection, manipulation, and

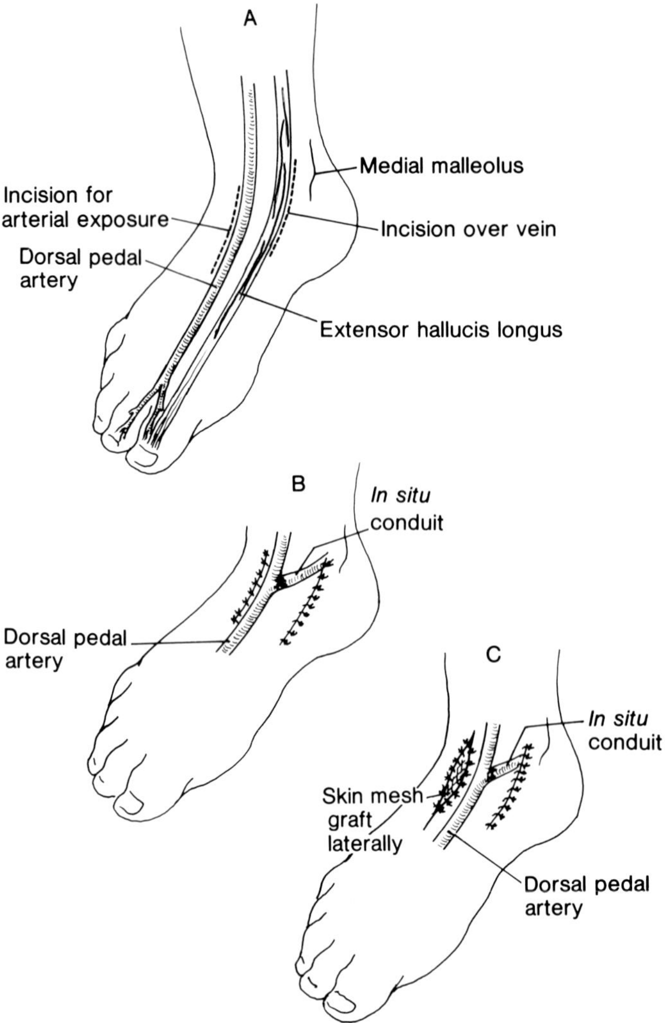

Figure 4 Incision placement for distal bypass to anterior tibial or dorsalis pedis artery. *A*: Note parallel incisions. The artery is exposed by an incision lateral to extensor hallucis longus. *B*: Closure of parallel flap. Note that the anastomosis is protected by lateral incision placement. *C*: Alternative method showing meshed skin graft applied laterally to minimize compression by skin enevelope. The anastomosis is protected by lateral incision placement.

Table 1 Revisions Among 53 of 59 Perioperative
Occlusions or Deterioration of Graft Flow

Early Revisions	< 30 Days
A-V fistula	13
Residual valve	10
Distal vein patch	12
Distal arterial outflow	9
Proximal arterial inflow	5
Proximal vein patch	2
Mid vein patch	2
Total	53

application of occluding clamps) (20). A particularly devastating injury is direct loss of the endothelium by abrasion, especially when circumferential. This form of injury is most likely to be caused by the use of coronary dilators, catheters, balloons, or cylindrical valve disrupters introduced through the distal divided end of the vein.

To prevent postoperative problems we recommend: (a) intraoperative use of papaverine hydrochloride injected percutaneously along the saphenous vein to prevent spasm, (b) rigid control of the pressure that is used to dilate vein segments, and (c) limitation of the warm ischemic time of the mobilized portions of the vein. These measures, together with strict avoidance of mechanical trauma as just indicated, are important technical details that affect long-term patency of these bypasses. In addition, the extreme ends of the mobilized segments are maximally exposed to mechanical endothelial trauma. Because this is particularly critical in the divided distal end of small veins, an excess of 2 cm in length of distal mobilized vein segment should be dissected. The excess distal vein segment can then be excised to construct the distal anastomosis with an uninjured vein segment.

Occlusion Due to Progression of Disease

Of particular interest is a small group of patients who have presented late with totally obstructed bypasses that remained patent and filled with liquid (unclotted) blood. There were 15 such late occlusions. Twelve were due to distal outflow occlusion, and three were due to complete inflow occlusion with no thrombus in the in situ conduit in spite of clearly delineated symptoms of occlusion for 3 to 10 days before reoperation (21). Examination of patients with distal occlusion revealed a strong pulse in the bypass, but a completely obstructive (pistol shot) Doppler signal. In this situation, angiography will fail to visualize the bypass because of the lack of flow within it. The angiographic observation may be interpreted as thrombotic occlusion, but these conduits are, in fact, filled with nonclotted fluid blood. These bypass conduits can be retrieved and patency preserved by performing appropriate inflow and outflow procedures. In distal occlusions, such bypasses will provide the necessary inflow source for revision to more distal patent arteries visualized arteriographically, usually by the addition of short segments of autogenous vein. These vein segments may be obtained from any of the following sources: the lateral accessory vein, the remaining half of a double saphenous vein, the lesser saphenous vein, a portion of distal greater saphenous vein, the cephalic vein, or the contralateral lower extremity. Ultrasound imaging preoperatively is of immense aid in finding and evaluating both the size and the length of available vein in either primary or redo operations.

Thus, it can be seen that, although the frequency of reoperation is low after properly performed in situ vein bypasses, the indications are well defined and differ somewhat from those usually associated with reversed vein or prosthetic grafts. Careful, systematic follow-up is often rewarded by the retrieval of an in situ bypass, even after occlusion has apparently occurred. This irreplaceable vascular asset might otherwise be lost. Failure to revise a retrievable in situ conduit may be associated with high probability of amputation, particularly in patients with distal bypasses to the tibial arteries.

References

1. Bush HL, McCabe ME, Nabseth DC: Functional injury of vein graft endothelium: role of hypothermia and distension. Arch Surg 119:770, 1984.
2. Hall KV: The great saphenous vein used in-situ as an arterial shunt after extirpation of the vein valves. Surgery 51:492, 1962.
3. Buchbinder D, Singh JK, Karmody AM, et al: Comparison of patency rate and structural change of in-situ and reversed vein arterial bypass. J Surg Res 30:213, 1981.
4. Bush HL, Graber JN, Jukobowski JA, et al: Favorable balance of prostacyclin and thromboxane A2 improves early patency of human in-situ vein grafts. J Vasc Surg 1:149, 1984.

5. Carney WI, Balko A, Barrett MS: In-situ femoropopliteal and infrapoplitel bypass: two year experience. Arch Surg 120:812, 1985.

6. Levine AW, Bandyk DF, Bonier PH, et al: Lessons learned in adopting the in-situ saphenous vein bypass. J Vasc Surg 2:145, 1985.

7. Leather RP, Shah DM, Karmody AM: Infrapopliteal arterial bypass for limb salvage: increased patency and utilization of the saphenous vein used "in-situ." Surgery 90:1000, 1981.

8. Corson JD, Karmody AM, Shah DM, et al: In situ vein bypasses to distal tibial and limited outflow tracts for limb salvage. Surgery 96:756, 1984.

9. Langeron P, Puppinck P, Cordonnier D: La technique de la greffe veineuse "in situ" dans la chirurgie arterielle restauratrice des membres inferieurs. J Chir 115:171, 1978.

10. Szilagyi DE, Hageman JH, Smith RF, et al: Autogenous vein grafting in femoropopliteal atherosclerosis: the limits of its effectiveness. Surgery 86:836, 1979.

11. Downs AR: Repair of late vein graft occlusions. Arch Surg 103:639, 1971.

12. Sladen JC, Gilmour JL: Vein graft stenosis: characteristics and effect of treatment. Am J Surg 141:549, 1981.

13. Farber C, Fitzgerald K, Karmody AM: Early detection of preocclusive lesions in in-situ saphenous vein bypasses by planned non-invasive testing. Bruit 8:168, 1984.

14. Corson JD, Leather RP, Shah, DM et al: In-situ vein branch angioplasty. Surg Gynecol Obstet 159:282, 1984.

15. Leather RP, Shah DM, Corson JD: Instrumental evolution of the valve incision method of "in-situ" saphenous vein bypass. J Vasc Surg 1:113, 1984.

16. Leather RP, Karmody AM: The in-situ saphenous vein arterial bypass. In Mannick J (Ed): Advances in Surgery. Chicago, Year Book Medical Publishers, 1985.

17. Spencer TD, Goldman MH, Hyslop JW, et al: Intraoperative assessment of in-situ saphenous vein bypass grafts with continuous-wave Doppler probe. Surgery 96:874, 1984.

18. LoGerfo FW, Quist WC, Crawshaw HW: An improved technique for preservation of endothelial morphology in vein grafts. Surgery 90:1015, 1981.

19. Abbott WM, Wieland S, Austen WG: Structural changes during preparation of autogenous vein grafts. Surgery 76:1031, 1974.

20. Schwartz SM: Vascular integrity. In Stanley JC, Burkel WE, Lindenauer SM, et al (Eds); Biologic and Synthetic Vascular Prostheses. New York, Grune & Stratton, 1982, p. 27.

21. Naraynsingh V, Karmody AM, Leather RP, et al: The nature of thrombosis in an obstructed autogenous vein bypass: observations on the in-situ vein. Br J Surg 71:391, 1984.

12

Arterial Reconstruction After Failed Femorotibial or Femoroperoneal Bypass

PAUL E. COLLIER,* ENRICO ASCER, ANSELMO A. NUNEZ,†
SUSHIL K. GUPTA, and FRANK J. VEITH
*Montefiore Medical Center - Albert Einstein College of Medicine,
New York, New York*

Patients with disease of the popliteal trifurcation who require bypasses to the tibial or peroneal arteries are at high risk medically and surgically. Such patients have a high incidence of diabetes mellitus and coronary artery disease and may exhibit severe manifestations of peripheral vascular disease with tissue necrosis. Because the arterial occlusive disease in these patients is peripheral, the reconstructive options available to the surgeon are limited.

Femorodistal (i.e., tibial or peroneal) bypasses have a high failure rate, most notable during the first 3 to 6 months after insertion (1-3). An aggressive surveillance program with frequent patient visits and noninvasive evaluations is essential, especially if subtle indications of impending graft failure are to be detected. In this way, appropriate interventions can be undertaken to prevent closure of these "failing grafts" (4).

When femoral-to-distal artery graft failure occurs, many but not all of these patients will again develop limb-threatening ischemia. Arteriography is essential in these cases to assess the status of the inflow and outflow vessels. Adjunctive percutaneous transluminal angioplasty can be employed to improve the inflow and thereby shorten the length of vein required for a new bypass procedure. Venography is often necessary to determine the presence and quality of the saphenous vein in the ipsilateral leg or in the other ex-

Present affiliations:
*Sewickley Valley Hospital, Sewickley, Pennsylvania
†University of Miami School of Medicine, Miami, Florida

211

tremities (5). When there is no usable vein available in either the leg or arms, prosthetic grafts can be utilized to salvage some of these patients' limbs (6).

Graft Surveillance and the "Failing Graft" Concept

Close follow-up of patients after femoral-to-infrapopliteal bypass grafting with both physical examination and noninvasive laboratory investigation is essential to detect stenotic, flow-reducing lesions before graft thrombosis (4,7). Anastomotic intimal hyperplasia, proximal or distal disease progression, or lesions within the graft itself can produce signs and symptoms of hemodynamic deterioration before graft thrombosis occurs. We have previously referred to this condition as a "failing graft" because if the lesion is left uncorrected, graft thrombosis will occur (4,7-9). The importance of the "failing graft" concept lies in the fact that many difficult lower extremity revascularizations can be salvaged for protracted periods by relatively simple interventions if the lesion responsible for the altered blood flow can be detected before graft thrombosis occurs.

During the last 2 years, we have increasingly utilized duplex scanning as an integral part of our follow-up protocol. Although graft insonation by Doppler techniques without direct visualization of infrainguinal bypass grafts has been reported to be predictive of impending graft failure (10), we have found that duplex scanning is more accurate and can locate with precision the lesion responsible for a "failing graft." Great care is taken to assess the inflow and outflow vessels and the entire length of the bypass graft. The proximal and distal graft anastomoses are directly visualized, and the midstream flow is sampled for the presence of hemodynamic disturbances.

The technique for Duplex examination of the distal graft anastomosis varies, depending on the outflow vessel. Grafts to the anterior and posterior tibial arteries are best imaged with anterior and medial approaches, respectively. Grafts that extend to the below-knee popliteal artery and tibioperoneal trunk are best visualized from a posterior approach with the patient in the prone position (11). Anastomoses to the peroneal artery are difficult to visualize because the artery is in a deep position and is obscured by bony structures. We have found, however, that with the patient in the prone position and with the ankle supported, the peroneal artery can be easily visualized if the duplex probe is placed one fingerbreadth medial to the posterior ridge of the fibula.

Duplex scanning is performed in the immediate postoperative period 1, 3, and 6 months postoperatively and then every 6 months thereafter. Normally functioning grafts have well visualized anastomoses without changes in Doppler flow velocities throughout the course of the arterial reconstruction. Vein graft walls are indistinct from the surrounding tissues, and normal polytetrafluoroethylene (PTFE) grafts have a residual lumen diameter at least 95% of that present at insertion. Normal graft peak systolic velocities vary greatly from 10.7 to 106 cm/sec (mean 70.7 ± 48.5). The anterior and posterior tibial arteries distal to the graft can be visualized to below the ankle, while the peroneal artery can be evaluated to its bifurcation above the ankle. Peak systolic flow velocities in the distal arteries are similar to those found in the distal graft segment. Failing grafts that have hemodynamically significant, flow-reducing lesions also have decreased luminal diameters ($<$ 1.9 mm), thickened graft walls, and peak systolic flow velocities of less than 30 cm/sec distal to the stenotic area. In some instances, duplex scanning has detected hemodynamically significant, flow-reducing lesions before any evidence of impending graft failure was detected by other means.

In 51 (75%) of our 68 failing grafts, percutaneous transluminal angioplasty corrected the lesion and prevented graft failure for prolonged periods; in the remaining cases, a simple proximal graft extension (2 cases), distal graft extension (12 cases), or patch angioplasty (3 cases) was required (4). The relative ease with which hemodynamic integrity can be restored to the "failing graft" as compared with the rigorous methods necessary to salvage an ischemic extremity once a graft has thrombosed mandates careful and frequent follow-up examinations for all patients with infrapopliteal bypasses. Any return of symptoms, change in pulse examination or hemodynamic deterioration as determined by noninvasive laboratory parameters is an indication for urgent arteriography and appropriate correction of new or progressive lesions. Failure to treat the failing graft aggressively will result in a higher incidence of acute graft thrombosis and increase the need for more complicated reoperations that do not achieve the same high rate of continued patency and limb salvage (4).

The Montefiore Experience with Thrombosed Distal Bypasses

From January 1979 to December 1984, 25* of our 184 reversed saphenous vein and 52* of our 207 PTFE infrapopliteal bypasses thrombosed and required reoperation for limb-threatening ischemia (1). Distribution of local

---

*These numbers do not include those patients with thrombosed grafts who did not develop recurrent limb-threatening ischemia and, therefore, did not require reoperation.

and systemic risk factors, techniques of initial operative and postoperative management, methods for patient observation and determination of graft patency, and lifetable patency rates have been previously reported (2,3,6, 12,13). Of the 77 failed infrapopliteal bypass grafts, 45 occluded within the first postoperative month and 32 occluded late (from 1 to 48 months after the initial operation). Thirty day operative mortality was 3% for all 77 re-operative procedures. Patency rates for these 77 reoperative cases were calculated from the time of first reoperation by the lifetable method (14).

Management of PTFE Graft Occlusion

Fifty-two patients with thrombosed PTFE femoral-to-distal artery bypasses underwent reoperation for recurrent limb-threatening ischemia. If graft occlusion occurred beyond the first postoperative month, femoral arteriography was performed with visualization of the arterial tree from the aorta to the forefoot. In this way, inflow problems proximal to the graft origin could be assessed and the character and patency of arteries distal to the graft insertion could be determined.

Under regional or general anesthesia, the distal incision was reopened. The graft was identified and traced distally until the anastomotic sutures could be seen. The recipient artery proximal and distal to the anastomosis was dissected beyond the area of perianastomotic scarring. Heparin was administered, and a 1.5 cm longitudinal incision was made in the hood of the graft to within 1 mm of the tip of its beveled end (Fig. 1). Through this incision, thrombectomy of the graft and arterial tree was performed using partially inflated balloon catheters (Fig. 2). The distal anastomosis and the arterial lumen were then inspected for intimal flaps, anastomotic intimal hyperplasia, or narrowing of the arterial lumen. In 47 (90%) of 52 cases it was possible to restore unimpeded proximal flow by this approach, while in 2 cases it was necessary to open the proximal incision to remove adherent clot or fibrin from the proximal graft without revision of the proximal anastomosis. In three of these reoperations, a totally new bypass was constructed because all fibrin and debris could not be removed from the graft.

In all but the last three cases, after all clot was removed and proximal flow was reestablished, attention was directed to the distal anastomosis to determine the cause of graft occlusion so that appropriate corrective measures could be taken. If *intimal hyperplasia* narrowed the recipient artery at or near the distal graft insertion (four cases), the graft incision was extended distally

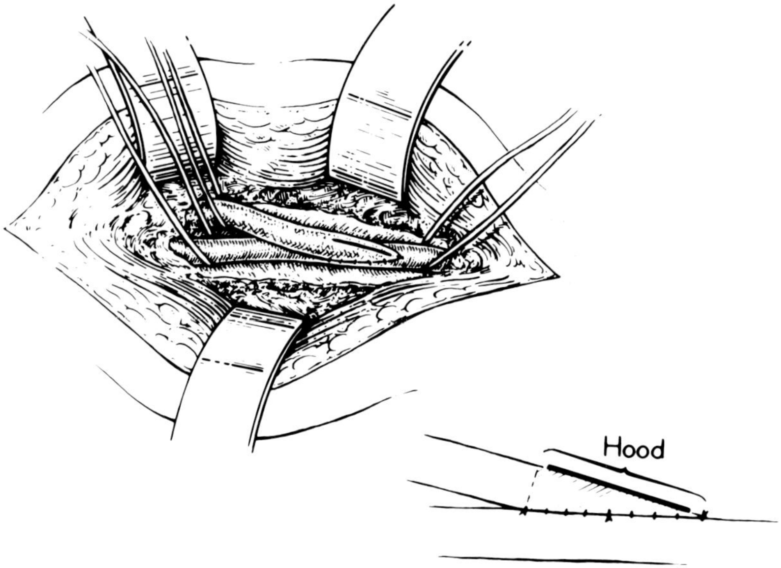

Figure 1 Operative exposure of the distal anastomosis. The incision in the hood of the graft is made to within 1 mm of the distal end of the graft. This provides optimal exposure of the distal anastomosis and facilitates thrombectomy.

across its apex and down the recipient artery until its lumen was no longer narrowed. A PTFE or vein patch was inserted across the stenosis to widen the lumen (Fig. 3), and an arteriogram was obtained to assure adequacy of the repair and outflow. If no intimal hyperplasia was present at or beyond the distal anastomosis, the graft incision was closed and operative arteriography and pressure measurements were performed. If these assessments revealed any stenotic lesion due to *distal disease progression* (11 cases), a segment of vein or PTFE graft was inserted side-to-end in the original graft to extend the bypass to a patent artery below the stenotic lesion (Fig. 4) or a new bypass to the same artery more distally was constructed when the original graft could not be effectively reopened. Often the preoperative arteriogram was helpful in identifying progressive atherosclerotic lesions responsible for graft thrombosis. If graft failure was due to *proximal disease progression* (four cases), a segment of PTFE was inserted to extend the bypass proximal to the lesion. If *no cause* of graft closure could be identified (30 cases) thrombectomy alone was performed. No postoperative anticoagulation was administered, although patients received 0.6 to 0.9 g of aspirin and 100 to

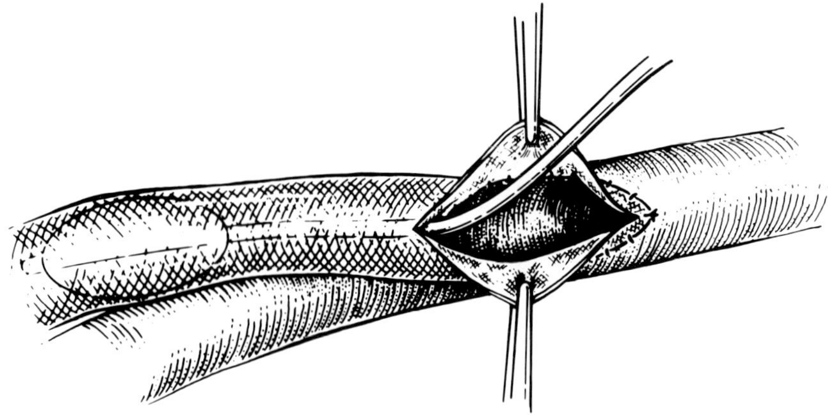

Figure 2 Thrombectomy alone is performed through the distal graft incision when no cause for graft failure is identified. Clot is removed from the graft and, if needed, from the artery both proximally and distally.

375 mg of dipyridamole daily while in the hospital and thereafter. Observation of graft patency by previously described, objective methods has been complete in 50 of the 52 patients. Two patients (4%) were lost to follow-up, 17 and 29 months, respectively, after their first reoperation. Both patients had patent grafts at the time of their last examination. Twenty-one (40%) of these 52 patients required more than one reoperation to prolong graft patency.

Following this plan of management, our overall 3 year patency rate from the time of first reoperation was 13% for failed femorodistal PTFE bypass grafts (Fig. 5). Whether the graft failed early (<1 month) or late (>1 month) did not affect the success of reoperation. Repetitive reoperations did not improve the patency rate if the graft thrombosed again. No reoperation was successful for longer than 9 months if runoff was not continuous to the foot. However, if continuous runoff was present, the 3 year reoperative patency rate was 31%. If no cause for graft thrombosis was identified and thrombectomy alone was performed, only 8% of the grafts remained patent for 3 years. When the cause of graft failure was identified and appropriate reoperation was performed, a 33% 3 year reoperative patency was achieved (1).

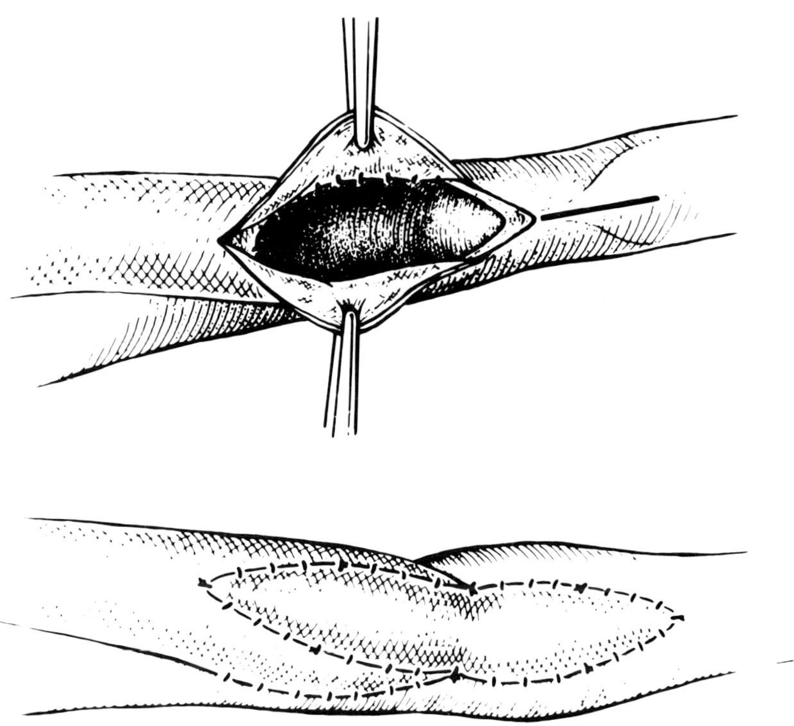

Figure 3 A stenosis caused by intimal hyperplasia or an unrecognized atherosclerotic lesion is corrected by extending the graft incision distally across its apex and down the recipient artery until its lumen is no longer narrowed. A patch of PTFE or vein is then inserted across the stenosis to widen the lumen. (From Ref. 1 used with permission.)

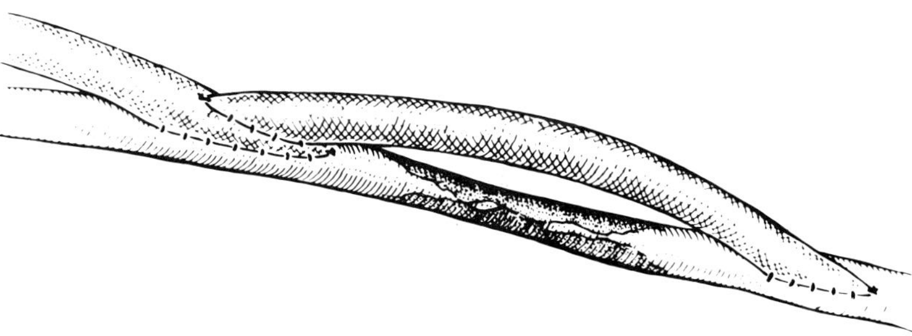

Figure 4 When graft failure is due to progression of atherosclerosis, a short graft extension is inserted from the graft incision to the artery distal to the atherosclerotic narrowing. (From Ref. 1, used with permission.)

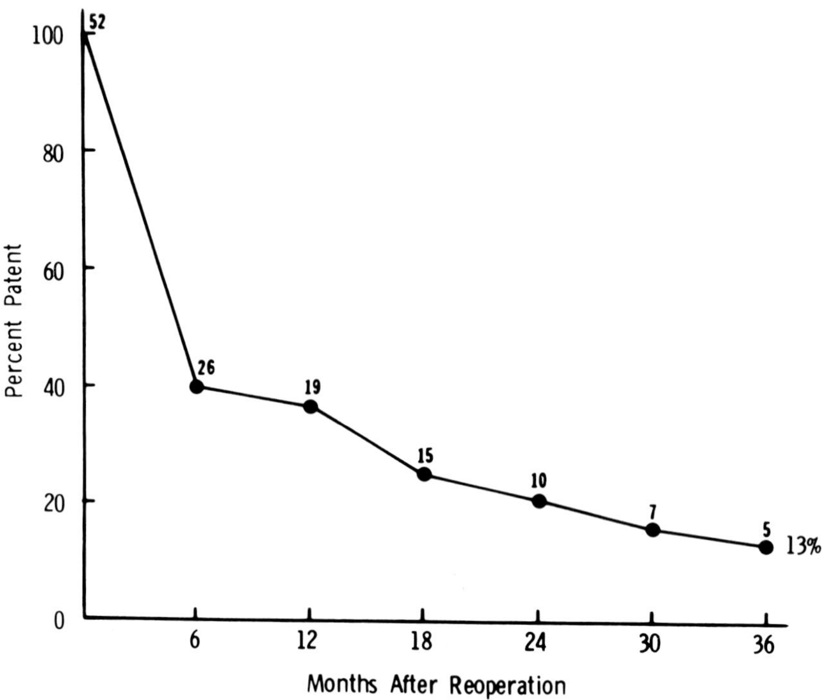

Figure 5   Three year lifetable patency rate after reoperation on 52 PTFE femorodistal bypasses. Reoperation consisted of thrombectomy of the original graft from a longitudinal incision over the distal anastomosis and the appropriate corrective procedure as indicated (see text).

Recent Modifications for PTFE Femorodistal Bypass Failure

Although we previously attempted to salvage all thrombosed PTFE bypasses by the techniques just described, we have been influenced by the relatively poor late patency rates of reoperations for failed infrapopliteal bypasses. Accordingly, we recently altered our management of failed infrapopliteal PTFE grafts and generally performed entirely new bypasses using either autologous vein or PTFE grafts anastomosed to virginal inflow and outflow arteries. Originally, we used this approach only when the original PTFE bypass was complicated by infection or was performed at another institution and the technical details of the primary operation could not be ascertained. For the last 3 years, we also performed entirely new bypass grafts when a femorodistal bypass failed and no cause of failure could be detected or when failure occurred for a second time. Although accurate and conclusive comparisons are not possible at present, this modified approach has resulted in a 3 year patency rate of 39% for all secondary operations after failure of a previous femorodistal PTFE bypass (1).

Management of Femorodistal Vein Graft Occlusion

The outlook for restoring patency to an autologous saphenous vein femorotibial or femoroperoneal bypass that fails after the immediate postoperative period has generally been poor. A completely new, secondary bypass is probably the best option for reversing ischemia (15), although more recently, some success with vein thrombectomy and graft revision has been reported by Whittemore and his associates (9), and this has been our experience. If reoperation is conducted within 24 hours after occlusion of the vein graft, simple thrombectomy with correction of defects in the vein or the inflow and/or outflow tracts is a method that can restore patency (9). Only when such defects are identified and repaired (ideally, before they cause graft thrombosis) can simple reoperative correction be performed with uniformly good results (4,7-9). We have performed thrombectomy of distal vein grafts in three cases and have achieved prolonged patency in two of them. In two of these cases, thrombectomy was delayed for 4 to 7 days after thrombosis of the vein graft had occurred.

Often, thrombosed saphenous vein grafts require the performance of a new bypass using virginal vessels for inflow and outflow and ectopically harvested autologous vein from the arms or contralateral leg or PTFE. If no autologous vein is available, a PTFE graft may be used, and such a bypass is certainly a better option than performing a major amputation (3). Preoperative arteriography is essential and preoperative venography is helpful in determining whether the ipsilateral saphenous vein or other veins are available and useful (5). We have achieved a 3 year patency rate of 48% for the 25 secondary femorodistal vein grafts that required operation because of a primary vein graft failure (Fig. 6). Sixteen of these new bypasses were constructed of PTFE alone, five were composite sequential (PTFE/vein) bypasses, and four were constructed completely with ectopic autologous vein obtained from the upper extremities or the opposite lower extremity.

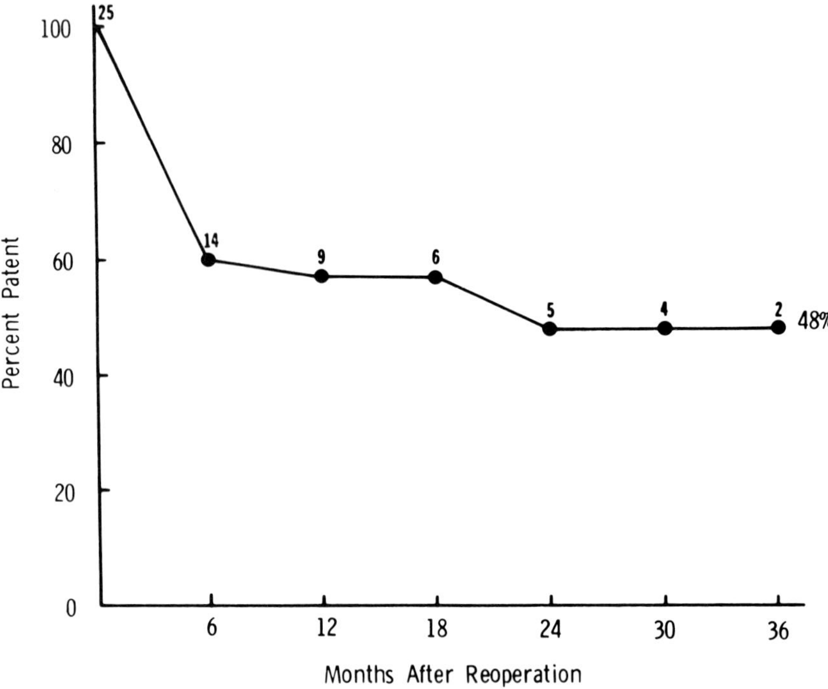

Figure 6   Three year lifetable patency rate after reoperation on 25 patients with thrombosed femorodistal vein grafts. Reoperation consisted of performing a new bypass using virginal vessels for inflow and outflow (see text).

Other Considerations in Our Present Approach to Failed Femorodistal Bypass

When femorodistal graft thrombosis occurs and limb-threatening ischemia develops, it is essential to know which conduit was used for the original reconstruction, the exact anatomic and physiologic status of the arterial tree in the involved limb, and the quality and length of usable vein that is available for the secondary arterial reconstruction. In general, these are carried out as a totally new bypass using previously undissected arteries for inflow and outflow whenever possible. The possible role for fibrinolytic agents and interventional radiology in treating failed grafts is controversial (16-18). We have abandoned the use of intra-arterial streptokinase infusions because of the frequency of distal embolization, which made usable distal arteries unsuitable for a secondary bypass and led to limb loss (19).

Currently, we construct both our primary and secondary femorodistal bypasses with autologous vein whenever possible. To maximize vein utilization, it is important in all infrainguinal operations, but especially in secondary operations, to minimize the length of vein used to perform the reconstruction. Our first step is to find an acceptable source of inflow as far distally in the leg as possible. We have shown that using the superficial femoral, popliteal, or even the tibial arteries as the source of inflow does not negatively affect patency and, in fact, may enhance patency rates (20,21). When the superficial femoral artery is unsuitable as an inflow source, we have also used the middle and distal portions of the deep femoral artery to provide inflow. A high quality multiplanar angiogram is essential to assess the adequacy of the iliac inflow and the proximal portions of the superficial and deep femoral arteries. In a limited experience, we have also found the duplex scanner to be accurate in determining the adequacy of the deep femoral artery.

When the superficial femoral artery is occluded, we evaluate the arteriogram carefully to see if the popliteal artery has any patent segment. When insufficient amounts of autologous vein are available and there is a patent, albeit blind, segment of popliteal artery, we do not hesitate to construct a composite, sequential bypass graft. A specific indication for this sort of operation is the presence of extensive infection or gangrene in the foot (22). We use PTFE for the proximal femoropopliteal bypass, and the tibial extension is constructed using the available vein as a bypass from either the distal-most segment of popliteal artery or the distal end of the PTFE graft, depending on the length of the vein available and the quality of the artery. We have noted in several instances that the distal vein graft thrombosed after the patients had healed their ischemic lesions. In all such cases, the leg remained viable because the PTFE bypass to the isolated popliteal segment remained patent.

Using delayed exposures and the hyperemic technique, our radiologists can usually demonstrate the distal arteries in the leg and foot. Rarely, when flow or cardiac output is extremely poor, digital subtraction angiography is required to demonstrate the vascular anatomy in the foot. We have almost never needed to perform intraoperative femoral or popliteal angiography to define an outflow vessel. However, although this technique may be useful in some settings (23), we often perform completion angiography after our isolated popliteal bypasses to assess the distal circulation in case the patient requires a subsequent distal extension to heal the ischemic lesion (22).

When there is no autologous vein available or when no suitable tibial vessel is found (conditions that are particularly common after a failed distal bypass), we construct a bypass with PTFE to an isolated popliteal artery segment if one is available. We have previously reported (22) excellent patency rates for these bypasses, and have found that bypasses to isolated popliteal artery segments can provide enough blood flow to the foot to control rest pain or heal small ischemic ulcers or areas of gangrene. However, bypasses to isolated popliteal segments provide insufficient flow to save extremities with advanced gangrene or extensive infection in the foot. In such cases, a sequential bypass or a direct tibial bypass is required for limb salvage.

Although it is our preference not to jeopardize the contralateral leg by harvesting its vein, we will consider use of that saphenous vein for secondary tibial bypass if that leg is not threatened and has near normal arterial flow and pressure as demonstrated by the noninvasive vascular laboratory. If the length of vein needed is kept to a minimum, venography may demonstrate a loop or major tributary of the saphenous vein that can be used, thereby preserving the main body of the vein. Otherwise, either a proximal or distal segment of the vein may be harvested so that the remaining vein is preserved in an undamaged condition.

Before a secondary tibial bypass, we also examine the patient's upper extremities both visually and with ultrasound, when necessary, to evaluate the patency and quality of the cephalic and basilic veins. Although aneurysmal dilation has been reported (24,25) when these veins have been used as an arterial substitute, overall results have been good. We have now followed one patient for 20 months with a cephalic vein bypass from his distal deep femoral to his peroneal artery after three previous ipsilateral arterial reconstructions had failed and his contralateral saphenous vein had been used for aortocoronary bypass. The cephalic vein dilated to a maximum diameter of 12 mm, but has remained stable at this diameter for more than 1 year. We have also had success joining two or more cephalic vein segments together and combining segments of cephalic and saphenous vein to increase the length of the available autologous vein.

When, after a primarily failed distal bypass, there is absolutely no autologous vein available and the popliteal artery is totally occluded, we construct a PTFE femorodistal bypass. Although the patency rates for prosthetic femorodistal bypasses are not as high as similar bypasses performed with autologous vein (3), occasionally long-term patency (up to 7 years) can be achieved. More importantly, limb salvage for more than 3 years can still be achieved in over half of these patients (3).

Conclusions

Patients with failed infrapopliteal bypasses and threatened limbs represent one of the greatest challenges in vascular surgery. The options available to the vascular surgeon to salvage these patients' limbs are often very limited. However, we believe that with proper preoperative assessment of the arterial and venous systems and with meticulous operative technique, more than half of these patients can have their threatened limb saved in a useful condition for prolonged periods of time.

References

1. Ascer E, Collier PE, Gupta SK, Veith FJ: Reoperation for PTFE bypass failure: the importance of distal outflow site and operative technique in determining outcome. J Vasc Surg (in press).
2. Veith FJ, Gupta SK, Samson RH, Scher LA, Fell SC, Weiss P, Janko G, Flores SW, Rifkin H, Bernstein G, Haimovici H, Gliedman ML, Spryregen S: Progress in limb salvage by reconstructive arterial surgery combined with new or improved adjunctive procedures. Ann Surg 194:386-401, 1981.
3. Veith FJ, Gupta SK, Ascer E, White-Flores S, Samson RH, Scher LA, Towne JB, Bernhard VM, Bonier P, Flinn WR, Astelford P, Yao JST, Bergan JJ: Six-year prospective multicenter randomized comparison of autologous saphenous vein and expanded polytetrafluoroethylene grafts in infrainguinal arterial reconstruction. J Vasc Surg 3:104-114, 1986.
4. Veith FJ, Weiser RK, Gupta SK, Scher LA, Samson RH, Ascer E, White-Flores SA, Sprayregen S: Diagnosis and management of failing lower extremity arterial reconstructions. J Cardiovasc Surg 25:381-384, 1984.
5. Veith F, Moss CM, Sprayregen S, Montefusco CM: Preoperative saphenous venography in arterial reconstructive surgery of the lower extremity. Surgery 85:253-256, 1979.
6. Veith FJ, Moss C, Fell SC, Daly V, Haimovici H: New approaches to limb salvage by extended extra-anatomic bypasses and prosthetic reconstructions to foot arteries. Surgery 84:764-774, 1978.
7. Berkowitz HG, Hobbs CL, Roberts B, Freiman D, Oleaga J, Ring E: Value of routine vascular laboratory studies to identify vein graft stenosis. Surgery 90:971-979, 1981.
8. O'Mara CS, Flinn WR, Johnson ND, Bergan JJ, Yao JST: Recognition and surgical management of patent but hemodynamically failed arterial grafts. Ann Surg 193:467-476, 1981.
9. Whittemore AD, Clowes AW, Couch NP, Mannick JA: Secondary femoropopliteal reconstruction. Ann Surg 193:35-42, 1981.
10. Bandyk DF, Cato RF, Towne JB: A low flow velocity predicts failure of femoropopliteal and femoro-tibial grafts. Surgery 98:799-809, 1985.

11. Bandyk DF: Postoperative surveillance of femoro-distal grafts: the application of echo-Doppler (duplex) ultrasonic scanning. In Bergan JJ, Yao JST (Eds): *Reoperative Arterial Surgery*. Orlando, Grune & Stratton, 1986, pp. 59-79.
12. Veith FJ, Moss CM, Fell SC, Montefusco CM, Rhodes BA, Haimovici H: Comparison of expanded polytetrafluoroethylene and autologous saphenous vein grafts in high risk arterial reconstructions for limb salvage. Surg Gynecol Obstet 147:749-752, 1978.
13. Bergan JJ, Veith FJ, Bernhard VM, Yao JST, Flinn WR, Gupta SK, Scher LA, Samson RH, Towne JB: Randomization of autogenous vein and polytetrafluoroethylene grafts in femoral-distal reconstruction. Surgery 157:437-442, 1982.
14. Colton T: Statistics in Medicine. Boston, Little, Brown, and Co., 1974, p. 237.
15. Szilagyi DE, Elliot JP, Smith RF, Hageman JH, Sood RK: Secondary arterial repair: the management of late failure in reconstructive arterial surgery. Arch Surg 110:485-493, 1975.
16. Hargrove WC III, Barker CF, Berkowitz HD, Perloff LJ, McLean G, Freiman D, Ring EJ, Roberts B: Treatment of acute peripheral arterial and graft thrombosis with low-dose streptokinase. Surgery 92:981-993, 1982.
17. Van Breda A, Robison JC, Feldman L, Waltman AC, Brewster DC, Abbott WM, Athanasoulis CA: Local thrombolysis in the treatment of arterial graft occlusions. J Vasc Surg 1:103-112, 1984.
18. Lang EK: Streptokinase therapy: complications of intraarterial use. Radiology 154:75-77, 1985.
19. Veith FJ: In discussion of Hargrove WC, et al. Surgery 92:990, 1982.
20. Veith FJ, Gupta SK, Samson RH, Flores SW, Janko G, Scher, LA: Superficial femoral and popliteal arteries as inflow sites for distal bypasses. Surgery 90:980-990, 1981.
21. Veith FJ, Ascer E, Gupta SK, White-Flores S, Sprayregen S, Scher LA, Samson RH: Tibiotibial vein bypass grafts: a new operation for limb salvage. J Vasc Surg 2:552-557, 1985.
22. Veith FJ, Gupta SK, Daly V: Femoropopliteal bypass to the isolated popliteal segment: is polytetrafluoroethylene graft acceptable? Surgery 89:296-303, 1981.
23. Flinn WR, Flanigan DP, Verta MJ Jr, Bergan JJ, Yao JST Jr: Sequential femoral-tibial bypass for severe limb ischemia. Surgery 88:357-365, 1980.
24. Kakkar VV: The cephalic vein as a peripheral vascular graft. Surg Gynecol Obstet 128:551-556, 1969.
25. Harris RW, Andros G, Dulawa LB, Oblath RW, Salles-Cunha SX, Apzan R: Successful long-term limb salvage using cephalic vein bypass grafts. Ann Surg 200:785-792, 1984.

13

Reoperative Procedures for Complications of Dialysis Access Fistulas and Grafts

HUGH H. TROUT, III
George Washington University Medical Center, Washington, D.C.

The increased number and survival rate of patients with chronic renal failure being treated with hemodialysis require maintenance of adequate hemoaccess. Though these patients have a shortened life expectancy, instances in which death results from lack of a suitable vascular access should be rare. For this to be so, each access constructed should last as long as possible and, when complications with the access occur, prudent efforts to salvage it should be made before constructing a new access at another site. Problems with hemoaccess procedures are outlined in Table. 1. This chapter discusses the reoperative management of complications related to *arteriovenous (A-V) fistulae* defined as an autogenous artery to vein anastomosis, and to *arteriovenous (A-V) grafts*, defined as synthetic vascular grafts interposed between an artery and a vein. External devices such as shunts and percutaneous catheters will be briefly described.

The access with the best long-term patency rate and the fewest complications is the A-V fistula first described by Brescia and co-workers (1). The next best, again with respect to both patency and complication rate, is the A-V graft constructed with expanded polytetrafluoroethylene (PTFE) material. Interposition grafts using Dacron, modified bovine carotid heterografts, human umbilical cord vein allografts, and autologous saphenous vein have all been employed in the past. But, because of a greater complication rate with these grafts than with PTFE, they are currently less frequently used.

Arteriovenous graft and fistula patency and complication rates vary considerably. Some of the relevant variables include the type of access con-

Table 1 Problems Associated with
Hemoaccess Procedures

External Devices
  Scribner shunt
  Percutaneous catheters

Local Access Problems
  Thrombosis
    A-V fistula—early
    A-V fistula—late
    A-V graft—early
    A-V graft—late
  Decreased flow
    A-V fistula or graft
  Aneurysm Formation
    Pseudoaneurysm
    Dilatation
  Graft infection or exposed graft
  Seroma formation

Extremity Complications
  Swollen extremity
  Painful extremity
    Distal ischemia
    Neuropathy

Systemic Complications
  Congestive heart failure

---

structed, access location (forearm, upper arm, thigh), access configuration
(looped, straight), size and adequacy of arterial inflow and venous outflow,
the presence of diabetes, and the experience and technical proficiency of the
operating surgeon. Certain general patency predictions are possible (2,3).
Arteriovenous fistulae at the wrist have about a 20% failure within 1 month.
Of those that are patent at 9 months, however, (about 65%), almost all
remain patent for 4 years. In contrast, PTFE grafts have a high early patency
rate that steadily falls, such that about 60 to 65% (including as patent those
who have successful revisions) are patent after 4 years. These figures
emphasize that, given the shortened life expectancy of patients with chronic
renal failure, careful attention to planning, construction, revision, and mainte-

nance of A-V fistulae and grafts is likely to be rewarding. Few patients should require unusual and sometimes awkward hemoaccess procedures, must discontinue hemoaccess for lack of a suitable access, or die of uremia for lack of a usable access.

External Devices

Scribner Shunt

This was one of the first methods of achieving hemodialysis. A plastic catheter is inserted into an artery brought through the skin, and connected to a similar catheter inserted into a vein. The most common site employed originally was the radial artery and cephalic vein. As the importance of the forearm and wrist for the construction of fistulae and grafts became apparent, however, the most frequent site for shunt placement has now become the leg. This procedure uses one of the arteries at the ankle and the greater saphenous vein. The complications of shunts are usually either thrombosis or infection. Thrombosis can often be successfully treated by balloon thrombectomy in the dialysis unit. On occasion, repositioning of one or both of the catheters to a more cephalad site may be necessary. Infection at one of the catheter exit sites through the skin can sometimes be treated for a short time with local drainage and systemic antibiotics, but definitive management almost always requires shunt removal. Though some shunts remain functional for prolonged periods, in general these are devices used relatively briefly while awaiting recovery from acute renal insults or until other more permanent accesses are constructed. At present, percutaneous venous catheters can usually provide both these functions and, as a consequence, the use of external A-V shunts has diminished considerably.

Percutaneous Catheters

These catheters, either single- or double-lumen, are inserted into the superior vena cava, most often by percutaneous subclavian vein cannulation. The complications are insertion related — pneumothorax, arterial or venous trauma — or occur after the catheter has been in place. The latter would include increased venous resistance, catheter thrombosis, infection around the catheter insertion side, catheter tip infection, or subclavian vein or superior vena cava thrombosis or stenosis. The insertion-related complications require immediate attention, with close observation, insertion of a chest tube, external compression, or, on rare occasion, direct operative exposure and repair of a lacerated vessel.

Increased venous resistance encountered while the catheter is being used may render effective hemodialysis difficult or impossible. In this situation, replacement of the catheter over a guidewire is usually necessary, though repositioning of the catheter is sometimes effective. Similarly, catheter thrombosis can be treated with irrigation and lytic agents, but again catheter replacement is frequently required. Infection, either systemic or around the exit site of the catheter through the skin, almost always requires catheter removal. The most ominous complication of these catheters, however, is subclavian vein or superior vena cava vein stenosis or thrombosis. The incidence and severity of either stenosis or occlusion are not known, but one major causative factor is almost surely directly related to the length of time the catheter is in position. As a consequence, when a more permanent hemoaccess route is anticipated at the time of catheter insertion, expeditious construction of the new access is wise in order to minimize the duration of percutaneous catheter use. The role of lytic agents for treatment of major vein thrombosis is still unclear and requires considerable judgment. The advantage of regaining venous patency must be balanced by the risks of releasing a potential fatal pulmonary embolus. Similarly, the role of balloon dilation of subclavian or innominate venous strictures is uncertain. The advantage of achieving reduced venous hypertension should be balanced by the potential complications and the unknown long-term success rate for major venous stricture dilatation.

Local Access Problems

Thrombosis

A-V Fistula—Early

Early thrombosis of an A-V fistula is almost always the result of using an inadequately sized vein or artery, usually the former, or is caused by technical error. When the size of the vein seemed adequate at the time of the original operation, then reoperation, looking for kinks, twists, anastomotic errors, hematomas, or other causes of internal stenosis or external compression, is warranted. Immediate reoperation is probably not highly critical, though revision should most likely be performed within 72 hours. If no cause for fistula failure is detected, a thrombectomy, using a balloon catheter through a small venotomy, can be attempted. If this is not successful, a more proximal fistula revision or construction of another access at some other site will be required.

A-V Fistula—Late

Late thrombosis frequently heralds the permanent failure of an A-V fistula. Nevertheless thrombectomy, local revision, or revision to a more cephalad level may succeed and may be warranted. Thrombectomy alone after late failure, however, is rarely successful; access salvage usually requires intra-operative angiography and revision or patching (4). Evaluation and attempts at revision are much more successful when, prior to thrombosis, venous hypertension is noted during hemodialysis. An arteriogram can be obtained to demonstrate a discrete stricture amenable to balloon dilatation or direct repair.

A-V Graft-Early

There are three main causes for early A-V graft thrombosis: (a) technical error, (b) choice of inadequate arterial inflow source, and (c) a patient with a hypercoaguable state or marked prolonged hypotension. When technical error is suspected, appropriate revision is warranted since salvage of a useful graft often provides excellent long-term access. If arterial inflow is in-adequate (such as might be found in a patient with diabetes mellitus who had a strongly palpable radial pulse preoperatively, but was found to have a small heavily calcified artery at operative exploration), repeated attempts to salvage such an access will likely fail. In addition, nerve innervation or arterial per-fusion to the hand may be compromised. In this setting, it is probably best to abandon the A-V graft and seek another site or method for dialysis. Thrombectomy is warranted in patients suspected of being hypercoaguable, though preoperative evaluation of the hematologic abnormality is of value in determining proper treatment to prevent rethrombosis. Thrombectomy in patients with prolonged hypotension will likely fail unless the hypotension is corrected. If percutaneous catheters prove inadequate, either peritoneal dialysis or a large single-lumen venous dialysis catheter (Hickman dialysis catheter, Evermed Inc., Kirkland, Washington) permits adequate dialysis while the cause of the hypotension is corrected.

A-V Graft—Late

A late thrombosis of an A-V graft is the most common cause of reoperation for failed hemoaccess conduits. A stricture at the arterial graft anastmosis can cause thrombosis, but the most common finding is a stricture, caused by pseudointimal hyperplasia, at the venous graft anastomosis (5). Angiography is not helpful in distinguishing between these two causes after thrombosis has occurred. Some (6) have advocated angiography, lytic therapy, and balloon dilatation. Though success has been reported (7), it is unlikely to be long-lasting because this stenotic venous graft anastomosis area is quite fibrotic and not amenable to successful long-term dilatation (8).

If the thrombosis is relatively recent, however, the finding of a pulsatile graft just distal to the arterial graft anastomosis points to the cause of the thrombosis being a venous graft stricture. Similarly, if the dialysis nurses cite a recent history of venous hypertension when the patient was on dialysis, this too suggests a venous graft stricture. In the absence of a history of decreased arterial flow while on dialysis, indicating arterial graft stricture, the etiology is most likely venous stenosis. In this setting, I make a longitudinal incision in the skin over the presumed venous graft stricture. This incision is carried down to the graft, 3000 to 5000 units of heparin are given systemically, and the graft is then opened with a longitudinal incision 1 to 2 cm proximal to the venous graft anastomosis. No attempt is made to gain circumferential control of either the graft or the vein. Attempts at controlling the vein are likely to injure the vein and are not necessary — internal control with balloon catheters is easily accomplished. Balloon catheters are passed cephalad, and the vein is cleared of the recent thrombus. At this time, a tight venous graft stricture will usually be noted. If any question of a stricture exists, the incision in the graft is carried cephalad through the anastomosis (and through the suture line) into the vein until a patent nonstrictured lumen is encountered. A patch graft (usually PTFE) is then sewn in place, taking care to make substantial bites at the lateral edges where the previous venous graft anastomosis had been (Fig. 1). Although it is an established belief that autogenous vessel graft anastomoses do not heal and, thus require an intact suture line, in this setting, one can cut across the old suture line and sew on a patch graft with little likelihood of a subsequent false aneurysm. This is so when polypropylene suture is used and it will likely be true with sutures made of PTFE material. After about two-thirds to three-quarters of the patch graft closure has been achieved, balloon catheters are then repeatedly passed toward the arterial graft anastomosis until brisk pulsatile arterial blood flow is achieved. The thrombus at the origin of the graft is distinctive and characterized by having a whitish cap and a concave surface (5). Removal of such a thrombus is a favorable prognostic sign with regard to the adequacy of the arterial inflow. Blood loss is controlled both proximally and distally with balloon catheters, and the patch closure is completed. The balloon cathers are removed just before the last suture or two.

If no venous graft stricture is detected with the cephalad passing of the balloon catheter, then and the longitudinal incision in the graft is carefully

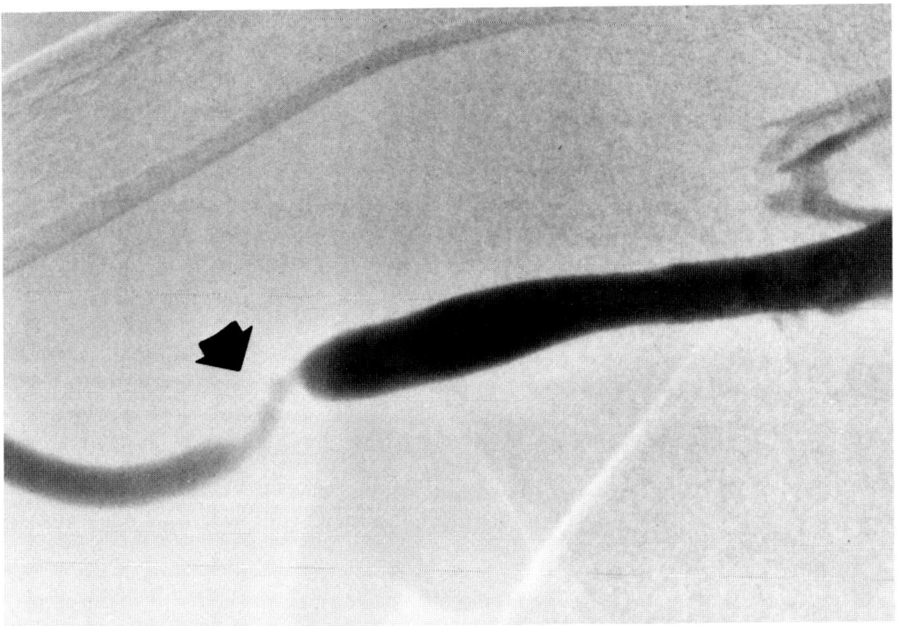

Figure 1   Arteriogram with a stricture at the venous anastomosis of an A-V graft.

closed. Again, blood loss is controlled with the use of internal balloon catheters. If this procedure is successful, then the same anatomic situation exists postoperatively as existed before the graft thrombosed. As a consequence, antiplatelet drugs or moderate postoperative anticoagulation is suggested.

If acceptable arterial flow cannot be achieved or if an arterial stricture is suspected from the beginning, an incision must be placed to expose the arterial graft anastomosis. If a venous graft anastomotic stricture was found and acceptable arterial inflow was not attained simply because the balloon catheter could not be adequately manipulated, the incision in the graft can be made 2 to 3 cm beyond the previous arterial graft anastomosis. In this circumstance, control of the graft both proximal and distal to the transverse incision in the graft will minimize blood loss once the obstructive thrombus is removed.

In contrast, if the primary problem is deemed to be at the old arterial graft anastomosis, either an incision in the graft quite close to the previous anastomosis or an incision through the old anastomosis with subsequent patch grafting will be necessary. In these circumstances, control of blood loss is a more challenging technical problem. The easiest method is to use a proximal tourniquet, thus controlling all blood flow to and from the extremity (9). This technique requires a good regional anesthetic block and adequate preoperative preparation. If a tourniquet is not used, either proximal and distal arterial control with encircling elastic bands or internal control with balloon catheters may suffice. Successful correction of an arterial graft anastomotic stricture requires careful preoperative planning of incisions and meticulous technique as local vessel control can be difficult to achieve without damaging the artery or adjacent nerves because of tissue scarring from the original operative dissection.

Emergent repair of a thrombosed PTEE A-V graft is not critical. Successful repairs are often obtained any time within 2 weeks of the thrombosis, though a prolonged interval between thrombosis and thrombectomy makes success less likely.

Decreased Flow

A-V Fistula or Graft

Flow-related problems during hemodialysis can be caused by decreased arterial inflow, a venous graft anastomotic stenosis, or a venous stricture. When it is difficult to maintain an adequate dialysis flow rate, compromised arterial flow is likely. High venous resistance is caused by a venous graft anastomotic stenosis or a venous stricture. In these situations, sonography (10) or duplex scanning (11) may be informative, though at present, angiography remains the diagnostic procedure of choice (12). This is accomplished by puncturing the graft or vein and injecting contrast medium while a tourniquet, tightened to a pressure above the patient's systolic pressure, is in position well cephalad to the entire access (13). Contrast medium will then fill both the arterial and venous tree and may reveal an arterial or venous stricture (Fig. 1) that may then be treated, on occasion, with balloon dilatation (14) or, more frequently, with patch angioplasty using autogenous vein or PTFE as the patch material.

After arteriography, the operative approach can be easily planned because the location of the stenosis is well delineated. If the stricture is at the arterial anastomotic site, tourniquet control of the entire extremity is employed. If a stricture is present in the graft or vein, internal balloon control of both the inflow and outflow vessels is carried out easily and expeditiously to permit repair.

Aneurysm Formation

Pseudoaneurysms

These may occur at the mid portion of the graft or vein secondary to repeated punctures in the same area. Though treatment of small pseudoaneurysms is not mandatory, if they enlarge, treatment is necessary. Direct repair with simple oversewing of the small defect or with a patch graft will usually suffice.

When a pseudoaneurysm is at an anastomotic site, concerns of occult infection are appropriate (this would almost always be at a graft vessel anastomotic site since an infected pseudoaneurysm at a A-V fistula anastomotic site is extremely rare). If an infection is not grossly evident, direct repair of the anastomotic breakdown with patch grafting is performed. Multiple cultures are sent in an effort to establish whether an occult infection exists.

If an infection is clearly present or if another pseudoaneurysm develops within 6 to 12 months, all prosthetic material should be removed and the artery ligated proximally and distally. If the brachial artery is involved, the profunda brachii is usually adequate to supply the extremity. If ligation of the brachial artery is contemplated, preoperative arteriography to confirm the presence and adequacy of the profunda branch is of value. If it is not considered adequate, autogenous reconstruction should be considered.

Graft Dilation

Though one manufacturer had early problems with PTFE dilatation, they altered their manufacturing process; this is now a rare occurrence with any PTFE graft currently available. Unfortunately, biological grafts such as bovine carotid artery and human umbilical cord vein allografts have an increased propensity to develop both false and true aneurysms (15-17). For this reason, their popularity has diminished in the United States; PTFE is preferred. Again, though small dilatations do not require immediate repair (the nurses, however, should not puncture these areas when placing the patients on hemodialysis), larger dilatations should be treated. Local repair of deteriorating biological grafts is not warranted since the aneurysmal process will continue in other portions of the graft. Replacement of the graft with a synthetic graft is the preferred treatment. If the aneurysm does not involve the arterial graft anastomosis, the preferred approach is to anastomose a new PTFE graft end-to-end to the old biological graft near the old arterial-biological graft anastomosis, to make a new subcutaneous tunnel for the new PTFE graft, and to anastomose the venous end of the PTFE graft end-to-end to a vein or to the old biological graft near the old venous graft anastomosis. Residual small segments of biological graft in continuity with arterial blood flow does leave a vulnerable segment that might subsequently deteriorate; however, this is not common. Perhaps this is so because the residual biological graft is not subjected to repeated needle punctures near the anastomoses and the short graft segments are generally well encased in scar tissue caused by the two operative procedures. The advantage of this approach is that the artery and veins, both of which are surrounded by scar tissue, do not require dissection and are less likely to be damaged. If the remaining small segments of biological graft subsequently dilate, they too must be resected.

Graft Infection or Exposed Graft

On occasion, it is possible to achieve healing of infected or exposed PTFE grafts without resorting to graft removal. When a suture line is exposed and infected, removal is usually indicated because of the increased risk of subsequent hemorrhage. When infection or skin necrosis occurs away from a skin suture line, however, cultures, appropriate systemic antibiotic therapy (usually anti-*Staphylococcus aureus* [18] and anti-*Staphylococcus epidermidis*) and local debridement therapy should be employed until no evidence of local or systemic infection persists. This local treatment may suffice (19) or a full-thickness skin flap might then be rotated to cover the defect (20). Either technique yields a high rate of successful repair. If resolution of the infection is unsuccessful, the main body of the graft is excised. Small uninfected graft remnants at the arterial anastomotic sites may be left in place to protect limb perfusion (21).

Seroma Formation

Perigraft fluid collections are caused by a reaction of the tissues to the graft material (usually Dacron) (22), a leak of serous fluid through the graft (usually PTFE) (23), or a leak from transected lymphatics (more common in the groin than in the upper extremity). Since Dacron is only infrequently used for dialysis access, tissue reaction is rarely encountered. If it does occur, replacement of the Dacron graft with PTFE is in order (24).

Perigraft serous collections occur because of a filtering action of PTFE. These can be extremely difficult to treat. Interestingly, the defect does not appear to be in the graft itself, but rather is in the patient's blood in that segments of excised PTFE have been repeatedly examined without revealing any intrinsic defect (23). It seems that in a few patients, the interstices of a portion of the graft do not fill with microthrombi as normally occurs at the time of graft insertion. The graft then becomes "wet," analogous somewhat to the nonpreclotted knitted Dacron graft, and serum leaks through. This phenomenon can be frequently observed at the time of graft insertion and is characterized by beads of clear fluid appearing on the outside of the graft. In most cases, the leak ceases and the graft becomes well incorporated in the surrounding tissues. When the leak continues, however, a perigraft collection of fluid accumulates. Once the process is started, it will almost always continue despite aspirations, evacuations, or topical application of enhancers of thrombosis.

The only successful treatment is removal of the involved segment and replacement with another graft. The replacement graft is usually Dacron, though I have had success by using an interposition segment of PTFE that had been washed out with absolute alcohol (which will "wet" the graft and make it porous), washing the alcohol out with saline, and then "preclotting" the PTFE with nonheparinized blood. This is not always successful, but it has worked on several occasions.

Leaks from transected lymphatics should be suspected when the access has been placed in an area of abundant lymph vessels. This is, however, a rare cause of perigraft fluid collection in areas other than the groin.

Extremity Complications

Swollen Extremity

After construction of an A-V fistula or graft, it is not unusual for an extremity to be swollen for 3 to 6 weeks. This swelling normally subsides without treatment. If the swelling persists or the extremity becomes swollen after the initial 3 to 6 week period, the diagnosis of venous hypertension is likely. In addition to edema, the extremity may develop a bluish discoloration and may become progressively painful or develop skin ulcerations.

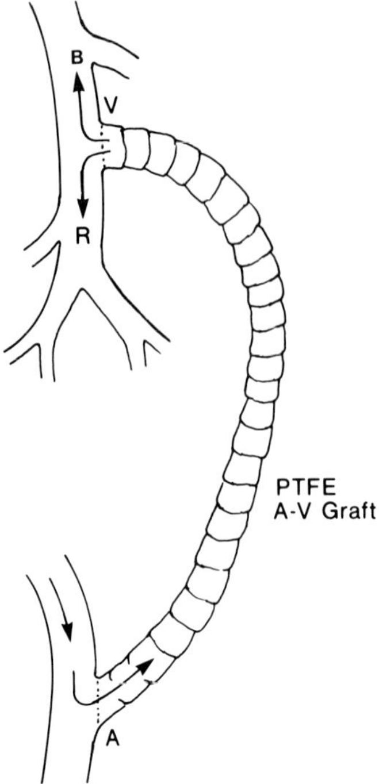

Figure 2 End-to-side anastomosis (*V*) of A-V graft, resulting in elevated venous pressures at *B* and also, because of retrograde flow, at *R*.

The cause of venous hypertension is usually venous dilatation, valve incompetency, and retrograde venous flow after arterialization of the venous system. One example is illustrated in Figure 2. This depicts an end-to-side anastomosis between the PTFE graft and the vein at *V*. In this configuration, the venous pressure is elevated at *B*, as it would be in an end-to-end anastomosis, but it is also elevated at *R* because of retrograde flow. Venous hypertension sufficient to cause chronic swelling may usually be prevented by constructing side-of-artery to end-of-vein A-V fistulae or end-of-graft to end-of-vein A-V grafts. If a chronically swollen extremity develops in spite of these measures, angiography should be performed. Either a large venous branch near the anastomosis that is delivering retrograde flow to the deep venous bed or a venous stricture that is causing venous outflow obstruction to the entire extremity may be found. Treatment of the former is ligation of the branch; of the latter, it is balloon dilation or patch angioplasty. If side-to-side A-V fistulae or end-of-graft to side-of-vein A-V grafts were constructed, the treatment of the chronically swollen extremity is ligation of the distal vein just distal to the venous anastomosis. When the venous stricture or occlusion is located in the subclavian vein (perhaps caused by prolonged use of a subclavian catheter), an axillary internal jugular vein bypass using PTFE may be considered. The increased flow generated by the A-V graft seems to preserve patency of the bypass; as a consequence, the swelling in the extremity decreases and the function of the A-V graft is prolonged (11). In rare situations where no correctable cause for the edema is found and yet the swelling is marked and persistent, ligation of the A-V fistula or A-V graft is necessary.

Interestingly, tieing off a major deep vein and using the more proximal end to construct a venous graft anastomosis does not cause marked distal extremity venous hypertension. Presumably, this hypertension does not develop because sufficient collateral veins exist and dilate enough to carry the necessary volume of blood, but do not dilate enough to make their venous valves incompetent. Consequently, retrograde flow of arterialized blood in the venous system is either infrequent or of insufficient volume or pressure to cause chronic edema.

Painful Extremity

Although venous hypertension with a chronically swollen extremity, as just discussed, can cause pain, the usual causes of extremity pain are distal ischemia and neuropathy.

Distal Ischemia

Ischemia of the distal upper extremity is characterized by burning and often severe pain of the fingers and hand, accompanied by cool or cold fingers and prolonged blanching. In severe cases, ulceration or gangrene of the finger tips occurs. The usual cause is reversal of arterial flow distal to the arterial anastomosis. A "steal" phenomenon is produced (e.g., arterialized blood in another vessel, usually the ulnar artery, is "short-circuited" via a major collateral, usually the palmar arch and, thus, never adequately perfuses the digital end arteries) (Fig. 3A). Treatment options include: arterial ligation just distal to the arterial anastomosis (Fig. 3B), banding of the graft or vein (Fig. 3C)

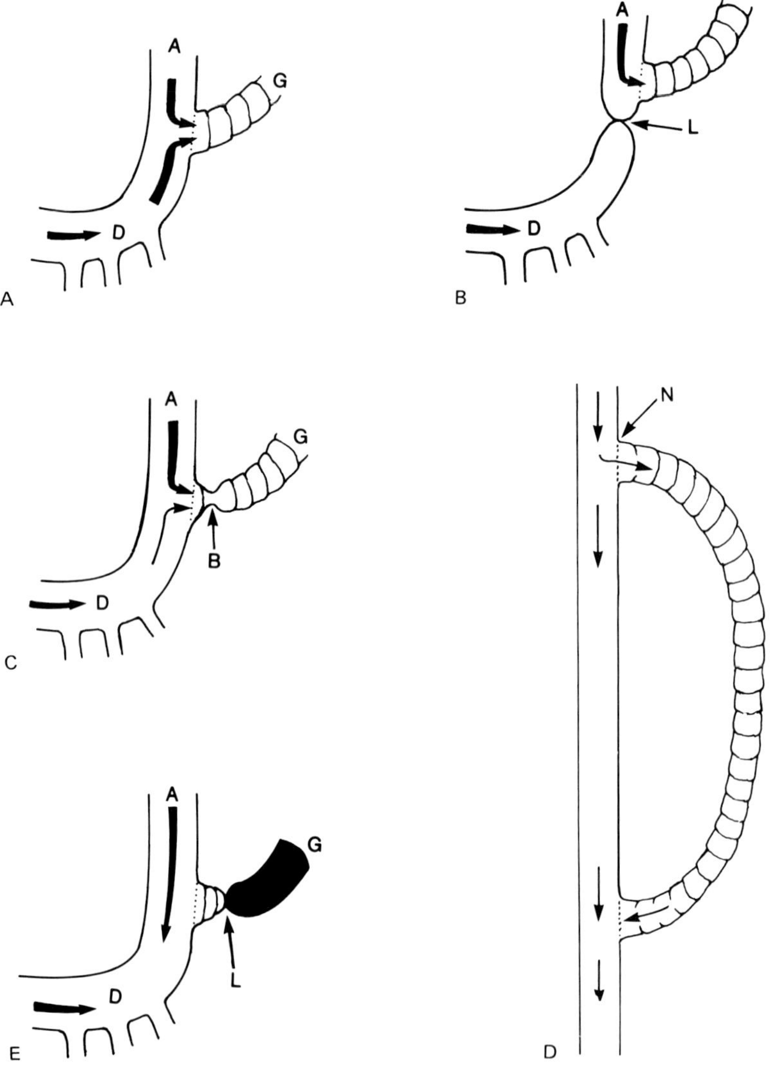

Figure 3 *A*: "Steal" phenomenon. Blood flow preferentially goes to the lower pressure system, the A-V graft (*G*), and away from the distal arteries (*D*). *B*: Ligation (*L*) of distal artery. Note that sufficient collateral flow must be available to prevent distal ischemia. *C*: Banding (*B*) of the A-V graft to increase resistance in the A-V graft and reduce flow away from the distal arteries (*D*). *D*: Construction of a new anastomosis (*N*) to convert an A-V graft into an arterio-arterial graft with parallel flow. No "steal" from the distal arteries is possible. *E*: Ligation (*L*) of the A-V graft.

238

taking down the venous anastomosis and constructing an arterio-arterial by-pass (Fig. 3D), and ligation of the graft or fistula (Fig. 3E).

Successful treatment is frequently achieved by ligating the artery just distal to the anastomosis and thereby preventing flow reversal (Fig. 3B). Caution must be exercised, however, to ensure that there is adequate collateral flow to the hand. If a palpable ulnar pulse or, at a minimum, an easily audible ulnar pulse is not present, an angiogram should be obtained before arterial ligation to confirm the presence of collateral arteries capable of adequate perfusion (25).

Another option is to reduce the flow in the graft or fistula by narrowing the lumen with an external cuff with plicating sutures or with a narrow lumen interposition graft (Fig. 3C) (26). In general, a flow of 300-700 ml/min is sufficient to maintain access patency while avoiding major "steal" or congestive heart failure.

Another interesting procedure that has been successful in patients with either the "steal" syndrome or in diabetics with severe vascular disease is construction of an arterio-arterial jump graft in the upper arm (Fig. 3D) (27,28). One end of the graft is anastomosed end-to-side to the axillary artery, the graft is tunneled laterally and then medially, and anastomosed end-to-side to the brachial artery just above the elbow. Parallel flow does not cause graft thrombosis, and the absence of a venous anastomosis prevents retrograde flow and "steal" into a low pressure system.

In situations where limb or digit viability is clearly threatened, it is probably best to ligate the access (Fig. 3E) to provide the best chance for minimizing tissue loss. Clearly, the urgency of attempted repair of a "steal" situation is much greater than that attendant with a thrombosed graft or fistula. Irreversible sensory and motor changes may occur if the ischemia is allowed to persist.

Neuropathy

Though uremic polyneuropathy can produce symptoms in the extremity with the dialysis access (this is usually symmetric, and the feet are the first to be affected), the more frequent cause of neuropathy is the carpal tunnel syndrome. The etiology for this unusual complication is not clear. Some (29) have postulated that swelling secondary to venous hypertension causes compression of the median nerve as it traverses the carpal tunnel. This theory, however, cannot account for the fact that patients with venous hypertension secondary to axillary vein thrombosis do not appear to have an increased propensity to develop the carpal tunnel syndrome. Others (30) postulate that the symptoms are elicited by ischemia secondary to a vascular steal, and they have reported partial relief of symptoms with ligation of the artery distal to a forearm A-V fistula.

Nerve conduction studies are useful in revealing typical slowing of median nerve conduction velocity across the wrist. Once the diagnosis is established, if the symptoms are severe or persistent, operative decompression usually provides relief.

Systemic Complications — Congestive Heart Failure

Though traumatic A-V fistulas have long been recognized to produce congestive heart failure (CHF), this complication is rare among patients with A-V fistulae and grafts constructed for chronic hemodialysis unless two patent hemoaccesses are present. Evidence obtained by Anderson and co-workers (31) suggests that the development of CHF is flow-related. The usual A-V fistula or graft has a flow range of about 250-600 ml/min. On occasion, however, the flow rates in patients with CHF may reach almost as much as 3000 cc/min.

When patients develop CHF or seem to have an elevated cardiac index with compromised cardiac function and two functioning hemoaccesses are present, one should be ligated. If only one is present, it should be explored and flows measured. Wilson (32) advocates banding of the fistula or graft with a Teflon cuff with progressive tightening until the flow rate is reduced to 300 to 400 ml/min. He cautions that reductions of less than 300 ml/min will result in thrombosis of the graft.

Summary

Multiple complications of A-V fistulas and A-V grafts have been reviewed, and general guidelines for successful management of each have been presented. Although failure of a single A-V fistula or graft is rarely catastrophic, repeated failures with loss of access sites will be disastrous for long-term patient care. Careful planning and well executed operations based on the principles outlined in this chapter should result in prolonged usefulness of each hemoaccess constructed. Only in the rarest instance should patients be forced to abandon hemodialysis for lack of suitable hemoaccess.

References

1. Brescia MJ, Cimino JE, Appel K, Hurwich BJ: Chronic hemodialysis using venipuncture and a surgically created arteriovenous fistula. N Engl J Med 275:1089-1092, 1966.
2. Anderson CB, Sicard GA, Etheredge EE: Primary and secondary operations for vascular access. In Evaluation and Treatment of Upper and Lower Extremities. Bergan JJ, Yao JST, (Eds): New York, Grune & Stratton, 1983, p. 279-305.
3. Palder SB, Kirkman RL, Whittemore AD, Hakim RM, Lazarus JM, Tilney NL: Vascular access for hemodialysis, patency rates and results of revision. Ann Surg 194:235-239, 1985.
4. Bone GE, Pomajzl MJ: Management of dialysis fistula thrombosis. Am J Surg 138:901-906, 1979.
5. Etheredge EE, Haid SD, Maeser MN, Sicard GA, Anderson CB: Salvage operations for malfunctioning polytetrafluoroethylene hemodialysis access grafts. Surgery 94:464-470, 1983.
6. Rodkin RS, Bookstein JJ, Heeney DJ, Davis GB: Streptokinase and transluminal angioplasty in the treatment of acutely thrombosed hemodialysis access fistulas. Radiology 149:425-428, 1983.
7. Zeit RM, Cope C: Failed hemodialysis shunts. Radiology 154:353-356, 1985.
8. Tortolani EC, Tan AHS, Butchart S: Percutaneous transluminal angioplasty. Arch Surg 119:221-223, 1984.
9. Babcock TL: A simplified technique for vascular access in the upper extremity. Surg Gynecol Obstet 155:563, 1982.
10. Scheible W, Skram C, Leopold GR: High resolution real-time sonography of hemodialysis vascular access complications. AJR 134:1173-1176, 1980.
11. Sidaway AN: Personal communication.
12. Reilly DT, Pearson HJ, Watkin EM. Wood RFM: Phlebography in the salvage of dialysis fistulae. Clin Radiol 33:569-575, 1982.
13. Anderson CB, Gilula LA, Harter HR, Etheredge EE: Venous angiography and the surgical management of subcutaneous hemodialysis fistulas. Ann Surg 187:194-204, 1978.
14. Hunter DW, Castaneda-Zuniga WR, Coleman CC, Young AT, Salomonowitz E, Mercado S, Amplatz K: Failing arteriovenous dialysis fistulas: evaluation and treatment. Radiology 152:631-635, 1984.
15. Guillou PJ, Leveson SH, Kester RC: The complications of arteriovenous grafts for vascular access. Br J Surg 67:517-521, 1980.

16. Mohaideen AH, Mendivil J, Avram MM, Mainzer RA: Arterio-venous access utilizing modified bovine arterial grafts for hemodialysis. Ann Surg 186:643-650, 1977.

17. Garvin PJ, Castaneda MA, Codd JE: Etiology and management of bovine graft aneurysms. Arch Surg 117:281-284, 1982.

18. Francioli P, Masur H: Complications of *Staphylococcus aureus* bacteremia occurence in patients undergoing long term hemodialysis. Arch Intern Med 142:1655-1658, 1982.

19. Bhat DJ, Tellis VA, Kohlberg WI, Driscoll B, Veith FJ: Management of sepsis involving expanded polytetrafluoroethylene grafts for hemodialysis access. Surgery 87:445-450, 1980.

20. Moosa HH, Peitzman AB, Thompson BR, Webster MW, Steed DL: Salvage of exposed arteriovenous hemodialysis fistulas. J Vasc Surg 2: 610-612, 1985.

21. Gifford RRM: Management of tunnel infections of dialysis polytetrafluoroethylene grafts. J Vasc Surg 2:854-858, 1985.

22. Kaupp HA, Matulewicz TJ, Lattimer GL, Kremen JE, Celani VJ: Graft infection or graft reaction? Arch Surg 114:1419-1422, 1979.

23. Bolton W, Cannon JA: Seroma formation associated with PTFE vascular grafts used as arteriovenous fistulae. Dialysis Transplant 10:60-63, 1981.

24. Blumenberg RM, Gelfand ML, Dale WA: Perigraft seromas complicating arterial grafts. Surgery 97:194-203, 1985.

25. Doscher W, Viswanathan B, Stein T, Margolis IB: Hemodynamic assessment of the circulation in 200 normal hands. Ann Surg 198:776-779, 1983.

26. Haimov M, Baez A, Martin N, Neff M, Martin N, Slifkin R: Complications of arteriovenous fistulas for hemodialysis. Arch Surg 110:708-712, 1975.

27. Geis WP, Giacchino J: A game plan for vascular access for hemodialysis. Surgical Rounds, January 1980, pp. 62-70.

28. Giacchino JL, Geis WP, Buckingham JM, Vertuno LL, Bansal VK: Vascular access: long-term results, new techniques. Arch Surg 114:403-409, 1979.

29. Warren DJ, Otieno LS: Carpal tunnel syndrome in patients on intermittent haemodialysis. Postgrad Med J 51:450-452, 1975.

30. Harding AE, Le Fanu J: Carpal tunnel syndrome related to antebrachial Cimino-Brescia fistula. J Neurol Neurosurg Psychiatr 40:511-513, 1977.

31. Anderson CB, Etheredge EE, Harter HR, Codd JE, Graff RJ, Newton WT: Blood flow measurements in arteriovenous dialysis fistulas. Surgery 81:459-461, 1977.

32. Wilson SE: Complications of vascular access procedures. In Wilson SE, Owens ML (Eds): Vascular Access Surgery. Chicago, Yearbook Medical Publishers, 1980, pp. 185-207.

14
Reoperation for Chronic Intestinal Ischemia

LARRY H. HOLLIER
Mayo Clinic, Rochester, Minnesota

Incidence and Etiology

Chronic intestinal ischemia is not often seen in most vascular surgical practices. However, this clinical syndrome poses a serious threat to life that is readily correctable by surgical intervention. Restoration of visceral artery flow dependably results in weight gain and relieves postcibal pain.

In a previous review of our experience with chronic intestinal ischemia at at the Mayo Clinic, my colleagues and I (1) identified 54 patients who had undergone visceral artery revascularization for postprandial pain and weight loss associated with visceral artery occlusive disease. Surgical revascularization resulted in relief of these symptoms in 96% of the patients. However, after a mean follow-up period of 3 years, symptoms had recurred in more than 25% of patients, usually in association with late occlusion of grafts. Furthermore, our study showed that the recurrence of symptoms was inversely related to the completeness of revascularization (Table 1). Among patients with multiple vessel stenoses, symptoms recurred in only 11% of those who had revascularization of all stenotic vessels, in 29% who had two of three stenotic vessels revascularized, and in 50% who had only one of three stenotic vessels revascularized. Other authors (2-5) reported similar recurrence rates.

In 1980, Zelenock and co-workers (2) reported 23 patients operated on for chronic intestinal ischemia. Their mortality rate of 17% was due to bowel infarction occurring after occlusion of a single graft placed to revascularize bowel in which all three visceral vessels had been occluded or stenotic. Also, in that series, the reoperation rate for recurrence of symptoms in patients

Table 1 Rate of Late Recurrence of Symptoms in Relation to Completeness of Revascularization of Occluded or Stenotic Visceral Arteries

No. of Vessels		
Involved	Revascularized	Recurrence (%)
3	1	50
2	1	50
3	2	29
3	3	11
2	2	11

Table 2 Visceral Revascularization Sequence

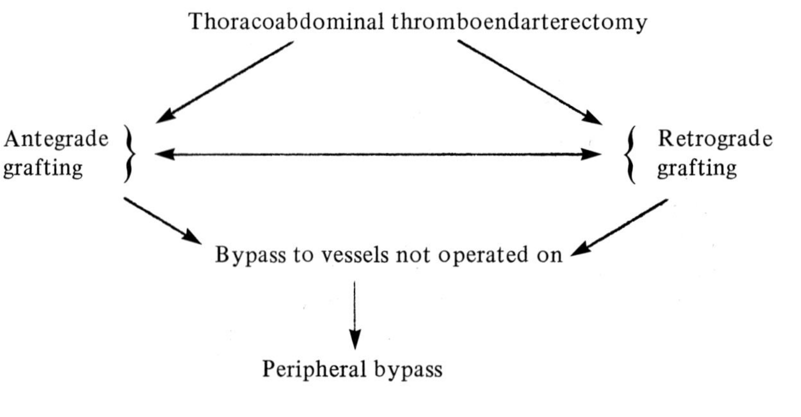

with incomplete revascularization was 25%. In 1974, Reul and associates (4) reported 25 patients (56% of their patients with stenosis of two or three of the visceral vessels) who had undergone single-vessel revascularization. The mortality was 8%, and long-term relief of symptoms persisted in only 50% of patients available for follow-up after 5 months to 8 years. In 1976, McCollum and colleagues (3) reported 33 patients who had revascularization of 87.5% of their stenotic visceral arteries. Although no mention was made of late recurrence rates, angiograms obtained in 13 patients demonstrated an 18% incidence of graft occlusion. Stoney and co-workers (5) quoted an exceptionally low incidence of symptom recurrence among patients who underwent transortic endarterectomy of both celiac and superior mesenteric arteries. Every series, however, regardless of technique or type of graft used, reported some late recurrence of symptoms.

Thus, although symptoms of chronic intestinal ischemia can usually be completely relieved with single-vessel revascularization, we generally recommend that all stenotic vessels be revascularized to minimize late recurrence of symptoms. Unfortunately, despite these precautions, recurrences are inevitable. This discussion, therefore, is an attempt to outline a long-term plan of management for recurrent ischemic symptoms in these patients. The schema of a stepwise visceral revascularization sequence is presented in Table 2.

Sequence and Technique of Operative Management

Optimal long-term management of patients with chronic intestinal ischemia ideally is planned at the time of the original revascularization procedure. As previously mentioned, I prefer to accomplish complete revascularization of all stenotic vessels. Data from Stoney and co-workers (5) suggest that in patients who are otherwise good risks, transaortic visceral artery endarterectomy is the most effective procedure and would be expected to provide good long-term patency. Revascularization of celiac, superior mesenteric, and inferior mesenteric arteries can easily be achieved by this extraperitoneal thoracoabdominal approach (Figs. 1 to 4).

First Recurrence

If late restenosis or occlusion of one or more visceral arteries occurs after this procedure, all the other options for visceral revascularization are still available because proximal endarterectomy does not interfere with late placement of a graft (Fig. 5). Conversely, if initial procedures include bypass

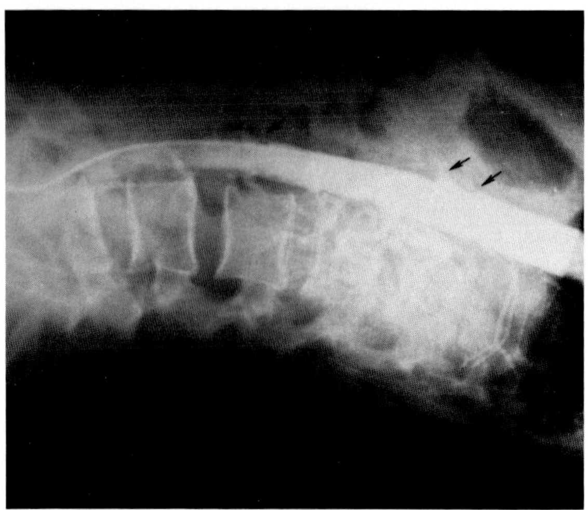

Figure 1 Preoperative aortogram, lateral view, showing high grade atherosclerotic occlusive lesions of celiac and superior mesenteric arteries in a 71-year-old woman.

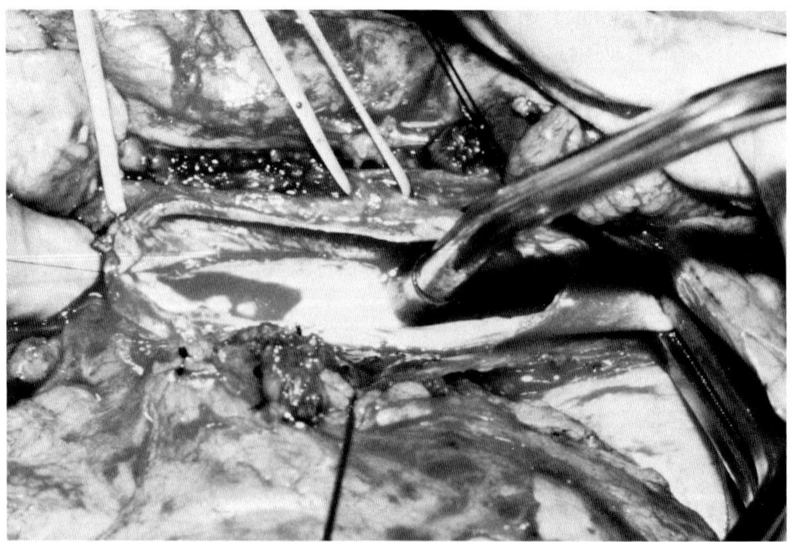

Figure 2 Operative photograph of "trap door" approach for transaortic endarterectomy of visceral vessels.

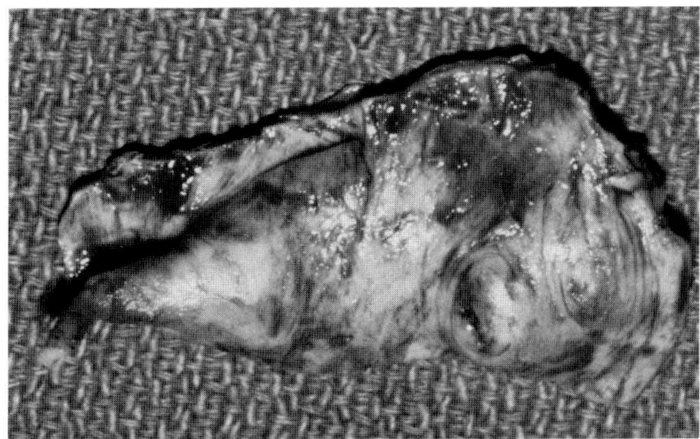

Figure 3 Specimen of atherosclerotic aortic plaque removed from orifices of celiac and superior mesenteric arteries.

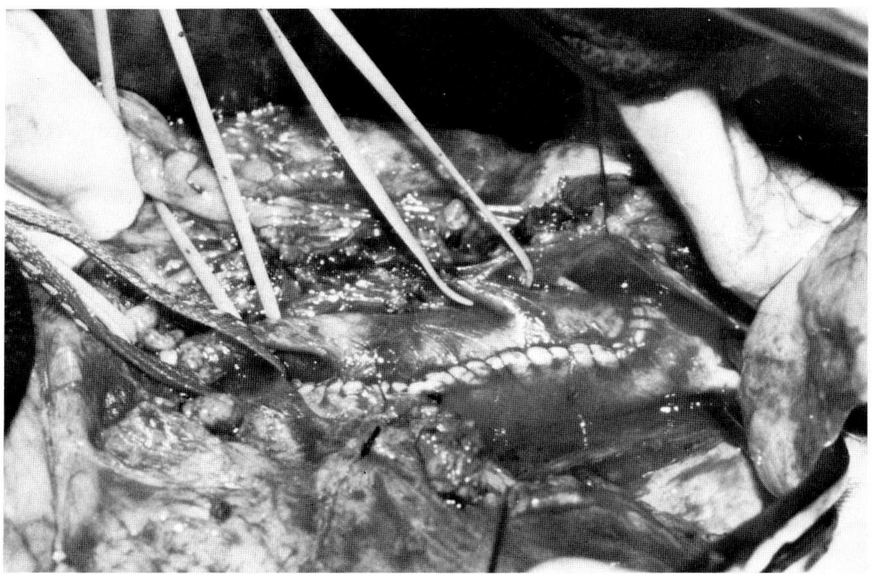

Figure 4 Operative photograph of completed closure of aortic "trap door." Running suture closure assures complete tacking down of intima in adjacent nonendarterectomized portion of aorta.

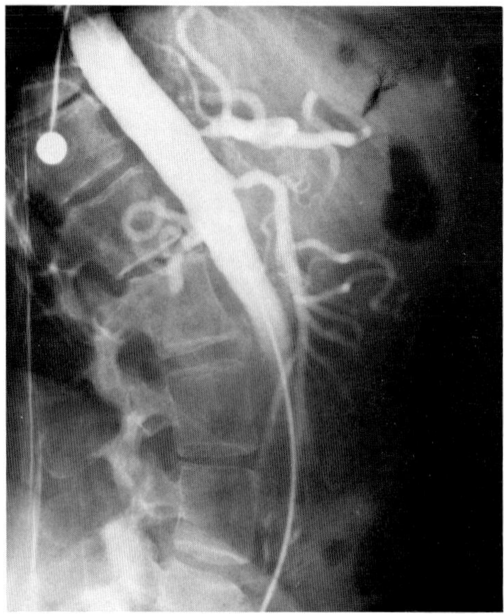

Figure 5   Visceral angiogram shows recurrent stenosis of celiac and superior mesenteric arteries 3 years after visceral artery endarterectomy.

grafting, endarterectomy usually cannot be done as a secondary procedure for restenosis, because the late stenosis is often related to neointimal hyperplasia at the distal anastomotic site. Therefore, in good risk patients, endarterectomy as the first procedure increases one's options in managing late recurrence of symptoms.

I prefer to manage primary recurrence of symptoms by transabdominal antegrade revascularization of celiac and superior mesenteric arteries. This is also our preferred choice as the first procedure in patients with chronic intestinal ischemia for whom thoracoabdominal transortic endarterectomy is unsuitable because of multiple medical risk factors. An antegrade bifurcation graft is generally placed on the supraceliac portion of the aorta; one limb is placed to the celiac artery and the other to the superior mesenteric artery. When gangrenous bowel needs resection, we prefer to use a pantaloon vein graft (Fig. 6) (6) in revascularization of acute ischemia. For the chronic prob-

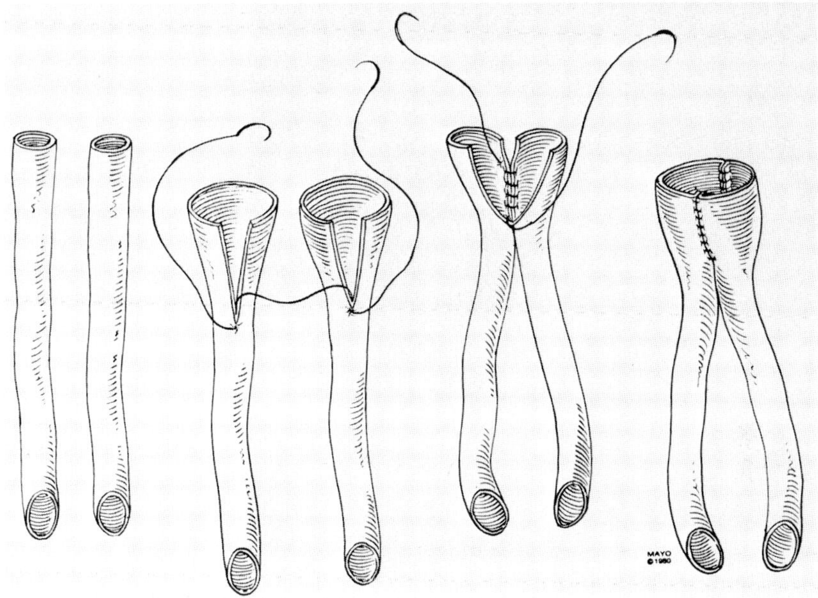

Figure 6 Steps in the creation of a pantaloon vein graft. (From Ref. 6, used with permission.)

lem, a bifurcated Dacron graft appears equally effective. I have found, however, that small grafts (i.e., limbs < 6 mm in diameter) have a higher rate of thrombosis. Because of this, if a prosthetic graft is to be used, I recommend a 14 by 7 mm bifurcated knitted Dacron graft. It has been effective and reliable, and I have not yet seen failure of any of these grafts that my colleagues and I have put in the antegrade position (Fig. 7).

Antegrade revascularization is performed by division of the crura overlying the supraceliac portion of the aorta and placement of a partial occlusion clamp for aortic control. After the straight portion of the bifurcation graft is sewn to the aorta at this level, one limb is cut short and preferably sutured end-to-end to the transsected celiac artery. If the celiac artery itself is occluded, the graft limb can be sutured to one of the proximal branches of the

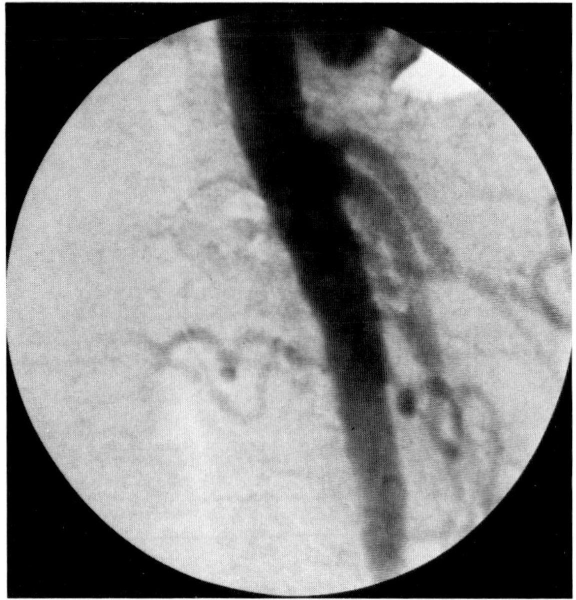

Figure 7   Postoperative angiogram in a patient who underwent secondary antegrade revascularization of celiac and superior mesenteric arteries with knitted double-velour graft.

celiac artery, preferably the hepatic artery. The other limb of the graft is usually tunneled behind the pancreas and sutured end-to-end to the proximal portion of the superior mesenteric artery. If the superior mesenteric artery has a long area of stenosis, the graft may be passed anterior to the pancreas and sutured end-to-side to the more distal portion of the superior mesenteric artery.

Antegrade revascularization is generally feasible even though the previous revascularization had been done in retrograde fashion. Because a retrograde graft to the celiac artery is usually placed to one of the branch vessels and a retrograde superior mesenteric artery graft to the posterior surface of the vessel, antegrade grafting can still be accomplished without great difficulty. The antegrade grafts can be placed on the trunk or unused branch of the celiac artery and on the anterior surface of the superior mesenteric artery.

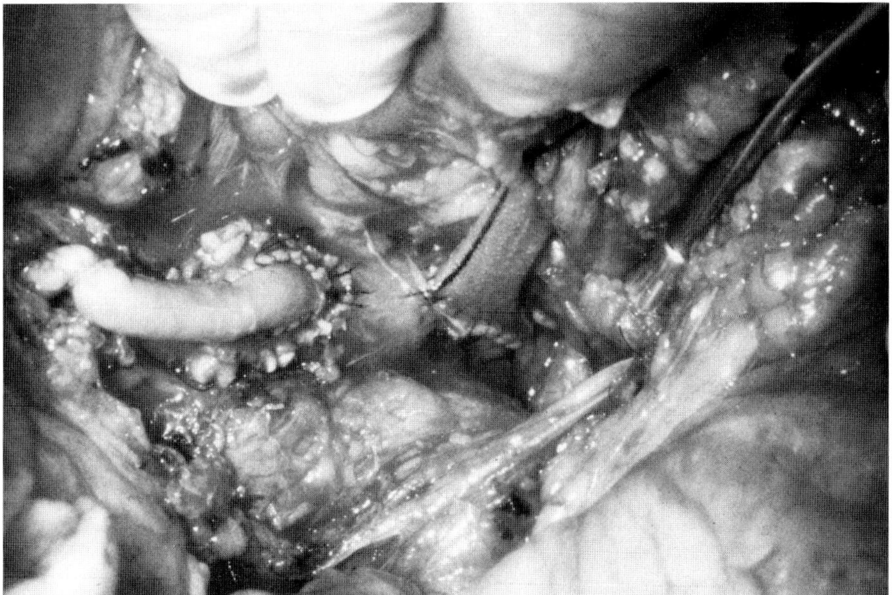

Figure 8 Operative photograph of retrograde aortosuperior mesenteric artery bypass after late failure of transaortic visceral endarterectomy.

Second Recurrence

Failure of multivessel antegrade grafts can also occur. In these cases, although repeat antegrade revascularization is possible, it entails dissection through the extensive scar tissue of the previous operation. Therefore, we prefer retrograde revascularization as the next procedure after failure of antegrade grafts. For retrograde grafts, the infrarenal portion of the aorta is exposed and the superior mesenteric artery is exposed just anterior and superior to the left renal vein. Isolation of the superior mesenteric artery so proximally allows interposition of a very short (2 to 3 cm) 10 mm knitted Dacron graft end-to-side between the aorta and the superior mesenteric artery (Fig. 8). If the splenic artery is patent, exposure of that vessel is obtained through the lesser sac. An 8 mm knitted Dacron graft is sewed end-to-side to the aorta-superior mesenteric artery graft, tunneled to the left of the superior mesenteric artery, and sutured end-to-side to this segment of the proximal portion of the splenic artery.

Third Recurrence

Graft occlusion after this extent of previous revascularization is managed by regrafting from the nearest accessible segment of aorta to any major visceral trunk remaining open. If all major trunks are occluded, revascularization can still be achieved by placement of a vein graft from the aorta or an iliac artery out to branches in the vascular arcade of the bowel. Because of the multiple branch occlusions in these cases, multiple vein grafts may be needed. Help in deciding whether additional grafts are required can be obtained by the use of a sterile Doppler probe to assess the character of flow in the peripheral vessels along the course of the bowel and in the hilus of the liver.

Perioperative Considerations

Postoperative management of the patient after repeat visceral revascularization is of critical importance. Careful monitoring of cardiac indices, including pulmonary capillary wedge pressure and peripheral vascular resistance, and an hourly assessment of urinary output are helpful. Because massive sequestration of fluid usually occurs in these patients, early and continuous replacement of these estimated losses should be undertaken. These losses occur by the development of marked postrevascularization edema of the bowel wall and, in some patients, by the actual transudation of fluid across the serosa of the bowel. Transudation may even result in the development of massive ascites or, as in two of our patients, life-threatening hydrothorax after spontaneous leakage from the abdomen into the chest. One of these patients required replacement of more than 1000 ml of fluid/hour for 3 days!

Although the mechanism for the edema and ascites is not fully clarified, we believe it is related to the loss of autoregulation in the vessels of the chronically ischemic bowel wall. This mechanism would be similar to that in massive revascularization edema of the foot after distal bypass for long-standing leg ischemia, and similar to that in the cerebral hyperperfusion syndrome that occasionally occurs after carotid endarterectomy (7).

We have also noted a similar, previously unreported, phenomenon of apparent vascular fragility in some patients. We have had two spontaneous splenic ruptures and one late mesenteric arteriolar rupture with resultant intramesenteric hematoma. Also, we have been told of an instance of delayed splenic rupture that occurred after visceral revascularization at another institution (8). Although one might suggest that these complications were the result of iatrogenic trauma, the surgeons in each case noted that no dissection had occurred in the involved areas. Each was convinced that the hemorrhagic event was the result of restoration of high pressure and flow in organ systems that had previously had long-standing severe ischemia. Why vessel rupture occurs only in some vessels and in so few cases are not known, but rupture may be related to the degree of ischemia. Regardless of the cause, the surgeon should be aware of these problems so that early intervention can be done if necessary.

Summary

Surgical revasculariation of the visceral vessels is highly successful in relieving symptoms of chronic intestinal ischemia. Symptoms can recur, however, and recurrence is almost invariably related to reocclusion of one or more visceral arteries. Reoperation is generally warranted, but may be complicated because of the previous revascularization. Thoughtful evaluation of each case before surgery simplifies the additional revascularization procedure and minimizes the inherent risks and complications.

References

1. Hollier LH, Bernatz PE, Pairolero PC, et al: Surgical management of chronic intestinal ischemia: a reappraisal. Surgery 90:940-946, 1981.
2. Zelenock GB, Graham LM, Whitehouse WM Jr, et al: Splanchnic arteriosclerotic disease and intestinal angina. Arch Surg 115:497-501, 1980.
3. McCollum CH, Graham JM, DeBakey ME: Chronic mesenteric arterial insufficiency: results of revascularization in 33 cases. South Med J 69:1266-1268, 1976.
4. Reul GJ Jr, Wukasch DC, Sandiford FM, et al: Surgical treatment of abdominal angina: review of 25 patients. Surgery 75:682-689, 1974.
5. Stoney RJ, Ehrenfeld WK, Wylie EJ: Revascularization methods in chronic visceral ischemia caused by atherosclerosis. Ann Surg 186:468-476, 1977.
6. Hollier LH: Revascularization of the visceral artery using the pantaloon vein graft. Surg Gynecol Obstet 155:415-416, 1982.
7. Sundt TM Jr, Sharbrough FW, Piepgras DG, et al: Correlation of cerebral

blood flow and electroencephalographic changes during carotid endarterectomy: with results of surgery and hemodynamics of cerebral
ischemia. Mayo Clin Proc 56:533-543, 1981.
8. Hertzer NR: Personal communication.

15

Recurrent Varicose Veins

J. LEONEL VILLAVICENCIO, JAMES M. SALANDER,
EDWARD R. GOMEZ, PAUL M. ORECCHIA, AND
NORMAN M. RICH
*Uniformed Services University of the Health Sciences,
Bethesda, Maryland; Walter Reed Army Medical Center,
Washington, D.C.*

Patients with some form of venous insufficiency constitute 10 to 35% of the general population (1,2). Venous diseases occupy seventh place in incidence among 28 chronic diseases according to a health survey in the United States (3). Widmer and co-workers (4) studied 4376 apparently healthy working persons from the Basle Chemical Industries, and found 22% with signs and symptoms of chronic venous insufficiency (19% men, 25% women).

Varicose veins constitute a disease the precise etiology of which remains unknown. The term includes any dilatation of the venous system in the extremities. They vary in size and distribution, ranging from tiny venules (venous stars, telangiectasiae) to large venous trunks. If all of these abnormal dilatations of the venous system are considered under the term "varicose veins," then more than half the world population have some form of varicose veins (5). In the Tecumseh Cummunity Health Study, Coon and associates (6) estimated that about 12% of the adult population in the United States have varicose veins of clinical significance. Bauer (7) calculated that there are 10 times as many sufferers from chronic venous disease of the lower extremities as from arterial disease with leg symptoms.

For a better understanding of the clinical problem of recurrent varicose veins, it is necessary to make certain considerations pertaining to the venous system and varicose veins, which we consider of importance. These considerations are:

1. The role of heredity in the genesis of varicose veins.
2. The considerable anatomic variation of the valves of the leg veins. These congenital variations are of great importance for the efficiency of the calf muscle pump mechanism.
3. The possible existence of biophysicochemical alterations in the venous system, with anomalies of the connective tissue, collagen, and elastin (named "dysmetabolism" by German and Swiss authors).
4. The importance of a careful investigation of the etiology of the varicose veins present.
5. The progressive and irreversible natural course of untreated varicose veins.
6. The deleterious role of thrombosis in the integrity and competence of the valvular mechanism.
7. The importance of a thorough knowledge of the surgical anatomy, physiology, and pathophysiology of the venous system.

All of the above considerations are of importance in explaining the recurrence of varicose veins in patients submitted to surgery for venous insufficiency.

The Role of Heredity

Reagan and Folse (8) found that the incidence of reflux in the femoral vein of children was twice as great if there were a family history (parents) of varicose veins. More than half of the patients seen at the Mayo Clinic (5) for problems of varicose veins have family members with similar problems. In 31 children younger than 10 years of age treated for varicose veins by our group (9), either mother or father, or both, as well as other members of the family were also afflicted. One of three female patients with varicose veins who have teenaged daughters, have asked us how to prevent the progression of varicose veins already present in their young daughters.

The Importance of Variations in the Anatomy of the Venous Valves of the Lower Limbs

In a series of 26 anatomic dissections of the veins of the lower limbs from the groin to the knee, the number and site of the valves were studied (10). The number of valves in the femoral vein varied from one to nine, with an average of five. All of the tributaries were valved, especially the muscular veins. The most constant valve was located just below the point where the deep femoral vein joined the superficial femoral vein to form the trunk of the common femoral vein. Other sites where valves were always present were in the mid-femoral vein and at the level of the Hunter's canal. A knowledge of the anatomic variation of these valves is of importance in understanding the information obtained by Doppler examination and the phlebographic images of reflux.

Of significant importance are the investigations of Eger and Casper (11) on the valves of the common femoral and external iliac veins, which revealed that nearly 40% of patients are prone to have varices of the long saphenous vein. They dissected the valves of the common femoral and external iliac veins in 38 cadavers. Findings revealed that no vein contained more than one valve. This is important because in all persons, only one valve protects the saphenous vein against the intra-abdominal pressures. (Fig. 1). This valve was absent bilaterally in nearly 8% of cases, and unilaterally in about 29%, for a total of 37%. If we consider that the common iliac vein and inferior vena cava do not have valves, we can assume that in individuals with these valve variations, the intra-abdominal pressures are directly exerted on the sapheno-femoral junction. This could help to explain the development of varicose veins in the long saphenous system.

If the only femoral valve becomes incompetent, the high orthostatic and thoracoabdominal pressures exert their constant and deleterious effects on the remaining valves of the superficial femoral and saphenous veins, rendering them incompetent sooner or later (Fig. 2).

The Possible Existence of Anomalies of the Connective Tissue in Patients with Varicose Veins

In a provocative study, Coget and Merlen (12) discussed the existence of a biophysicochemical alteration of the venous system in patients with essential varicose veins (known by Swiss and German authors as "dysmetabolism") in whom there are disorders of the connective tissue, collagen, and elastin. They considered that venous insufficiency develops as a consequence of a systemic metabolic disease of the connective tissue, which is progressive and ir-reversible, and that patients with this problem deserve periodic surveillance. Although not proven, this theory deserves careful consideration and further investigation. If properly documented, it could provide the basis to support the genetic tendency for varicosities observed clinically by every physician interested in venous disorders.

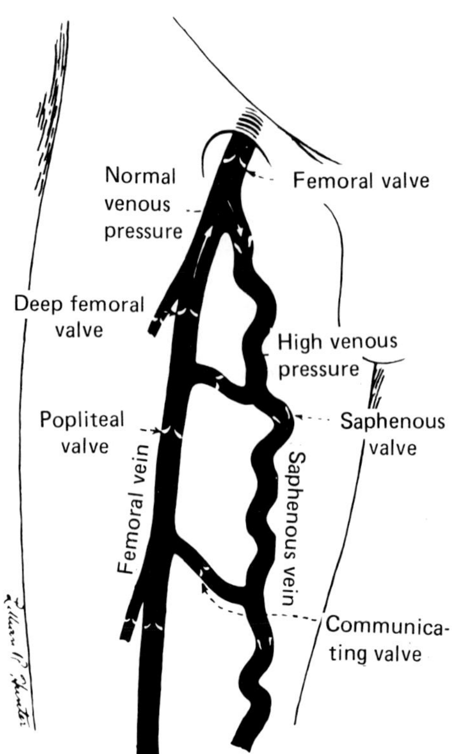

Figure 1 Presence of a competent valve in the common femoral vein. A competent valve in this region is a protection against the intra-abdominal pressure. This valve is absent in nearly 40% of all persons. Its importance is magnified by the fact that the inferior vena cava and common iliac veins do not have valves. Isolated incompetence of the long saphenous vein, as illustrated in the diagram, is present in a small percentage of the cases. In familial varicose veins, the combination of saphenous plus other valvular defects is a common finding. (From De Takats G (Ed): Venous insufficiency of the lower extremities. In: Vascular Surgery. Philadelphia, WB Saunders, 1959, p. 325, used with permission.)

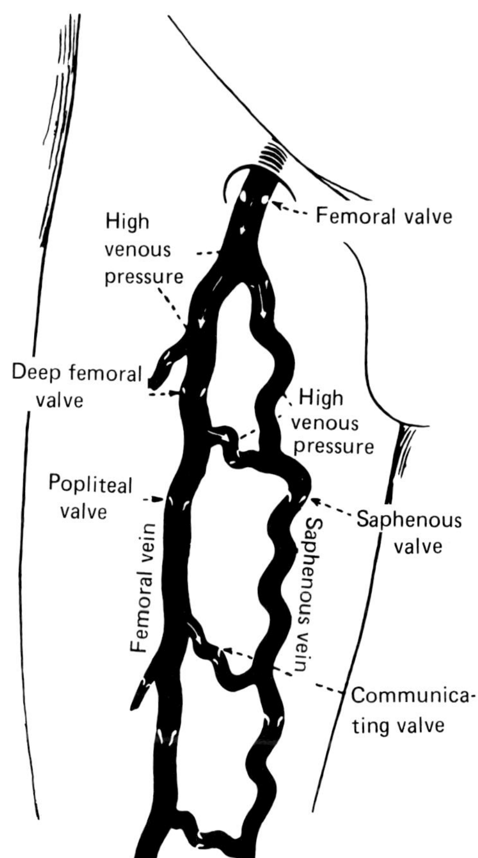

Figure 2   In this diagram, the only valve in the common femoral vein is incompetent. The high intra-abdominal pressure is transmitted directly to the long saphenous and superficial femoral veins, rendering them incompetent also. Doppler examination with a Valsalva maneuver will demonstrate a loud and prolonged reflux that can be heard down the saphenous vein as far distally as the lower leg. (From De Takats G (Ed): Venous insufficiency of the lower extremities. In: Vascular Surgery. Philadelphia, WB Saunders, 1959, p. 338, used with permission.)

Importance of Establishing the Diagnosis of the Clinical Type of Varicose Veins

Dilated venous trunks on the surface of the skin could indicate one or more of several different pathologic entities. Treatment of the problem varies considerably, depending on the etiology and magnitude of the clinical manifestations, type of varicose veins present, and the general condition of the patient. The clinical types of venous problems seen most often are as follows:

1. Congenital, essential, familial, or primary varicose veins are all terms being used for the same problem, namely, varicose veins that appear early in life, sometimes during childhood, and that are usually present in one or more members of the family.
2. Acquired, secondary, or postphlebitic varicose veins are the late consequences of an episode of thrombophlebitis. The clinical manifestations of these sequelae are usually severe and vary widely, depending primarily on the extent and location of the initial damage to the valvular mechanism of the deep and/or superficial venous systems and the degree of incompetence of the perforating or communicating systems (Fig. 3).
3. There are congenital anomalies of the venous system with or without arteriovenous (A-V) fistulae. Klippel-Trenaunay syndrome is the typical example of patients with congenital venous anomalies without obvious A-V fistulae (Fig. 4). Patients with this syndrome have congenital varicose veins, cutaneous hemangiomas, and hypertrophy of soft tissue and bone with overgrowth of the extremity (13). This type of venous malformation should not be confused with the Parkes Weber syndrome (14,15), wherein the major pathologic difference seems to be the presence of A-V fistulae.
4. In acquired, iatrogenic, or traumatic A-V fistulae, varicose veins are secondary to the venous hypertension occurring on the venous side of an A-V communication. The hemodynamic effects on the venous system depend, to a great extent, on the location, size, and the duration of the abnormal A-V communication.
5. Venous stars, spiders, telangiectases, venous lakes, and venules are all ordinary small veins in the skin that are present wherever there is elevation in venous pressure and stasis. They appear especially in women on the medial, posterior, and lateral aspects of the thigh and less often in the lower leg and calf. These type of blemishes have a striking familial tendency.

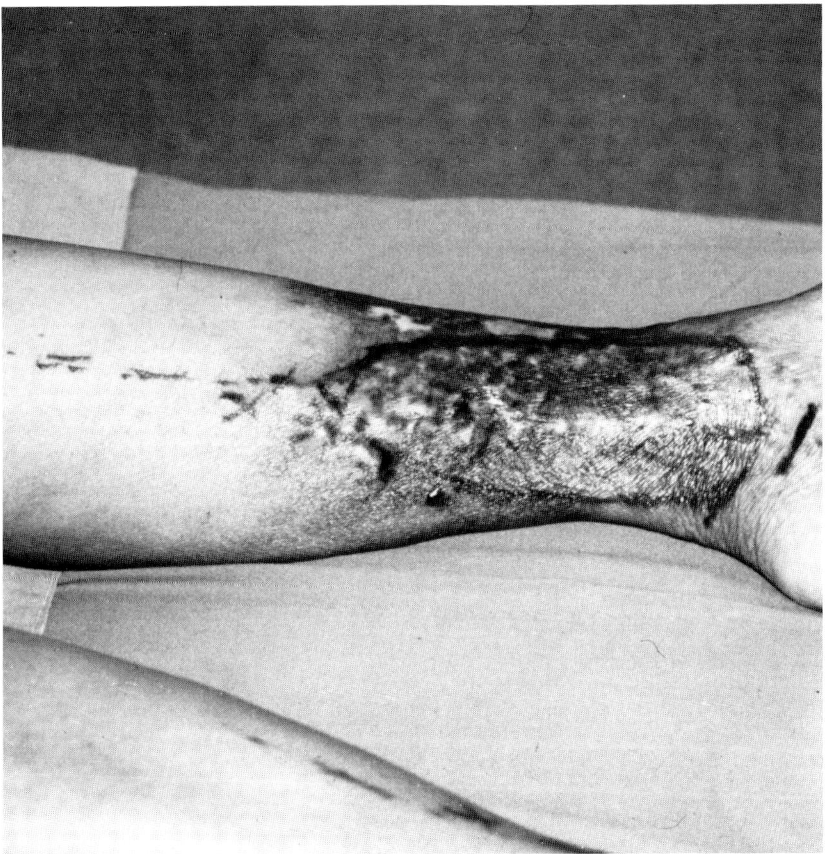

Figure 3 The devastating sequelae of an old deep venous thrombosis are
illustrated. Edema, dermatis, hyperpigmentation, and induration are part
of the incapacitating postphlebitic syndrome. These changes appear 2 to 30
years after the acute episode of venous thrombosis. In the final stages, painful ulceration complicates the clinical picture and is closely related to the
extensive damage to the valvular mechanism.

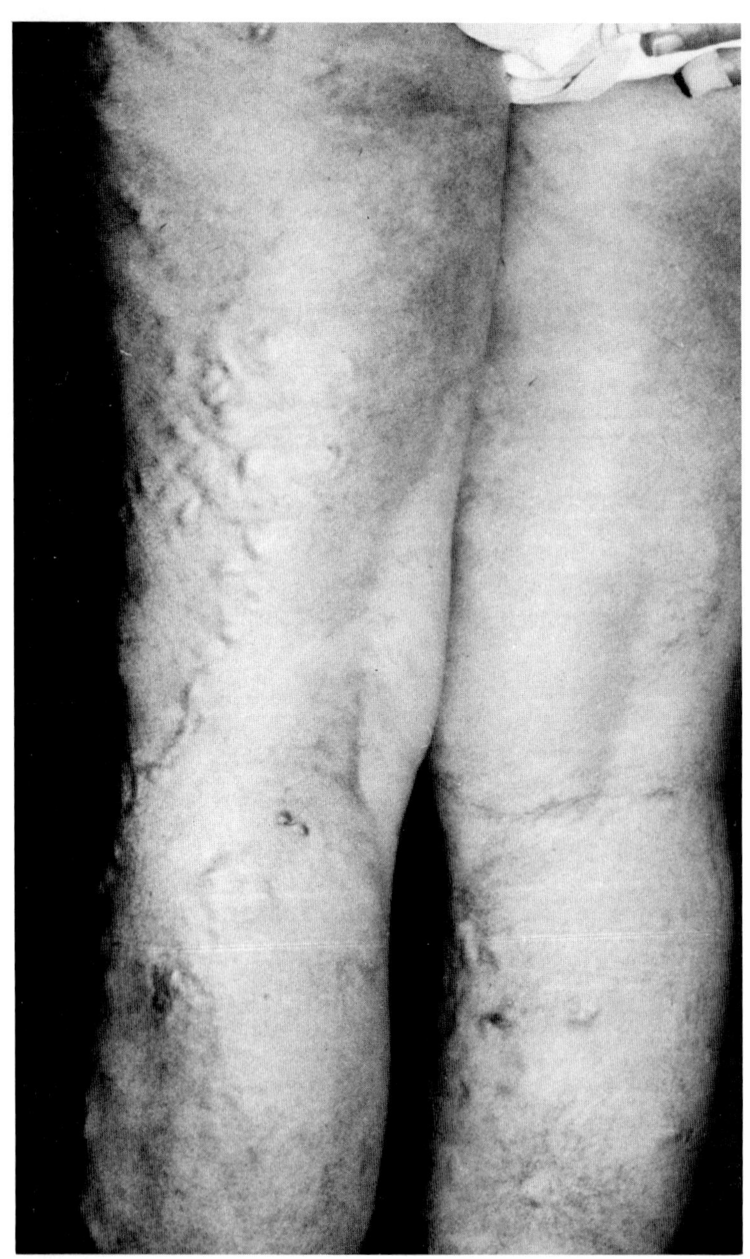

Figure 4

Each of the clinical types of varicose veins described has a distinct and specific type of treatment. Recurrences may occur if a patient with post-phlebitic syndrome is treated as if it were a case of primary varicose veins. Brunner (16) described recurrent varicose veins in a patient who had a mild unrecognized case of Klippel-Trenaunay syndrome. Varicose veins are certain to recur after surgery if they are secondary to unrecognized AV-fistulae, either congenital or acquired.

The Progressive and Irreversible Natural Course of Untreated Varicose Veins

The progressive nature of varicose veins deserves to be emphasized, and constitutes the basis for recommending periodic surveillance of patients with venous disorders. Recurrent varicose veins may appear in other territories after an apparently successful treatment, when a new source of venous hypertension appears or becomes enlarged as a consequence of pregnancy or advanced age. Veins that become varicose will continue to grow slowly as long as a source of venous hypertension is present. This source should be eliminated either by surgery or sclerotherapy. The only instance of spontaneous regression of varicose veins occurs in some pregnant women after delivery. Subsequent pregnancies may produce permanent damage to the valvular mechanism.

The Deleterious Effect of Thrombosis on the Valvular Mechanism

In 1917, Homans published his work on thrombosis of the deep veins of the lower limbs and established that recanalization with valve destruction was a common occurrence after an episode of deep venous thrombosis, and that skin changes of the leg, including ulceration, were closely related to the thrombotic episode. It is now common knowledge that more than 50% of patients with ulcers of the legs have had a previous history of deep venous

---

Figure 4   Young woman with bilateral Klippel-Trenaunay syndrome. This distressing congenital anomaly of the venous sytem is a challenging problem. The patient has extensive venous dilatations on the lateral aspect of the legs, port wine hemangioma, increased soft tissue growth, and stenotic areas in the deep venous system.

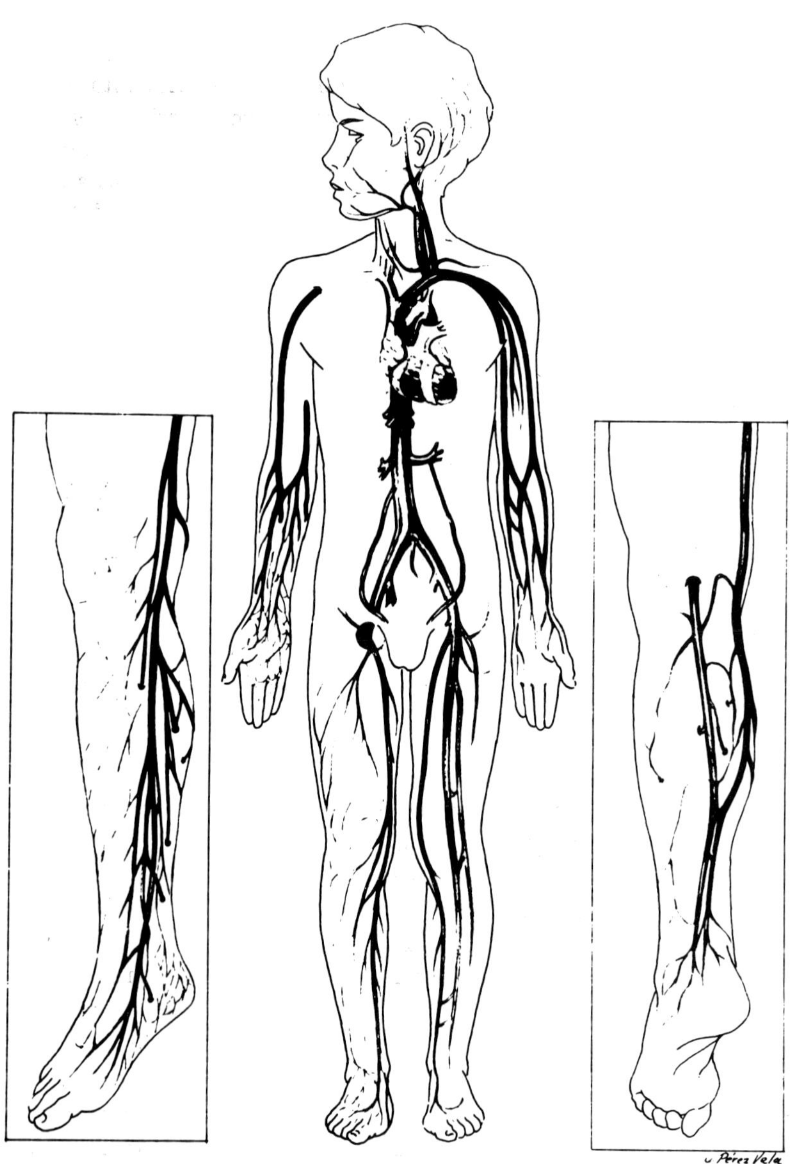

Figure 5 Artist's rendering of the anatomy of the venous system. The superficial venous system is illustrated in the two lateral drawings. In the central illustration, the superficial system has been drawn on the right side of the body and the deep system on the left. Note the multiple perforating veins in the lower extremities and the communications between the short and the long saphenous veins in the posteromedial aspect of the leg.

thrombosis. The unpredictable course and location of the venous thrombi, with the subsequent damage to the valves of the different venous territories involved by the phlebitic process, explain the widespread areas of venous hypertension observed in patients with the postphlebitic syndrome.

These type of patients constitute a challenge because it is quite difficult to locate with accuracy every site of venous hypertension present in an extremity. A missed perforator, no matter what size, will eventually be a source of recurrence.

The Importance of a Thorough Knowledge of the Surgical Anatomy, Physiology, and Pathophysiology of the Venous System

The anatomy of the venous system differs from the anatomy of the arterial system basically in the relatively large incidence of variations. There are multiple variations of a basic anatomic pattern in the venous system. This contributes to the rich and varied clinical distribution of the lesions in patients afflicted with venous insufficiency. The physician caring for patients with venous disorders needs to have a thorough knowledge of the anatomy of the venous system (Fig. 5). This is particularly true in the case of the surgeon. He or she should be aware of the possibility of duplication of the greater saphenous vein, the presence of constant communicating veins at the level of the medial aspect of the thigh (17), as well as in the inner and lateral aspects of the distal third of the leg. The surgeon also should be familiar with the anatomic variations of the short or lesser saphenous vein, whose importance in recurrent varicose veins has been well recognized by our group and other investigators (18-21). The widespread use of the Doppler examination and the availability of phlebography have contributed a great deal to the better understanding of venous disorders. The interpretation of the information provided by these methods, however, requires a thorough knowledge of the physiology and pathophysiology of the venous circulation.

Incidence

It has been stated that "no combination of methods is proof against recurrence" (22). This statement reflects the experience of a number of frustrated physicians who deal with a disease the inherent trait for recurrence and refractory nature of which are borne out by the many different methods of treatment described.

Puncturing (23), ligation, and ligation and division of the saphenous vein in the thigh (24-26) have been some of the methods performed during the past few centuries. In modern times, surgical techniques carefully tailored for each type of venous problem, either alone or supplemented with sclerotherapy have provided lasting relief to a high percentage of patients. It is unfortunate, as Dodd and Cockett (7) stated, that a widespread concept exists that the surgeon may choose one of two treatments for varicose veins: surgery or sclerotherapy. Surgery of the veins is not the favorite procedure for many vascular and general surgeons. Sclerotherapy is an excellent alternative method of treatment. It has, however, very definite and limited indications. There is a happy medium, and the methods can and should be used to complement one another to give the patient lasting relief. It has been generally accepted that surgery is the best type of treatment for varicose veins. The use of sclerotherapy has been the center of controversies from two groups of advocates. On one side are physicians who use the method as the only type of treatment for varicose veins of all sizes and etiologies. On the other side is a group of investigators who believe that sclerotherapy is a method with definite indications but limited applications in this field.

The incidence of recurrences varies with each method. In an effort to elucidate the real place of sclerotherapy and surgery in the management of these problems, Hobbs (27) carried out a random trial of the treatment of varicose veins by surgery and sclerotherapy at St. Mary's Hospital in London. He treated 404 legs by injections and 275 legs by surgery, and followed up his patients during a 6 year period. At the end of the sixth year, fewer than 10% of the injected legs were cured (an incidence of recurrence of more than 90%). Of the patients treated by surgery, 84% were cured or improved when the proximal vein was incompetent; there was an even higher incidence of cure and improvement when the proximal vein was competent. In the remainder of this chapter, we will refer only to recurrences secondary to surgery for primary or essential varicose veins.

The reported incidence of recurrences after surgical procedures for essential varicose veins varies widely among different authors. It is difficult to assess the true incidence of recurrences of a procedure that has as many variants in pathophysiology, clinical presentation, and surgical techniques as there are individual surgeons. The surgical literature contains a considerable number of references in regard to the incidence, diagnosis, and management of recurrent varicose veins. In Table 1, we have analyzed the incidence of recurrences after surgical treatment for essential varicose veins as reported by several authors. The figures range from 0.53% at 32 years reported by Frileux and colleagues (28) to 40% in the series of Doran and Barkat (29). The latter found that defective operation techniques and diagnostic studies

Table 1   Recurrent Varicose Veins (Essential) After Surgical Treatment

Author	No. of Cases	Follow-Up Period (Years)	% Recurrences
Doran (29)	662		40%
Larson (30)	1000	10	15%
Lofgren[a] (31)	440	20	32%
Frileaux (28)	6000	32	0.53%
Elbaz (32)	2129	12	5.12%
Villavicencio (21)	1000	2-8	4.8-11%
Villavicencio[b] (33)	534	8-20	13-17%
Hobbs	275	6	14-16%

[a]Patients of the same group reported by Larson but followed up for 20 years.
[b]Patients of the same group reported earlier, who had a 20 year follow-up. Patients operated on by unsupervised residents had a 17% recurrence rate. When residents were supervised or patients were operated on by senior staff, the recurrence rate was 13% during the same period.

were the most common causes of recurrence. At the Mayo Clinic, Larson and co-workers (30) evaluated 1000 consecutive patients 10 years after the operation. There were 656 patients who were evaluated by a letter questionnaire and 278 who returned for an examination. In the letter questionnaire, 86% of patients considered the results were good to excellent. Of the 278 examined at the Mayo Clinic, 85% were judged to be in good to excellent condition by someone who did not do the operation. Fifteen percent of the patients had varices of such magnitude that surgery was advised. Some patients of this same group were similarly studied 20 or more years after the operation (31). Sixty-three percent of 440 patients who responded to the questionnaire considered the results to be good to excellent. Of these, 140 were examined at the Mayo Clinic; 32% had varices of surgical significance.

In 1982, Frileux and colleagues (28) reported the results of the large experience of his group. Among 6000 patients operated on, 35% had had sclerotherapy as the only treatment, and all of them recurred. He considered that sclerotherapy alone is not a definitive treatment for valvular insufficiency. Among the 6000 patients submitted to surgery, 51 (0.53%) were recurrences operated on by Frileux's group between 1949 and 1981. There were 281 recurrences in patients operated on elsewhere. It is of interest that in 96% of his series of recurrences, the lesser saphenous system had been neglected.

In 1982, Elbaz (32) reported his experience with 109 recurrences among 2129 patients operated on and followed up for 12 years. He stressed the importance of the perforators as a source of recurrences. Approximately 50% of a group of patients suffering from recurrent varicose veins observed from 1977 to 1981 had incompetent perforators in the lower leg ("Cockett perforators") or at the upper third of the leg (32).

The incidence of recurrent varicose veins in our series of 1000 cases followed up from 1962 to 1971 was reported earlier (33). The highest incidence (11%) of recurrences corresponded to patients operated on by residents without senior supervision. The incidence (4.8%) of recurrences in the series of patients operated on by the senior staff or by residents under supervision was significantly lower. An updated 20 year follow-up of 534 of these same patients was carried out in 1982 through questionnaires or by direct examination of the patient. The results are summarized in Table 1. It can be observed that the incidence of recurrences was 17% in patients operated on by residents without senior supervision, and 13% in patients operated on by senior staff or adequately supervised residents. The importance and significance of these findings and other educational factors will be discussed later.

In a series of 275 patients, reported by Hobbs (27) and followed up for a period of 6 years, there was an incidence of recurrences of 16% when the proximal vein was incompetent (saphenofemoral or saphenopopliteal junctions), and an even lower incidence when the proximal vein was competent.

Etiology

Some of the factors involved in the recurrence of varicose veins have already been discussed at the beginning of this chapter. Aside from the important and ever-present influence of gravity, which exerts its deleterious effects on all two-legged, erect-walking human animals, there are other well identified causes for recurrence of varicose veins in an apparently well operated patient. They can be summarized as follows:

1. Incomplete identification of incompetent territories.
2. Wrong operation for the type of varicose veins.
3. Defective surgical technique.

Incomplete Identification of Incompetent Territories

This is an error in physical examination. It may become apparent as early as
during the first week after surgery in those cases of grossly missed perforators
or, most often, during the first 4 years of the postoperative period. In only a
few areas of surgery can one see so clearly, the results of a careful and pain-
staking preoperative examination, as in the field of venous surgery. Good
results are usually the results of good surgery!
   Recurrences occur most frequently in the following sites:

1. Site of incompetent perforating veins. Incompetent perforators may be
    present in any place of the limb. The most common places for recur-
    rences, however, are the perforators in the perimalleolar area and distal
    two-thirds of the leg on its medial aspect (Cockett perforators). Other
    less frequent sites for recurrence are the lateral ankle perforators and
    the adductor canal communicating veins.
2. The saphenopopliteal junction and posterior calf perforators (gastroc-
    nemius and soleus veins).
3. The saphenofemoral junction and its tributaries.
4. The venous tributaries of the internal iliac vein (varices of the vulva and
    inner and posterior aspects of the proximal thigh).

Site of Incompetent Perforating Veins

Recurrences always occur at the site of communication between the deep and
superficial systems. In these places, the normal direction of venous blood
flow, which is from the superficial to the deep system, is pathologically
reversed. This high pressure leak may occur in one or more perforating veins.
The severity of symptoms of venous insufficiency is in direct proportion to
the number and size of the incompetent perforators. A relatively large
number of incompetent perforating veins are present in cases of postphlebitic
syndrome, and are responsible for the widespread damage to the adjacent
superficial circulation and tissues submitted to constant and severe venous
hypertension.
   Significant incompetent perforating veins were found in 29% of 82 patients
with recurrent varicose veins (34), and were the most frequent cause of recurrences in another series of 662 patients (29).
   Incompetent perforators were present in nearly 50% of Elbaz's patients
(32) (Table 1), in a 6.7% of 90 cases of recurrent varicose veins studied by

Gedeon and co-workers (35), and in 40% of a series of 157 patients examined by Rettori (17). In Rettori's cases, recurrences appeared most frequently in the territory of the long Hunterian communicating veins of the thigh (17). Incompetent perforators were the most significant cause of recurrences in our series. They accounted for 33% of the total number of recurrences analyzed (Table 1).

Comment

From the analysis of the reported data, we may conclude that incompetent perforators play a significant role in the development of recurrent varicose veins. The exact localization of a perforator is not an easy task. It requires experience and a good knowledge of the anatomic location of the main perforators of the limb. It stands to reason that leaving this task to the un-experienced member of the staff is an open invitation to recurrence.

Localization of incompetent perforators can be accomplished by one or more of the following methods:

Careful inspection.   Areas of pigmentation, capillary dilatation, and bulging veins are often associated with the presence of an incompetent perforator. One should look carefully for these signs of venous hypertension.

Palpation of the fascial defect produced by the "perforating" vein. This method, often called the "sliding finger method," requires experience, knowledge of the anatomic location of the perforating veins, and a suitable patient. Patients with thick or fatty legs give a higher incidence of errors than thin, muscular patients.

To locate the perforating veins with this method, the patient must be lying in the supine position for the identification of the medial ankle and thigh perforators, and in the prone position to locate the posterior and lateral calf perforators. To facilitate "sliding" of the finger, we apply a thin layer of aqueous transmitting gel (Doppler gel) on the skin, and elevate the leg to produce emptying of the veins. A depression is clearly felt by the examining finger whenever a fascial defect is encountered. It is wise to perform this study after marking the varicose veins to avoid mistaking a large empty vein for a fascial defect. It is well known that varicose veins of long-standing may leave a depression in the subcutaneous tissue, which is easily palpable on elevation of the leg. This method has a 60% mean incidence of success, but it can be as high as 85% in thin individuals examined by experienced hands (36).

Doppler ultrasonic flowmeter. Introduction of the Doppler ultrasound method for detecting blood flow transcutaneously (37,38) has been a remarkable step forward in the diagnosis of vascular disorders. In experienced hands, Doppler ultrasound has been shown to be very accurate in the diagnosis of the diseases of the venous sytem (39). There are two basic methods of recognizing incompetence of the valvular system. In the first one, the patient performs a Valsalva maneuver. If the veins proximal to the site of the probe are incompetent, a Valsalva maneuver will cause blood to rush in a retrograde manner from the abdomen toward the probe. This response is easily observed at the saphenofemoral junction and at the level of the common femoral vein. A loud and prolonged surge of blood will be heard in cases of valve incompetence at the saphenofemoral junction. The reflux can be heard down the saphenous vein as far distally as the lower leg.

Another method consists of compression of the leg above the probe. A light tourniquet should be placed proximal to the probe site to prevent reflux from the superficial system. The patient should be supine. If the perforator's valve is incompetent, a surge of blood will be heard. When compression is released, blood returns quickly up the leg, producing a to-and-fro sound. In this manner, the entire leg can be mapped, and the suspected perforator sites carefully marked. A comparison of the degree of success obtained by different investigators in the localization of incompetent perforators with the methods of palpation and Doppler examination is summarized in Table 2. The results were compared with the findings reported at the time of surgery. Careful Doppler examination was better than palpation in the hands of most investigators. A combination of diagnostic methods may produce better results. There are some patients in whom palpation cannot be performed in a satisfactory manner. These are patients with thick legs and soft tissue induration. Doppler and phlebography and/or varicography should be the methods of choice.

Thermography and fluorescence venography are two other methods that have been used mostly by European investigators (40,41) in the search for incompetent perforators. The success rates reported for thermography range from 39 to 94%, and for fluoresceine from 16 to 94%. There is little experience with these methods in the United States.

Phlebography and varicography. Ideally, every patient with recurrent varicose veins should submit to phlebography. Ascending phlebography is a good method to assess the deep venous system and detect incompetent perforators. The presence of contrast material in the superficial system, after an injection has filled the deep system, is evidence of retrograde flow and incompetence. The addition of the Valsalva maneuver to ascending phlebography has been reported by Hach (42). This author (42) stated that this technique allows the visualization of varicosities and the differentiation between true recurrent varicose veins and residual varices.

Varicography has been shown to be more accurate than ascending phlebography in detecting incompetent perforating veins in the calf and, especially, incompetent gastrocnemius veins. In the thigh, direct injection of dye under fluoroscopic control into a prominent varicosity has been highly successful in demonstrating the extent and communications of the varicose veins (43, 44).

In patients with recurrent varicose veins, we recommend the use of all the methods just described. Doppler ultrasound investigation should confirm the clinical examination, and the findings should be compared with the findings of phlebography and/or varicography.

The Saphenopopliteal Junction and Posterior Calf Perforators

In most of the reported series of recurrent varicose veins, the short saphenous vein territory appears to be an important source of recurrences. In Lofgren's series (34), the distal saphenous vein was dilated and incompetent in 39 of 136 extremities. Frileux and colleagues (28) found that in 96% of their cases, the short saphenous vein had been "neglected." In 90 cases of recurrent varicose veins studied by Gedeon and co-workers (35), the short saphenous vein was responsible for 33.3% of the recurrences. Davy and Ouvry (45) reported that among 1341 patients who had short saphenous stripping, there were a 16% recurrence rate when stripping had been performed in a systematic manner (routine stripping of short saphenous vein) and a 5% recurrence rate when the stripping was done selectively (only where incompetence was present). There were 34 short saphenous recurrences among 212 cases of recurrent varicosities reported by Devambez and associates (46). The latter authors recommended routine use of Doppler and phlebography in cases of recurrences. One of the reasons for the high recurrence rate in the short saphenous vein territory is the wide variation in the pattern and level of the saphenopopliteal junction. This variability has been well documented by several investigators (18,19,20,47). In our experience, the anatomic variations of the short saphenous vein and especially the communications with an incompetent long saphenous vein in its distal two-thirds have been responsible for 12% of the recurrences. In these cases, the saphenopopliteal junction may be competent, but the distal two-thirds of the vein becomes incompetent through its communications with an incompetent long saphenous vein and/or a large gastrocnemius perforator. Recognizing the difficulties involved in the precise localization of the saphenopopliteal junction, some investigators (48,49) have recommended the routine use of peroperative phlebography to localize the junction and other variations that could be of importance for the surgeon. This method has been found to be very useful in the identification of incompetent calf perforators.

Comment

It is clear that the short saphenous vein has been the source of an important percentage of recurrences in most of the series reported. Therefore, surgeons should make every effort to ensure accurate localization and division of the saphenopopliteal junction and posterior calf perforators. Together with a good clinical assessment of the extent of incompetence of the short sapehnous vein and its communicating veins, careful Doppler examination and perioperative phlebography should be performed in every case of incompetence of the short saphenous territory. We have not performed routine perioperative phlebography during the primary operation. However, we are convinced of its usefulness and recommend its use in every case of recurrent short saphenous varicosities. We have used a sterile Doppler probe to identify incompetence of the saphenopopliteal and saphenofemoral junctions in the intraoperative period (Fig. 6). With the Doppler probe accurately placed over the saphenous vein just distal to its junction with the femoral or popliteal vein, a Valsalva maneuver is elicited to test for incompetence of the saphenofemoral junction. A short compression of the thigh proximal to the probe will produce an audible reflux down the short saphenous vein in the cases of incompetence. Another useful intraoperative maneuver to identify incompetence of the saphenopopliteal junction is the compression of the distal calf with the probe over the proximal short saphenous vein. A to-and-fro sound is evidence of incompetence (this sound has a similar hemodynamic pathophysiology as the systolic-diastolic murmurs heard in cases of incompetence of the cardiac valves).

The Saphenofemoral Junction and Its Tributaries

The saphenofemoral junction, unlike the saphenopopliteal junction, has fairly constant anatomic relationships (Fig. 7). It is located at the groin, medial to the femoral artery, and about 2.5 cm lateral and below the pubic tubercle. At this level, there are several terminal tributaries of the saphenous vein that are of surgical importance. They are the superficial and deep external pudendal veins (the deep pudendal veins are more often found as direct tributaries of the femoral vein or the saphenofemoral junction), the

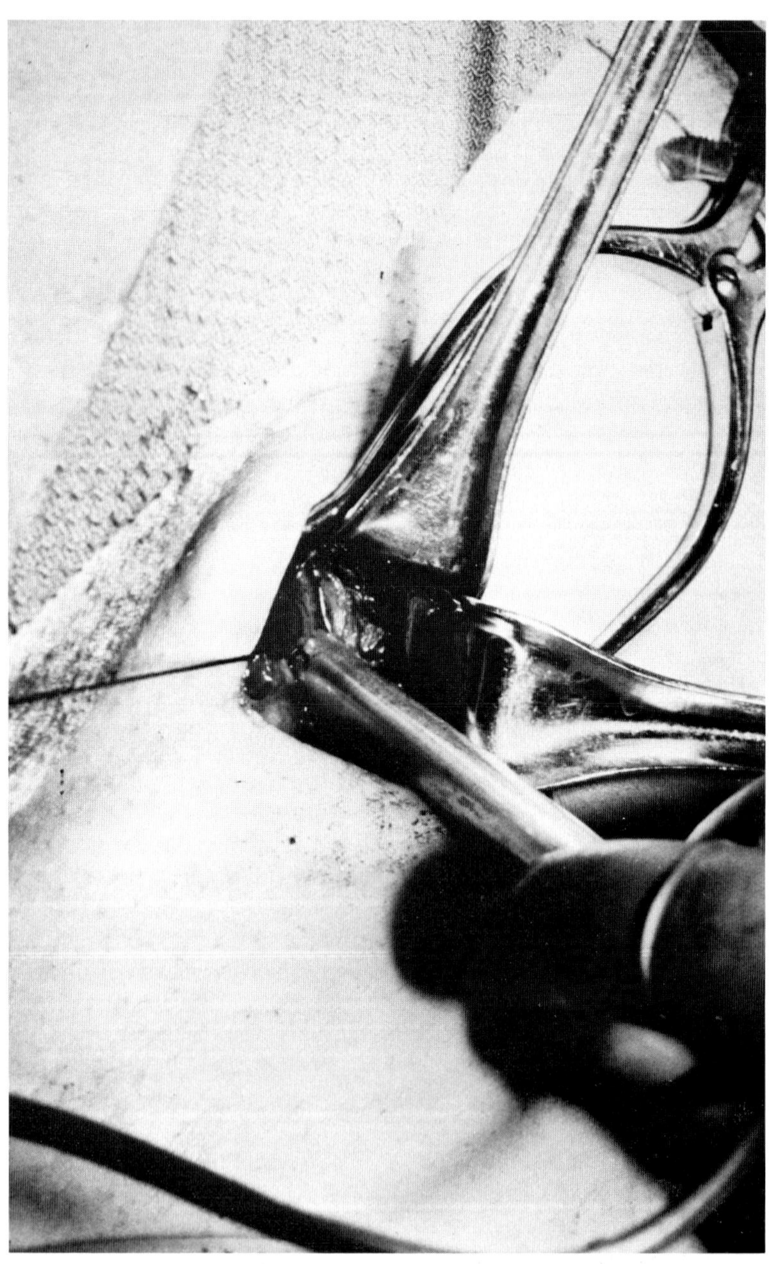

Figure 6

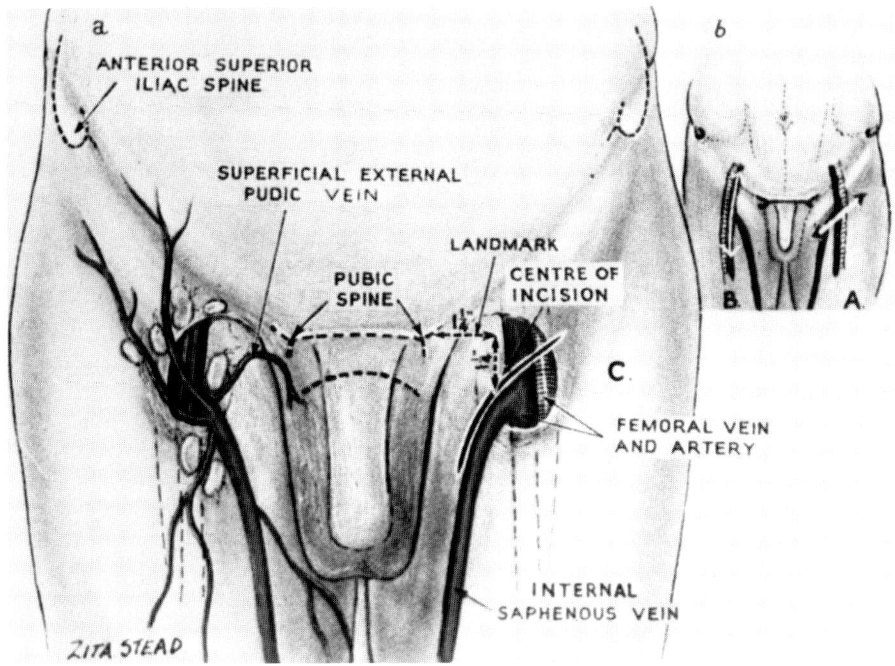

Figure 7 The saphenofemoral junction and its tributaries. The saphenofemoral junction has fairly constant anatomic relationships. It is located 2.5 cm lateral and below the pubic spine, medial to the femoral artery. This bony reference is very useful in obese patients. Inadequate ligation of the saphenous vein at the saphenofemoral junction and failure to ligate tributaries of this region account for most of the recurrences reported. (From Dodd H, Cockett FB: Surgery of varicose veins in Dodd H, Cockett FB (Eds): Pathology and Surgery of the Veins of the Lower Limb. 2nd Edition. Edinburgh, London, New York, 1976, p. 117, used with permission.)

Figure 6 Diagnosis of incompetence of the saphenofemoral junction by intraoperative Doppler examination. A 9.1 MHz gas-sterilized Doppler probe is placed on the saphenous vein 2 to 3 cm distal to the saphenofemoral junction. A Valsalva maneuver will cause a loud surge of blood, which can be heard on the saphenous vein in cases of valvular incompetence. Investigation of competence of the femoral vein at different sites can give valuable hemodynamic information about valve competence. If no incompetence is detected, the saphenous vein is not stripped. Similar investigation can be performed at the saphenopopliteal junction.

275

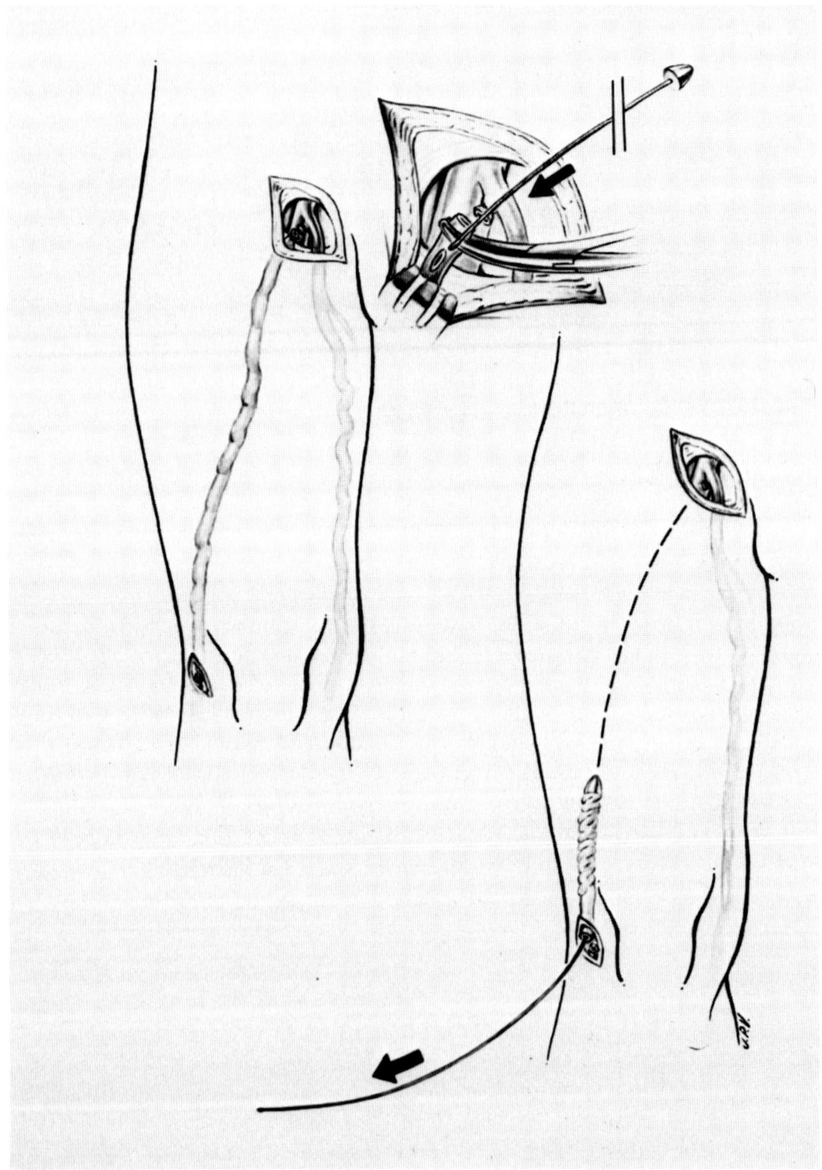

Figure 8

superficial epigastric vein, and the superficial circumflex iliac vein. These veins have considerable variations in their manner of termination in the saphenous vein. Two other tributaries of the saphenous vein at the groin are worth mentioning. One is the anterolateral tributary that drains into the main saphenous trunk 1 or 2 inches below the saphenofemoral junction and, in cases of incompetent saphenous vein, gives origin to large varices on the anterolateral aspect of the thigh (Fig. 8). The other is the posteromedial tributary that is formed by the vein of Giacomini at the level of the sapheno-popliteal junction and runs up and medially to join the long saphenous vein at the level of its upper third in the thigh. In about 15 to 20% of the cases, the short saphenous vein does not terminate at the popliteal vein, and drains into the long saphenous vein through the posteromedial tributary (18).

Inadequate or incomplete ligation of the saphenous vein at the sapheno-femoral junction and failure to ligate tributaries of the long saphenous vein account for most of the recurrences reported by Lofgren (34), Devambez and associates (46), Gedeon and co-workers (35), and many others. "Main channel stripping," leaving many tributaries untouched, was the procedure performed in many hospitals during the 1940s and 1950s. Strange as it may seem, and indeed, as a consequence of the lack of interest in the field of venous disorders, we continue seeing patients in our vascular clinics who have recurrent varicose veins secondary to a simple operation that was poorly performed.

Comment

Flush ligation at the saphenofemoral junction and complete excision of all incompetent and dilated tributaries of the long saphenous vein are the goal. Careful Doppler examination is especially useful in diagnosing incompetent saphenofemoral junction or residual connections between the recurrent varicose veins and a residual saphenous trunk. Occasionally, a duplication of the saphenous vein may be unrecognized and be the source of recurrences. In

---

Figure 8 Anterolateral tributary of the long saphenous vein. This drawing illustrates the large anterolateral tributary of the long saphenous vein, which is often responsible for large clusters of dilated veins over the anterior and lateral aspect of the thigh, knee, and upper third of leg. It drains into the saphenous vein about 4 cm distal to the saphenofemoral junction. A short stripper can usually be passed from the groin as far distally as the knee. If unrecognized, it is an importance source of recurrences.

STRIPPER A
S.E.V.
S.E.P.V.
S.E.P.ART.
S.C.I.V.
A.L.V.
INTERNAL
SAPHENOUS
VEIN
(DUPLICATED)
STRIPPER B
S.C.I.V.
S.E.V.
S.E.P.V.
ANT LAT
VEIN
INT
SAPHENOUS
VEIN
(DUPLICATED)
ANT
VEIN of the
LEG
POST ARCH
VEIN of the
LEG

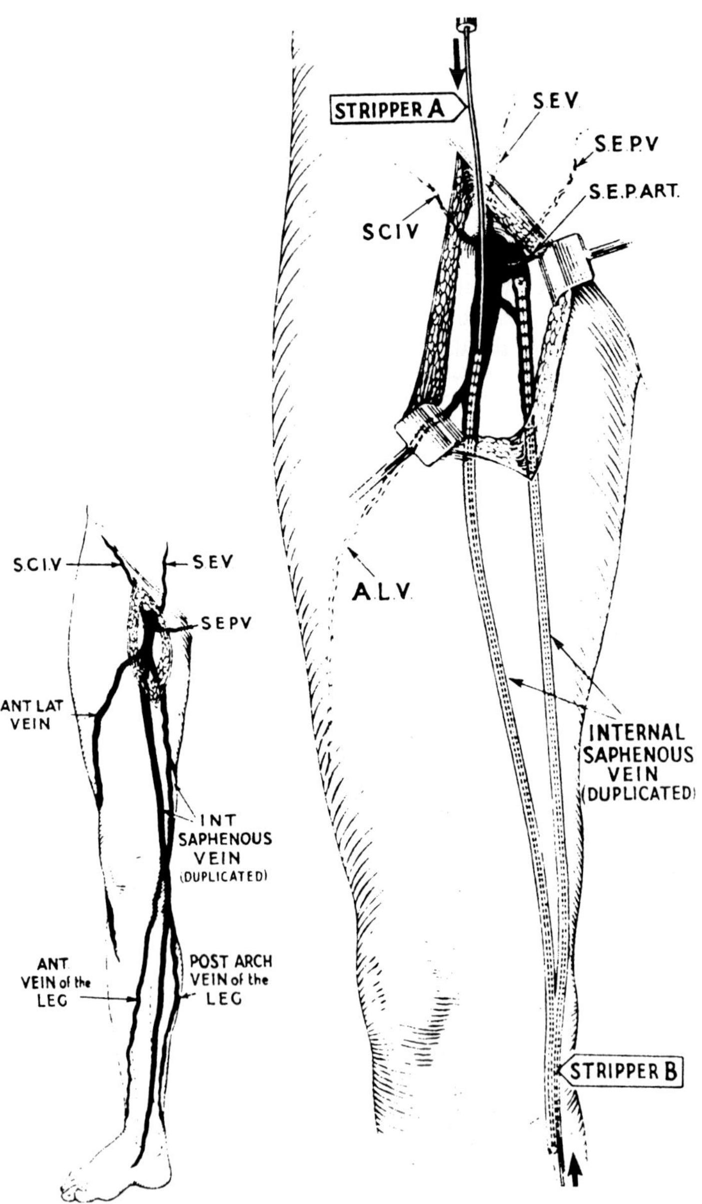

Figure 9

some of these cases, the posteromedial tributary may mimmick a true duplication of the long saphenous trunk (Fig. 9). After a thorough clinical and Doppler examination, varicography and/or ascending phlebography should be recommended for every case of recurrent varicose veins. Intraoperative Doppler studies as described in the previous section have been found very useful in diagnosing incompetence of the saphenous vein at the saphenofemoral junction. Stripping of the long saphenous vein should be performed in cases of overt saphenofemoral incompetence. Selective venous surgery is indicated when there are isolated segments of dilated, tortuous, and incompetent veins. In these cases, only the diseased segments are excised. The current trend to preserve the long saphenous vein for possible later use as an arterial substitute is not justified if the vein is diseased and there are varicosities due to incompetence of that territory. A diseased vein should not be used as a substitute conduit in the arterial system (50).

The Venous Tributaries of the Internal Iliac Vein

The internal pudendal, obturator, and gluteal veins are tributaries of the internal iliac vein and drain the venous territories of the buttocks, upper and medial aspect of the thigh, and perineum. Within the pelvis, the iliac vein is joined by the pelvic visceral veins (uterine veins). Of great interest is the communication of this system with the long saphenous vein through the deep external pudendal veins. They may dilate significantly, producing pelvic and vaginal varicose veins, which are observed in some women during and after pregnancy.

   Reflux from the internal iliac system through the gluteal, sciatic, and isquiatic veins produces varicosities on the posterior aspect of the thigh.

Figure 9 Duplication of the long saphenous vein. We have encountered this variation of the saphenous vein quite often in the course of femoropopliteal bypass surgery with autogenous vein. In cases of incompetence of the saphenofemoral junction, both segments of vein should be removed as shown in the drawing. The posteromedial tributary may drain into one of the two segments. This tributary should be recognized and removed since it may be a source of recurrence. (From Dodd H, Cockett FB: Operative treatment of varicose veins. In Dodd, H, Cockett FB (Eds): The Pathology and Surgery of the Veins of the Lower Limb. Edinburgh, London, E. & S. Livingstone Ltd, Baltimore, 1956, Williams and Wilkins Co. p. 242, used with permission.)

These veins often communicate with the femoral system (profunda femoris) through perforating veins on the back of the thigh.

Comment

Recognition of reflux in the territory of the internal iliac vein is important to avoid recurrences. Retrograde phlebography has been very useful to demonstrate reflux from the internal iliac vein into the thigh and labia. Doppler ultrasound has also been of assistance in identifying reflux into the vulval varices during the Valsalva maneuver. In these cases, retroperitoneal ligation of the veins responsible for the reflux has been utilized by our group with success.

Wrong Operation for the Type of Varicose Veins

Varicose veins will recur if the operation performed is not an adequate operation. We have described the five types of varicose veins that may be present clinically. Each one should be treated differently. Long saphenous stripping is erroneously performed as the only treatment in the postphlebitic syndrome. The recurrence rate is high in these cases. Patients with varices secondary to A-V malformations need embolization and/or resection of the A-V communications if permanent cure is desired (16). Reconstruction of an acquired or traumatic A-V fistula is mandatory in patients with venous hypertension and varicose veins after trauma to the vascular system and arteriovenous shunting. Patients with postphlebitic sequelae and multiple incompetent perforators, hyperpigmentation, edema, eczema, and ulcers need a very special type of surgical procedure to interrupt the leaking veins and heal the ulcers (Fig. 3). In these patients, recurrences develop if an important perforator is missed.

Comment

Patients with varicose veins need a thorough history and physical examination to establish an accurate diagnosis of the etiology of the problem. The non-invasive vascular laboratory, phlebography, and arteriography have contributed greatly to our ability to establish an accurate preoperative diagnosis.

Defective Surgical Technique

Failure to perform a flush ligation of the long or short saphenous veins at their point of junction with the femoral and popliteal veins, respectively, constitutes one of the most common technical errors in varicose vein surgery. Recurrences are bound to occur if the surgeon fails to ligate an incompetent perforating vein flush to its fascial orifice, especially if there is a tributary between the point of ligature and the point of entrance to the fascia. The best method to prevent recurrences is to perform a good operation the first time! Most technical errors occur because of a lack of familiarity with the anatomy and characteristics of the venous system.

The normal anatomy of the long saphenous vein at the saphenofemoral junction is depicted in Figure 7. Each one of the tributaries described should be identified and divided.

Because the anatomic pattern of termination of the tributaries of the long saphenous vein is variable, it is important to recognize that sometimes there are tributaries that drain directly into the femoral vein. Failure to expose the femoral vein above and below the saphenofemoral junction may lead to missing these veins and, thus, establishing the path for recurrences.

Mistaking a dilated posteromedial tributary for the trunk of the saphenous vein is another potential error leading to recurrences. The surgeon should be aware of this possibility and always identify this important tributary.

Flush ligation of the short saphenous vein is a difficult procedure because the termination of this vein is not constant. In only 42% of the cases does the short saphenous vein terminate at the level of the knee joint (18). Careful localization of the saphenopopliteal junction should always be attempted either by Doppler examination or perioperative phlebography. This allows for a well placed incision (48,49). We have found that the most common mistake performed during the surgical exploration of the short saphenous vein is to try to expose it with the patient in the supine position. It is practically impossible to visualize the junction in this position. About 50% of the patients with short saphenous varicosities have added incompetence of calf perforators that cannot be adequately operated on in the supine position.

Recurrent varicose veins of the short saphenous vein are illustrated in Figure 10A; this patient had been operated on twice before. The preoperative photograph shows the sites of previous incisions at the level of the knee joint and a few centimeters above. Preoperative ascending phlebography demonstrates a dilated segment of residual short saphenous vein and a very dilated posteromedial connection, with the long saphenous vein originating from the popliteal vein a few millimeters above the saphenopopliteal junction (Fig. 10B). Incompetent midcalf perforators complicated the clinical picture.

Management of Recurrent Varicose Veins

Not all recurrent varicose veins need to be operated on. As stated previously, sclerotherapy is an excellent alternative method of treatment. It has, how-

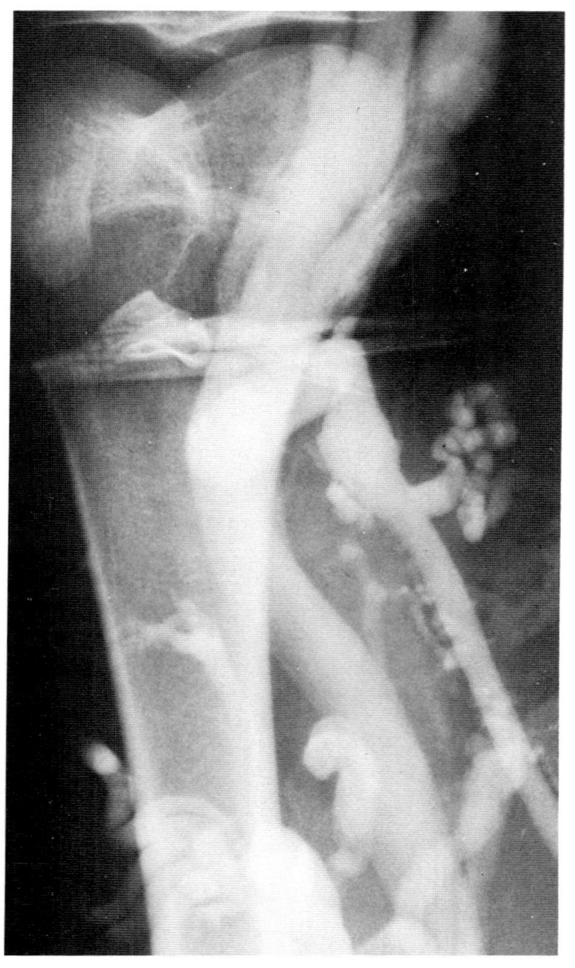

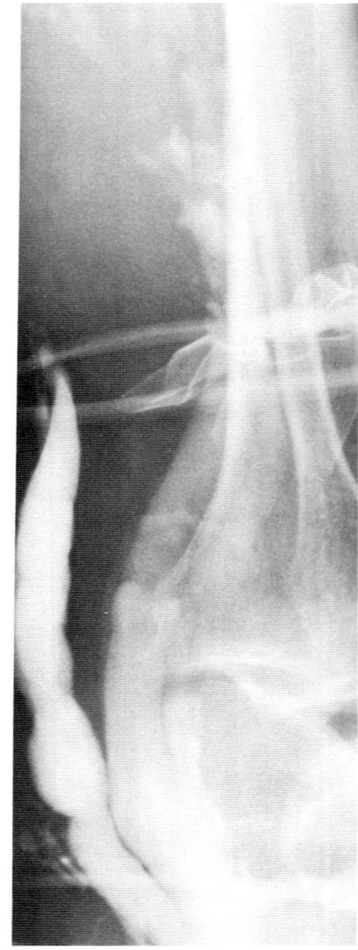

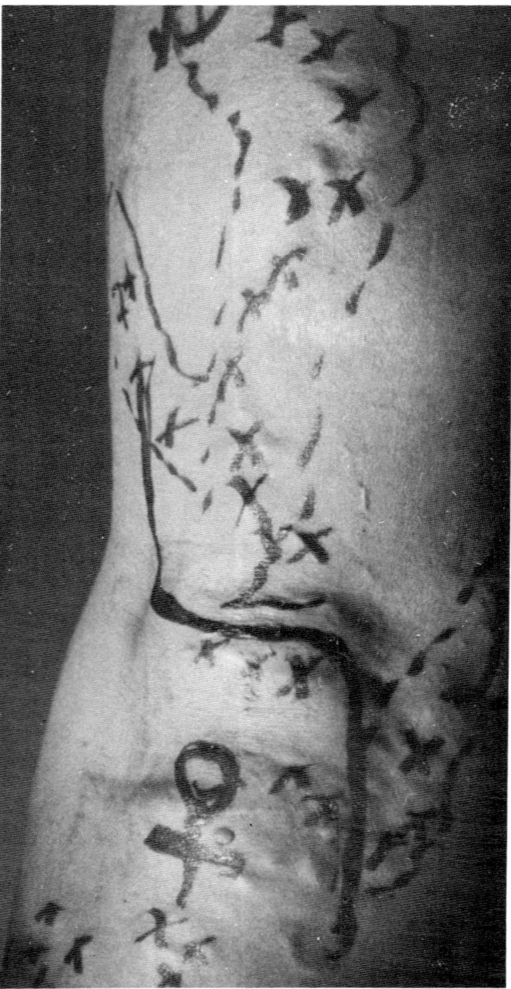

B

ever, very definite and limited indications. Mild recurrences in older people may be best treated with sclerotherapy and other nonoperative measures such as elevation of the extremities, daily wash with a mild soap and water, skin lubrication, and good elastic support. There are, however, many distressed patients who have had from one to four operations for varicose veins and still come back with a leg that seems to be worse than ever. These patients need to be carefully evaluated and reoperated on.

Reoperation may be limited to a single perforator that can be removed through one or more small incisions, often under local analgesia as an office procedure, or it may require a formal operation, which requires hospital admission. We will refer to the latter.

Preoperative Evaluation

On the patient's initial visit to the clinic, a comprehensive clinical history and physical examination should be done. A good history often provides the physician with a presumptive diagnosis. Every effort should be made to establish an accurate diagnosis because the surgical technique will vary according to the etiology of the varicosities. It should be determined whether the problem is congenital (essential or primary) or acquired (secondary). If it was noticed during the first years of life, we may think about a whole group of diseases that are characteristically congenital (e.g. A-V malformations or other vascular anomalies, hemangiomas, and primary

---

Figure 10 *A*: Preoperative photography of patient with recurrent short saphenous varices. This patient had been operated on twice before for recurrences at the popliteal fossa. A loud reflux could be easily heard from with the Doppler probe 5 cm above the knee line. There was associated incompetence of posterior calf perforators (Gastrocnemius). A "Z" incision offered excellent exposure of sapheno-popliteal junction and a large communicating vein between the short and the long saphenous veins in the thigh. *B*: Preoperative ascending phlebography, lateral view. A long segment of incompetent short saphenous trunk and saphenopopliteal junction are clearly observed on the left. On the right, a large incompetent vein of Giacomini communicated the short saphenous system with the upper third of the long saphenous vein in the thigh. It can be seen just above the sapenopopliteal junction. This vein was responsible for large clusters of varicose veins in the thigh.

varicose veins). Often the history reveals that the mother, father, or other members of the family have had varicose veins.

If the problem appeared later, one should inquire about trauma, infectious process, previous history of operations, and invasive studies. All of these factors may produce venous thrombosis and, thus, the type of varicose veins may be secondary or postphlebitic. It is very important to try to rule out deep venous thrombosis since we have quite often seen patients with post-phlebitic legs who have had long saphenous stripping as if they had primary varicose veins. In these cases, recurrences are the rule.

Certain diseases have a specific affinity for the vascular endothelium, namely, rickettsiasis and salmonella. Patients with these diseases may apparently recover without signs or symptoms of venous thrombosis. Vein damage is discovered some time later (often several years) when a typical postphlebitic syndrome becomes evident.

Physical Examination

Physical examination will usually confirm the clinical impression obtained during the interview. The patient should be examined while standing on a firm examining table and under good illumination. We have found tangential illumination to be extremely valuable in demonstrating the varicose veins. The patient is asked to turn around gradually to observe the distribution of the recurrent veins. At this time, old surgical incisions are examined to note their anatomic position. A low incision at the groin, with varicose veins originating around the incision, may suggest a faulty saphenofemoral ligation; varicose veins around the medial aspect of the thigh may tip the examiner towards a missed Hunterian perforator. Recurrent veins located on the posterior and upper medial aspect of the thigh, especially if vulvar varices are present, strongly suggest incompetence of the tributaries of the internal iliac vein system.

Inspection of the short saphenous vein territory may reveal recurrent veins originating above a previous surgical scar or coming from a midcalf perforator (Fig. 10A). One should keep in mind that varicose veins distributed on the lower two-thirds of the posterior aspect of the calf are often the result of communications between an incompetent long saphenous vein and the distal short saphenous vein.

Recurrences originating at the medial or lateral aspects of the calf are the unmistakable sign of missed incompetent ankle perforators. At this level, the characteristic changes of hyperpigmentation, dilated venules, chronic edema, eczema, induration, and skin necrosis speak for themselves, relating to the often obscure history of an episode of deep venous thrombosis that occurred many years before (Fig. 3).

Palpation of the affected venous territories should be performed to detect the degree of venous hypertension and communications between the different venous trunks. Percussion (Schwartz test) of the proximal trunk may reveal incompetence when the impulse is felt over the distal territories. The best method of exploration is the combination of gentle proximal percussion and a Doppler probe placed over the distal veins. If a signal is heard distally, the diagnosis of incompetence of the venous segment located between the finger and Doppler probe, can be made with certainty. This method is particularly useful to identify communications between the different venous territories.

No operation should be performed if there is active inflammation or any evidence of infection in the extremity. Operation should be deferred until the leg is in the best condition. In patients with induration, eczema, cellulitis, and other sequelae of chronic venous insufficiency it may take several months of preparation before the skin and subcutaneous tissues can be improved enough to withstand successfully the surgical trauma. Waiting is worthwhile!

Noninvasive Vascular Examination

Great progress has been made in the field of noninvasive vascular diagnosis. In venous diseases, the most important noninvasive tests are phleborheography (PRG), photoplethysmography (PPG), light reflecting rheography (LRR), strain gauge or impedance phlethysmography (SPG and IPG), and Doppler ultrasound. All of these tests are useful in establishing the diagnosis of venous thrombosis and/or venous incompetence. Photoplethysmography has been especially useful in establishing the diagnosis between essential varicose veins and postphlebitic or secondary varicose veins (51-53).

Doppler ultrasound examination has been very valuable in the preoperative demonstration of the presence or absence of reflux at the saphenofemoral (SF) and saphenopopliteal junction (SP). In 110 consecutive patients preoperatively assessed for SF and SP reflux by Doppler ultrasound and compared with the findings at surgery, Hoare and Royle (49) found that Doppler ultrasound was superior to clinical assessment. Doppler ultrasound detected 100% (two false positives) of incompetent SF junctions and 100% of SP junctions (six false positives) as compared with the clinical detection of 72% (no false positives) and 64% (five false positives), respectively.

Saphenofemoral reflux is assessed in the standing position. A 4 MHz nondirectional ultrasound probe is placed over the saphenous vein and superficial femoral vein distal to SF junction. Saphenopopliteal reflux is assessed with the examiner behind the standing patient. The examined leg should be slightly flexed. Bearing of body weight should be on the opposite limb. Reflux is assessed by compressing the calf and then releasing it. Incompetence is diagnosed if reflux is heard during the release of distal calf compression provided that digital control of short saphenous vein abolishes reflux. If reflux is not abolished, incompetence of popliteal valves is diagnosed.

Confirmation of the presence or absence of reflux can be made at the time of surgery by observing free reflux of blood from the proximal end of the divided long or short saphenous vein 2 to 3 cm from its junction or by placing a sterile Doppler probe directly over the vein and eliciting a Valsalva maneuver as previously described in this chapter (Fig. 6). If there is no incompetence of the long or short saphenous veins, surgery is limited to excision of dilated varicose veins and division of incompetent perforators. Localization of incompetent perforators by palpation and Doppler ultrasound has been previously discussed (Table 2).

Table 2   Value of Palpation and Doppler Ultrasound in Diagnosing Incompetent Perforators

Author	Year	Palpation		Doppler	
		No. Legs	% Hits	No. Legs	% Hits
Knospe	1978	85	34	88	55
Myrhe	1971	20	35	20	95
O'Donnell	1977	39	60	39	62
Burnand	1975	32	53	32	67
Voori	1972	68	63	N/A	N/A
Miller	1974	N/A	N/A	30	89
Villavicencio (9)	1985	378	78	275	87

Source: Modified from Wienert V. Diagnosis of incompetent perforating veins: value of methods. In May R, Partsch H, Staubesand J (Eds): Perforating Veins. Munchen, Baltimore, Urban & Schwarzenberg, 1981, pp. 184-188, used with permission.

Phlebography and/or Varicography

Every patient with recurrent varicose veins should have ascending phlebography and/or varicography. The value of these methods in detecting incompetent perforators and revealing valuable anatomic information cannot be overemphasized. Ascending phlebography can only assess the status of the valve system in a very generalized fashion. Descending phlebography provides a means of identifying the physiologic status of the iliac and femoral vein valves and offers a means to assess venous insufficiency. Herman and co-workers (54) and Kistner (55) described details of interpretation and a grading reflux system. The findings, however, should be correlated with ascending phlebography and Doppler examination. Intraoperative phlebography should be used in cases of recurrent short saphenous varicosities. Varicography has been previously discussed in this chapter. It should be performed in case of complex problems to help clarify the origin of difficult areas of recurrence.

As soon as the decision to reoperate has been made, the patient should have routine blood and urine analysis, electrocardiogram, chest films, and any other examination that may be pertinent to complete the preoperative assessment.

Preoperative Marking

We are convinced that aside from an adequately technical performance of the operation, preoperative marking (Fig. 11) is the single most important technical step in varicose vein surgery. The examiner must have experience, skill, thorough knowledge of anatomy, physiology, and pathophysiology, and perform a careful physical and Doppler examination.

Inadequate preoperative marking is not usually listed as a causative factor in recurrent varicose veins. It stands to reason, however, that an improperly and carelessly marked extremity is an open invitation for recurrence.

Preoperative marking must conform to the following rules:

1. The patient must have had the extremity (or extremities) washed daily with an antiseptic soap and water for at least 3 days before surgery.
2. The extremity and pubis (if groin exploration is contemplated) should be carefully shaved before marking.
3. Marking should be done before the administration of any preanesthetic medication. Tracing the veins requires the patient to be standing on a

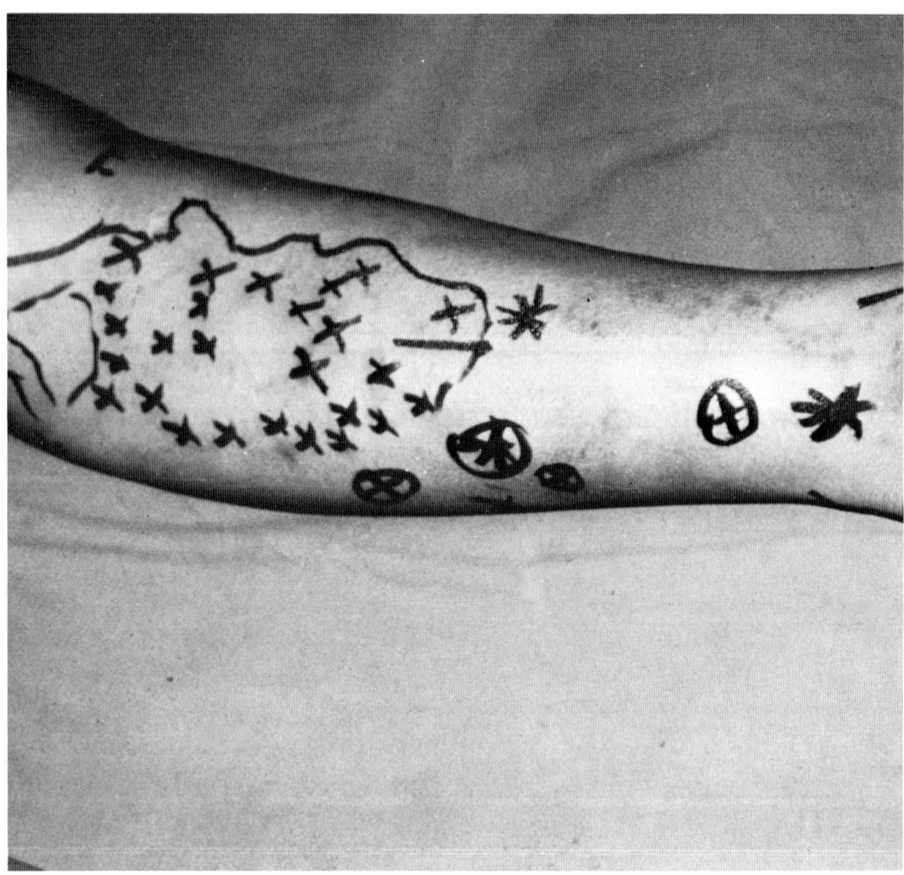

Figure 11 Preoperative marking. Aside from an adequate surgical technique, preoperative marking is the single most important technical step in surgery of varicose veins. Inadequate marking should be considered a causative factor in recurrent varicose veins. The surgeon who marked the patient should perform the operation.

platform under a good light (we employ tangential illumination) and completely awake. This is not possible if the patient is under the effects of a sedative. We have seen surgeons trying to mark the varicose veins on a patient who is half asleep and sitting up at the edge of the operating table. Marking and examining the patient under these circumstances should be condemned.

4. During the last 12 years, we have used a water-resistant black marker that can be purchased in any shop selling artist's supplies (Pantone). It does not come off during skin prepping.

5. After marking, the patient is advised to wear pajama pants and avoid direct contact of one extremity with the other since this may lead to ink smearing.

6. Each surgeon develops his or her own technique for marking, utilizing keys and clues and different signs and tracings to identify perforators and clusters of veins. For this reason, surgery must be performed by the surgeon who marked the patient! (In teaching centers, the senior surgeon must be present during marking and assist the resident or fellow with the operation.)

Anesthesia

Continuous epidural or spinal anesthesia has been our choice in more than 3000 procedures for venous insufficiency. This type of anesthesia has been utilized in 99% of our patients. General anesthesia with endotracheal intubation has been used extensively in other centers. We have only used general anesthesia when there is no surgery planned on the posterior aspect of the extremity, or in extremely apprehensive patients.

Technical Considerations

A reoperation for recurrent varicose veins is a surgical challenge. It should always be performed by experienced individuals or by residents or vascular fellows under senior supervision. Good surgical instruments are essential. The surgeon must have a complete assortment of instruments for vein surgery. Good instruments are the surgeon's most valuable asset (Fig. 12A and B).

There are three areas of recurrence that deserve special consideration:

1. Recurrences at the saphenofemoral junction at the groin.
2. Recurrences over the popliteal fossa (short saphenous recurrences).
3. Recurrences over areas of incompetent perforating veins (pudendal veins, mid thigh, medial and lateral leg perforators, posterior calf perforators).

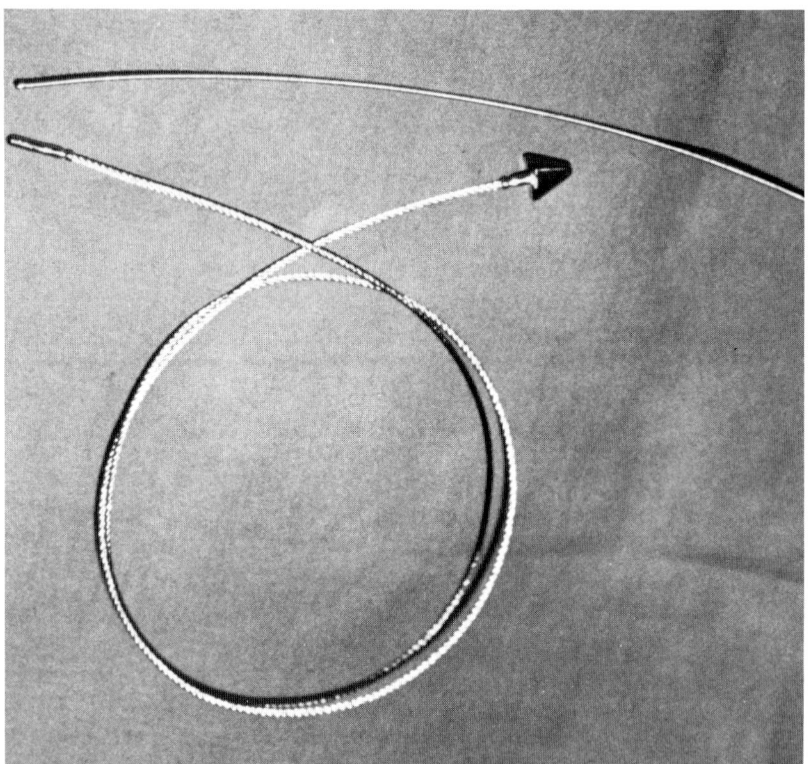

Figure 12 A

Figure 12   *A*: Instruments for surgery of varicose veins. No surgical procedure can be properly performed without adequate instruments. These are
the instruments for surgery of the venous system. A flexible intraluminal
stripper with detachable conic olives is shown. Also demonstrated is a short
and thinner stripper utilized to remove small tributaries of the saphenous
vein. *B*: In this photograph, we have illustrated from top to bottom a set of
Samuels vein strippers. There are three short rigid strippers utilized for
removing short segments of veins and the lesser saphenous vein. The fourth
and larger instrument is a flexible stripper employed to excise the long saphenous vein. Two extraluminal Mayo strippers are shown in the center, and the
Babcock rigid strippers are shown on the bottom. All have special indications
in surgery for varicose veins.

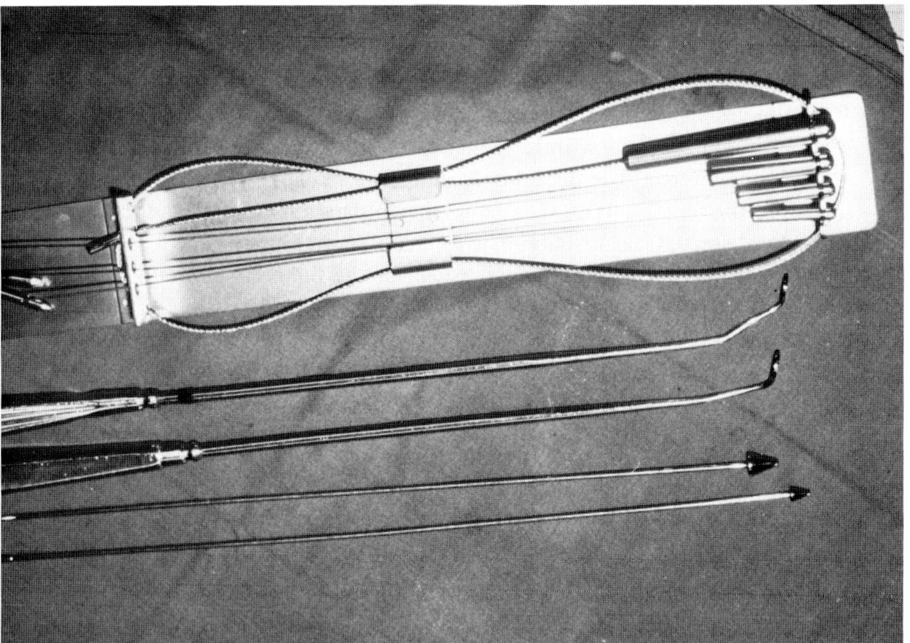

Figure 12 B

Recurrences at the Groin

Position.   Supine with operating table in Trendelenburg position.

Skin preparation.   Skin is prepared with a 2% iodine-alcohol solution from umbilicus to the tip of the toes, including the pubis. A glove is placed over the forefoot to keep the toes isolated from the surgical field. A folded sheet is placed under the distal third of the leg, immediately above the ankle.

Procedure.   The correct incision for exploration of the saphenofemoral junction should be made 2.5 cm lateral and below the pubic tubercle and centered on the femoral artery (feel the arterial pulse) (Fig. 7). One should try to avoid the highly vascular fibrous tissue that surrounds the previous surgical scar. If the scar is too low (which is most often the case), an incision should be made in the correct place, passing through subcutaneous tissue and the superficial fascia. The two edges of the incised superficial fascia are grasped with Kelly clamps and lifted. This maneuver separates the fatty tissue from the vessels and helps to identify the deeper vascular structures. Dissection should continue with Metzenbaum scissors, tying or cauterizing any vessels encountered. The deep fascia should be opened with a scalpel just medial to the femoral pulse. The femoral vein sheath is opened, and the vein carefully dissected out distally. The saphenofemoral junction will soon be encountered over the anteromedial aspect of the femoral vein. Often the saphenous vein is intact and can be easily dissected out. In these cases, the saphenofemoral junction is gently teased away from the surrounding tissues, and a 2-0 ligature is passed around it with a blunt-tip right angle vascular clamp. If the vein has been divided distally to some of its tributaries, the divided stump of the saphenous vein will be seen attached to the matted, fibrous, and scarred tissues. In these cases, the right angle clamp can be gently slipped between the femoral artery and the saphenous stump. To facilitate this maneuver, it is helpful to hold the fibrous stump with atraumatic DeBakey tissue forceps, trying gently to separate it from the artery as the right angle clamp is insinuated between the vessels. The ligature should be placed flush to the femoral vein. The varicose veins previously connected to the stump can be treated with sclerotherapy 4 to 6 weeks later.

In cases where the previous scar has been placed correctly, an oblique incision parallel to the groin is made just distal to the fibrous cicatricial tissues. Do not worry about the previous scar! Resecting the previous scar and going through fibrous scarred tissue intermingled with varicose veins and regenerated lymphatic vessels will frequently result in further damage to the lymphatics of the groin and development of secondary lymphedema. In these cases, dissection of the femoral vein is carried out proximally, and the procedure performed in a similar manner as just described.

Recurrences over the Popliteal Fossa
(Short Saphenous Recurrences)

Anesthesia.   Spinal or continuous epidural.

Position.   Patient prone with the operating table tilted in the Trendelenburg position. Place a folded sheet under the distal leg (the knee should be semiflexed).

Skin preparation.   Skin is prepared as described previously, from upper thigh to the tip of the toes.

Procedure. In cases where the saphenopopliteal junction has been accurately localized by any of the methods already described, a 5 cm transverse incision is made over the junction. If there is any need for wider exposure (patients with two or three previous operations and/or complex phlebographic image), a "Z" incision will provide the necessary exposure (Fig. 10A). The incision is carried through skin and subcutaneous tissue, ligating or cauterizing any vessels encountered. At this time, we have found it useful to elevate the skin flaps with fine-pronged retractors (Miller-Semb) and carefully dissect with Metzenbaum scissors under the subcutaneous tissue, trying to separate it from the underlying fascia. Often one can see the incompetent perforating vein coming from under the fascia and feeding the subcutaneous varices. This vein connects the short saphenous segment or the popliteal vein with the recurrent veins. At this time, the popliteal fascia is opened, and the subfascial segment of the perforating vein is followed towards its point of origin and ligated flush from the popliteal vein. Direct exposure of the popliteal vein should be carried out above the knee line in cases where no perforating vein can be found above the fascia. A vein of Giacomini draining into the proximal saphenous stump or directly into the popliteal vein has been found in 6% of our recurrences at the popliteal fossa. Any veins connecting the poplital vein with the recurrences must be ligated flush from the popliteal. Once the high pressure reflux has been interrupted, the remaining superficial varicosities should be excised through multiple small incisions.

One must keep in mind that more than 50% of the recurrences on the short saphenous territory are accompanied by incompetent posterior calf perforators (gastrocnemius, soleus). They should be dealt with at this time.

Recurrences over Areas of Incompetent Perforators

Stripping of the long and short saphenous veins does practically nothing to get rid of the incompetent perforators connected to their systems. This is especially true in the case of the perforators at mid thigh and distal third of the leg over its medial aspect. Recurrences are frequent in these areas. Reoperation for incompetent perforators has been performed in 30 to 60% of the reported series, including our own.

Procedure. Assuming that the site of reflux from an incompetent perforator has been identified, the incision is made directly over the marked area. There is no place here for small incisions. The average length of the incision is 4 cm and should be extended as necessary. The best cosmetic results are obtained when the incision is carried out with the scapel straight through the subcutaneous tissue and down to the fascia. Do not fall into the temptation to dissect out the transversing veins with a mosquito forceps! This will only lead to destruction of the subcutaneous tissue and depressed unsightly scars. If the subcutaneous tissues appear normal, a little undermining can be safely done under the incision to localize the perforator. If tissues are indurated and the skin has suffered from chronic venous hypertension, it is best to search for the perforator under the fascia. In these cases, it is convenient to lengthen the incision. Do not pick the skin edges with pick-ups! Use pronged retractors.

Perforators must be dissected out to the point of entrance through the fascia and ligated flush with it. Often there are tributary veins connecting perforators with segments of either short or long saphenous veins. These should be stripped using short strippers (Fig. 8). Varicose vein clusters that develop over incompetent perforators should be excised through separate small incisions, away from the main incision. Vein hooks specially designed by one of us have been found extremely useful to excise various sizes of tortuous varicose veins through 2 to 3 mm incisions, which become invisible a few months after the operation (Fig. 13).

Wound closure. Most patients, especially women, are more worried about the cosmetic effects of the surgical procedure than about its long-term results. To avoid wide unsightly scars, it is necessary to place a few approximating subcutaneous sutures using 4-0 absorbable material. This allows for early removal of skin sutures, usually during the second postoperative day. At this time, steri-strips are used to secure the wound. They are kept in place for 7 to 10 days. Placing of subcutaneous sutures requires the surgeon's patience and a little more time for surgery. However, a satisfied patient makes it worthwhile!

Dressings. Compression pads are placed over each surgical incision except the groin. Small pads should also be placed in the retromalleolar spaces to prevent swelling of this hard to compress area. Before wound closure, all blood should be evacuated to prevent hard, cordlike, painful hematomas. This is done by gently kneading and squeezing over the areas of dissection. Pads are held in place with thick gauze bandages. A firm 6 inch elastic bandage is applied from the toes to groin. Groin wounds are dressed with a simple 4 x 4 sterile gauze held with adhesive paper.

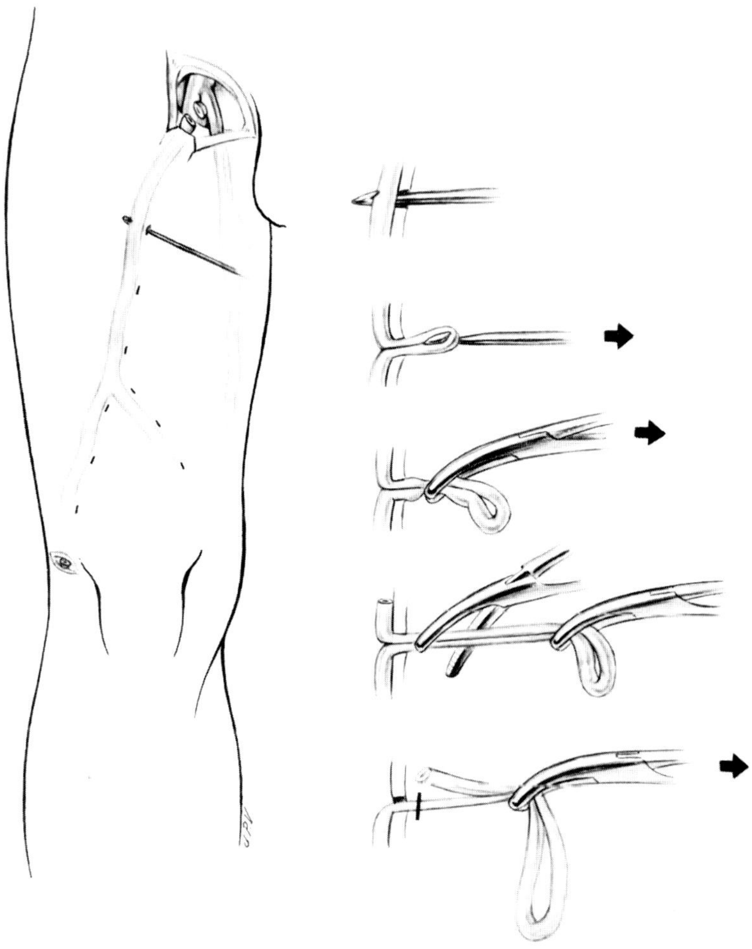

Figure 13 Varicose vein removal with vein hooks. In this drawing, the removal of a tortuous anterolateral tributary of the long saphenous vein is illustrated. Especially designed vein hooks (American V. Mueller Co., Chicago, Illinois) are introduced parallel to the vein through 2 to 3 mm skin incisions. The vein is carefully hooked and pulled out through the incision. Long segments of veins can be excised with this method. After a few months, the scars are undetectable.

Postoperative Management

The most serious complications in surgery for varicose veins are infection and deep venous thrombosis. The former can be avoided by good preoperative preparation of the skin (as described) and by observing strict asepsis during the operative procedure. Antibiotics are not used routinely for varicose vein surgery. In prolonged and complicated procedures, however, prophylactic antibiotics are advisable. The latter complication can be prevented by adhering to the following postoperative measures:

During the immediate postoperative period, the bed should be in the Trendelenburg position (foot of the bed elevated on 6 inch blocks).

Bed rest is advised on the operative day. The patient is encouraged to move the legs in bed. Check bandages for excessive tightness or bleeding. A small amount of bleeding may stain the dressings and is considered normal. Analgesics are given as necessary.

On the first postoperative day, stop intravenous fluids as soon as the patient tolerates oral intake. Unwrap bandages and reapply from foot to knee. The thigh should be wrapped, leaving knee area free or under slight compression. Patients should sit up at the edge of the bed to dangle their feet every hour for increasing periods of time (from 1 to 3 minutes). They may faint if asked to get up and walk after being on Trendelenburg position for prolonged periods. After the third hour, walking should be encouraged for 5 to 10 minutes of every hour, walking should be vigorous, lifting feet 20 to 30 cm from the ground. No sitting down is allowed during the first week.

On the second postoperative day, dressings should be changed and wounds inspected. Walking time is increased to about 15 minutes of every hour. With fresh dressings and firm elastic bandages, patients walk with little or no pain.

On the third postoperative day, in females, skin sutures are removed and wound edges supported with steri-strips (spraying tincture of benzoin is advisable before applying steri-strips). Walking is encouraged every hour for as long as desired. The patient is discharged and asked to return in a week. Elastic bandages are recommended for 1 month. We have observed that wounds heal better when the extremity is free of edema. Bed blocks are removed after the second week.

During the late postoperative period after the first week visit, the patient is asked to return in 1 month. At that time, the legs are examined for residual varicosities that the surgeon purposely chose to treat with sclerosing agents. If sclerotherapy is necessary, it should be started during the eight postoperative week. At this time, no echhymosis are present, healing is complete, and residual veins can be clearly seen.

Patients operated upon for varicose veins have an inherent disease that needs to be followed for an indefinite period. A careful follow-up is essential to maintain the patient free of disease and recognize an early recurrence that can usually be managed with sclerotherapy. We recommend postoperative visits at 6 months, 1 year, and every year therafter.

It is known that pregnancies exert an adverse effect on varicose veins. If possible, no more pregnancies are advisable. However, if the varicose patient is young and desires children, we strongly recommend them to have an operation as soon as the veins become symptomatic or prominent, rather than to wait as some recommend until the patient finishes having her family. At that time, the operation required is more complex than if performed when the patient was first seen. Also, it is our experience that if the operation has been adequately performed, the patient can tolerate one or two subsequent pregnancies. Sclerotherapy is the method of choice to control the varicosities that may appear as a consequence of pregnancy in an operated extremity.

Results

Despite our refinements in diagnostic methods, the statement by Matas (22) that "no combination of methods is proof against recurrence" is still valid. In this chapter, we have analyzed the results of experienced surgeons from different parts of the world in their struggle against recurrent varicose veins. The recurrence rates reported vary considerably. It is difficult to analyze the results of an operation that has so many variants and that is performed by surgeons who are proud of their individual differences. Because we assume that the published reports are an honest and careful analysis of the surgeon's experience, we find it difficult to explain the disparate results obtained with surgery.

From the reviewed experiences, we can state with all fairness that the surgical treatment of primary varicose veins offers the best chances for long-term control. If we exclude the excellent series of Frileux and co-workers (28) (0.53% at 30 years), the recurrence rates vary from 13 to 40%, with a mean of 17.5% at 15 years.

Our own results do not differ greatly from those of the reported series. From a group of 3000 patients operated on, we analyzed 1000 patients (1285 extremities) followed up for a mean period of 18 years (range 8 to 24). Information about the patient's condition was obtained by one of the following methods: personal examination, a questionnaire sent to the patient when personal examination was not feasible, questionnaire sent to the physician caring for the patient in the area of residence, or telephone interview.

The hospital charts and operative report of each patient were analyzed and correlated to obtain information about the type of operation and nature of the disease, the identity of the surgeon and surgical team, and the long-term results of the operation.

Information was obtained through personal interview in 80% of the patients, and through questionnaires in 12%. Therefore, information was obtained in 92% of the cases. This high follow-up figure was possible because of the captive nature of military personnel and dependents.

The incidence of recurrent varicose veins was analyzed per year. The highest incidence (17%) was observed during the years 1965 to 1967. These patients had been operated on by surgical residents without supervision. The incidence of recurrences in patients operated on by surgical residents under senior supervision was 13.7% during the same period of observation (mean 18 years). Similar results were observed when the operation had been performed by senior surgeons (14.3%). An interesting observation was made when we analyzed the duration of the operation. The mean operative time was 3.2 hours for surgical residents under supervision and 2 hours for senior surgeons. The operative time (recorded from the anesthesia records) of surgical residents without supervision was 1.2 hours! This group of patients had the highest incidence of recurrences.

Conclusions

Prevention of recurrences is the best management. This can be achieved by adhering to the following principles:

1. Identify the etiology of varices present.
2. Perform the necessary preoperative studies to localize the source of venous incompetence.
3. Mark the veins carefully, preferably the night before surgery.
4. Perform an adequate operation for the type of varices. Have a complete set of surgical instruments available.
5. Maintain a close follow-up of patients. Control with sclerotherapy as necessary.
6. Varicose vein surgery requires experience. Do not leave an unexperienced surgeon alone. Surgery for recurrences is always more complicated than the first surgery.

References

1. Bobek K, Cajzl L, Cepelak V: Etude de la frequence des maladies phlebologique et de l'influence de quelques facteurs etiologiques. Phlebologie 19:218, 1966.
2. Widmer LK, Mall TH, Martin H: Epidemiology and sociomedical importance of peripheral venous vein disease. In Hobbs JT (Ed): The Treatment of Venous Disorders. Philadelphia, JB Lippincott, 1977, p. 3.
3. Borschberg E: The Prevalence of Varicose Veins in the Lower Extremities. Basel, Karger, 1967.
4. Widmer LK, Kaufmann L, Hartmann G: Organization der Basler Studie uber Arterien, Venen und Herzkrankheiten. Schwaiz Med Wschr 97:99, 1967.
5. Lofgren EP: Treatment of long saphenous varicosities and their recurrence: a long-term follow-up. In Bergan JJ, Yao JST (Eds): Surgery of the Veins. Orlando, Grune & Stratton, 1985, pp. 285-299.
6. Coon WW, Willis PW III, Keller JB: Venous thromboembolism and other venous diseases in the Tecumseh Community Health Study. Circulation 48:839, 1973.
7. Bauer G: In Dodd H, Cockett FB (Eds): Introduction. The Pathology and Surgery of the Veins of the Lower Limb. Baltimore, The Williams and Wilkins Co., 1956, p.3.
8. Reagan B, Folse R: Lower limb venous dynamics in normal persons and children of patients with varicose veins. Surg Gynecol Obstet 132:15, 1971.
9. Villavicencio JL, Collins GJ, Youkey JR: Non-surgical management of lower extremity venous problems. In Bergan JJ, Yao JST (Eds): Surgery of the Veins. Orlando, Grune & Stratton, 1985, p. 323-345.
10. Cockett FB: Pathology and treatment of venous ulcers of the leg. MS Thesis, London, 1953.
11. Eger SA, Casper SL: In Dodd H, Cocket FB (Eds): Surgical anatomy of the veins of the lower limb. The Pathology and Surgery of the Veins of the Lower Limb. 2nd Edition. New York, Edinburgh, London, Churchill-Livingstone, 1976, pp. 33-35.
12. Coget JM, Merlen JF: Reflexions a propos des varices recidivantes. Phlebologie (France) 35:529-532, 1982.
13. Klippel M, Trenaunay P: Du naevus varique osteohypertrophique. Arch Gen Med (Paris) 3:641, 1900.
14. Parkes-Weber F: Angioma formation in connection with hypertrophy of limbs and hemihypertrophy. Br J Dermatol 19:231, 1907.
15. Parkes-Weber F: Haemangiectatic hypertrophy of limbs — congenital phlebarteriectasis and so-called congenital varicose veins. Br J Child Dis 15:13, 1918.

16. Brunner UV: Recidives essentielles sur la base des angiodysplasies mecconues Phlebologie 35:485-488, 1982.
17. Rettori R: Le role des perforantes de la face interne de al cuisse dans la recidive variqueuse. Phlebologie 35:475-483, 1982.
18. Kosinski C: Observations on the superficial system of the lower extremities. J Anat 60:131, 1926.
19. Haeger K: The surgical anatomy of the sapheno-femoral and saphenopopliteal junctions. J Cardiovasc Surg 6:420, 1962.
20. Mercier R, Fouques P, Portal N, Vanneuville G: Anatomie chirurgicale de la veine saphene externe. J Chir 93:59, 1967.
21. Villavicencio JL: Evolucion a larg plazo (1-8 anos) del tratamiento quirurgico de la insuficiencia venosa de las extremidades inferiores. Direccion General de Educacion Militar, Escuela Medico Militar de Mexico. Mexico City, Mexico, GISA Publishers, 1969, pp. 77-87.
22. Matas R: Cited by Ochsner A. and Mahorner H. Varicose Veins. St. Louis, C.V. Mosby Co., 1939.
23. Hippocrates: The Genuine Works of Hippocrates. Volume 2. (Translated by F. Adams). New York, William Wood and Co., 1886, p. 305.
24. Aegineta P: The Seven Books of Paulus Aegineta. Volume 2. (Translated by F. Adams). London, The Sydenham Society, 1846, pp. 406-409.
25. Malgaigne JF: Oeuvres Completes de Ambroise Pare'. Volume 2. Paris, JB Bailliere et Fils, 1840, p. 269.
26. Trendelenburg F: Uber die Unterbindung der Vena Saphena Magna bei Unterschenkel Varizen. Brusn Beitr Klin. Chir 7:195-210, 1890.
27. Hobbs JT: The management of varicose veins. Surg Annu 12:169, 1980.
28. Frileux C, Guillot C, Le Baleur A, Pillot P, Cosson J Ph: La Recidive variqueuse: opinion d'une equipe. Phlebologie 35:471-473, 1982.
29. Doran FS, Barkat S: The management of recurrent varicose veins. Ann R Coll Surg Engl 63:432-436, 1981.
30. Larson RH, Lofgren EP, Myers TT: Long-term results after vein surgery: study of 1000 cases after 10 years. Mayo Clini Proc 49:114, 1974.
31. Lofgren EP: Treatment of long saphenous varicosities and their recurrence: a long-term follow-up. In Bergan JJ, Yao JST (Eds): Surgery of the Veins. Orlando, Grune & Stratton, 1985, p. 298.
32. Elbaz CL: A propos des perforantes. Phlebologie 35:551-559, 1982.
33. Villavicencio JL: Incidence of recurrent varicose veins. A direct index of the hospital level of surgical teaching. International Vascular Symposium, London, Abstract 437, September 1981.
34. Lofgren KA: Recurrent varicose veins after stripping. Helv Chir Acta 39: 463-470, 1972.
35. Gedeon A, Barret A, Pradere B, Parent Y: Considerations sur le traitment chirurgical des recidives postoperatoires de varices. Phlebologie 35:519-521, 1982.

36. Wuppermann TH, Knospe E, Keiss HD, Mellmann J: Diagnosis of incompetent perforating veins: the ratio of hits of different methods of investigation in primary varicosis. In: May R, Partsch H, Staubesand J (Eds): Perforating Veins. Munchen, Baltimore, Urban and Schwarzenberg, 1981, pp. 177-192.
37. Satomura D: Study of the flow patterns in peripheral arteries by ultrasonics. J Acoust Soc Japan, 15:151, 1959.
38. Satomura S, Kaneko Z: Ultrasonic blood rheograph In The 3rd International Conference on Medical Electronics. London, 1960, pp. 254-258. Cited by Sumner, D. S. in Doppler Ultrasound. In: Bergan JJ, Yao JST (Eds). Venous Problems. Chicago, Yearbook Med. Publishers, 1978, p. 185.
39. Barnes RW, Russell HE, Wilson MR: Doppler Ultrasound and Evaluation of Venous Disease. A Programmed Audiovisual Instruction, 2nd Edition. Iowa City, University of Iowa Press, 1975, pp. 1-225.
40. Patil KD, Williams JR, Williams KLL: Thermographic localization of incompetent perforating veins in the leg. Br Med J 1:195-197, 1970.
41. Elem B, Shorey BA, Williams KLL: Comparison between thermography and fluorescein test in the detection of incompetent perforating veins. Br Med J 4:651-652, 1971.
42. Hach W: Diagnostic de la maladic variqueuse de recidive postoperatoire par la phlebographie ascendante avec manoeuvre de Valsalva. Phlebologie 35:493-496, 1982.
43. Thomas ML, Bowles JN: Incompetent perforating veins: comparison of varicography and ascending phlebography. Radiology 154:619-623, 1985.
44. Barabas AP, MacFarlane R: The usc of varicography to identify the sources of incompetence in recurrent varicose veins. Ann R Coll Engl 67: 208, 1985.
45. Davy A, Ouvry P: Place de la chirurgie dans le traitement de la varicose essentielle de la saphene externe. Phlebologie 35:317-326, 1982.
46. Devambez J, Mosca P, Jeu JF: Interet Du Doppler dans les recidives de varices operees. Phlebologie 35:497-505, 1982.
47. Kandel R: Chirurgisch-anatomische Eigentum lichkeiten bei der Behandlung der Varicosen vena Saphena Parva. Zbl Phleb 6:313, 1967.
48. Hobbs JJ: A new approach to short saphenous vein varicosities. In Bergan JJ, Yao JST (Eds): Surgery of the Veins. Orlando, Grune & Stratton, 1985, pp. 301-321.
49. Hoare MC, Royle JP: Doppler ultrasound detection of sapheno-popliteal incompetence ligation. Aust NZ J Surg 54:49-52, 1984.
50. Houser SL, Hashmi FH, Jaeger VJ, Chawla SK, Brown L, Kemler RL: Should the greater saphenous vein be preserved in patients requiring arterial outflow reconstruction in the lower extremity? Surgery 95:467-472, 1984.

51. Barnes RW, Collicot PE, Mozersky DJ: Noninvasive quantitation of venous reflux in the postphelbitic syndrome. Surg Gynecol Obstet 136: 769-773, 1978.
52. Abramowitz HB, Queral LA, Flinn WR: The use of photoplethysmography in the assessment of venous insufficiency: a comparison of venous pressure measurements. Surgery 86:434-441, 1979.
53. Norris CS, Beyrau A, Barnes RW: Quantitative photoplethysmography in chronic venous insufficiency. A new method of non invasive estimation of ambulatory venous pressure. Surgery 94:758-764, 1983.
54. Herman R, Neiman HL, Yao JST: Descending venography: a method of evaluating lower extremity venous valvular function. Radiology 137: 63-69, 1980.
55. Kistner, RL: Surgical repair of the incompetent femoral vein valve. Arch Surg 110:1936, 1975.

16

Reoperation for Microvascular Procedures

MARY H. McGRATH
*George Washington University Medical Center,
Washington, D.C.*

Clinical microsurgery deals with blood vessels less than 1.5 mm in external diameter. In this size range, the allowable margin of surgical error is small, and decreases further as vessel size approaches the present limits of technical competence at 0.3 to 0.4 mm diameter. A 0.5 mm of narrowing in a proximal posterior tibial artery might be tolerable, but it is catastrophic in a 0.8 to 1.0 mm vessel. A small tag of adventitia in a femoral artery is undesirable because it is a site for thrombus formation (although it can be relatively insignificant); the same tag and thrombus will fill the lumen of a digital artery.

Not only is the microvessel technically unforgiving, it also has a lower intraarterial pressure and a lower critical closing pressure. Moving from the aorta through arteries to arterioles, capillary bed, and venules produces a decremental change in intravascular pressure; a systemic value of 120 mmHg will decrease to 20 mmHg as the distal circulation is approached. At this level, a small elevation in extravascular tissue pressure can collapse the microvessel, and as a consequence, perivascular conditions assume enormous importance. Tissue edema due to compressive dressings, tight skin closure, or dependent positioning of an extremity can obstruct flow, but in general these conditions can be controlled. It is the edema due to direct injury or ischemia that is more problematic since it initiates a cycle of increased capillary permeability, even greater edema, higher extravascular tissue pressure, and further reduction of perfusion.

In light of the small sizes and low pressure conditions of microsurgery, vascular complications would not be unexpected, and do occur in a significant proportion of cases. Two major clinical applications for microvascular surgery are the reimplantation of amputated distal parts and the free transfer of skin or musculocutaneous flaps and vascularized bone or nerve. Currently, the average survival of reimplanted digits worldwide is between 70 and 90% (1), depending largely on patient selection criteria. For microvascular free flaps, an overall success rate of 94% was found in a multinational survey of 2233 flaps done in 21 microsurgery centers (2). While these statistics are much improved over those of a prior decade, the failure rate is still high for surgery where failure means complete loss of a body part or necrosis of an entire transplant.

Among the lessons of the past decade is the recognition of the frequency with which vascular complications occur in microvascular surgery. This recognition has been accompanied by the observation that many of these complications can be corrected surgically. Good results with early reoperation in cases with circulatory embarrassment have made reexploration a requirement; improved methods for monitoring vessel patency postoperatively are critical to this success.

Incidence and Results of Reoperation

At present, approximately 10 to 20% of replanted digits and free flaps develop postoperative vascular compromise and require reexploration. If the vessels are explored and problems corrected promptly, salvage is possible in about 50% of reoperated replanted digits. In surveying the medical literature on free flaps, it appears that 75% or more can be salvaged by reoperation (Table 1) (3-9).

The free tissue transfer has a significantly better chance of a successful outcome after reexploration than does the replanted digit. There are several reasons for this, primary among them is that the blood vessels of the amputated part are more likely to be damaged by mechanical trauma and prolonged ischemia, while the part is in transport to the surgical center and the operating room. Before 1976, the chances of an ultimately successful replantation were in the range of 40%; this has now risen to 90% in some centers (10). These statistics reflect, in part, an acceptance that contraindications to replantation do exist, and some parts and patients are not suitable for a replant effort. However, the improved results also reflect the

Table 1 Incidence of Reoperation and Salvage Rate in Microvascular Surgery

Author (Date)	Number of Cases	Number of Reoperations	Number of Cases Salvaged By Reoperation	Percent of Reoperated Cases Salvaged
Morrison et al. (3)/1977	100 replanted digits	25 (25%)	10	40%
Schlenker et al. (4)/1980	64 replanted thumbs	10 (16%)	5	50%
Tamai (5)/1982	293 upper extremity replants	15 (5%)	7	46%
Shaw (6)/1983	2233 free flaps	223 (10%)	90	40%
Daniel and Lidman (7)/1984	42 free flaps	8 (19%)	6	75%
Jones (8)/1985	15 free flaps	4 (26%)	2	50%
Lineaweaver and Buncke (9)/1986	72 free flaps	5 (7%)	5	100%

evolution of principles for the handling of microvessels and their anastomoses in the "zone of injury" of a traumatized part. That a larger number of replants have immediate and enduring success, that it has become axiomatic that the replant with vascular problems requires reexploration, and that something can be done differently at the time of reexploration to salvage about half of these replants are largely due to increasing use of vein grafts. It is important in replantation to place the anastomoses *outside* the zone of injury and incorporate only *undamaged* vessel ends. With the 10 to 25% of replants that require early reoperation, simple anastomatic revision is rarely successful and use of a vein graft generally is necessary.

Etiology of Vascular Complications

Clotting in the Microcirculation

Platelet aggregation and release mechanisms are more important in effecting microvascular patency than are the subsequent blood coagulation pathways (11). Long before a "red clot" has time to form, a small vessel can be occluded by the "white clot" created when platelets, which are approximately 2 μm in diameter, aggregate and adhere to the vessel wall. The stimulus for platelet aggregation appears to be collagen, a major component of the vascular media and adventitia. When vascular connective tissue is exposed at the cut edges of vessels, endothelial gaps, needle tracks, and denuded media in a crushed vessel, collagen fibers in combination with adenosine diphosphate (ADP), serotonin, epinephrine, and thromboplastin cause primary aggregation or the formation of bridges linking certain sites on the platelet surface (12). Aggregation initiates a secretory process, during which platelet granules release both ADP and the lipoproteins responsible for the further joining of platelets into larger, irreversible aggregates along with activation of the blood coagulation pathway via the lipoprotein complex and platelet factor III (12). Larger platelet aggregates alone in microvessels may occlude the lumen completely, as documented by scanning electron microscopy.

The Timing of Thrombosis

Studies of the healing of microvascular anastomoses have shown that intimal continuity is a key factor, because distortion, endothelial flap elevation, or poor endothelial approximation expose the subendothelial collagen surfaces where platelet aggregation begins. Large platelet plugs can be seen at sites of endothelial gaps where anastomotic bleeding occurred or where vasospasm has caused endothelial fragmentation and sloughing (13). When the intima is well approximated and endothelial healing progresses smoothly, a pseudo-intima covers the site of injury within 5 days, sutures are covered by re-generating endothelium within 7 days, and the intima is completely healed in approximately 2 weeks (14). The deeper layers of the muscular wall continue to regenerate with fibroplasia, collagen deposition, and myointimal thick-ening for months. Late problems due to medial discontinuity and resultant pseudoaneurysmal or aneurysmal changes can develop, but reoperative vas-cular problems in microsurgery are overwhelmingly those of the early post-operative period.

The morphologic evidence that the pseudointima is complete within 5 days correlates neatly with the clinical and laboratory findings that thrombosis of microvascular anastomoses occurs within the first 3 to 5 days. Clinical ex-perience with microvascular free flaps shows rare or no losses after 3 days (7,15,16), while most replant failures are observed during the first 24 to 48 hours (although later losses can occur occasionally) (3). In the laboratory, the critical period for occlusion is the first 72 hours for vessels 0.8 to 1.2 mm (17) or with an average 0.9 mm in diameter (18). These observations have led clinical microsurgeons to conclude that patency rates in vessels measuring 1.0 mm in diameter can be determined accurately immediately after the first week and in contrast to macrovascular anastomoses, if patency is maintained beyond 72 hours, permanent patency is practically assured (17).

The importance of the first 5 days of endothelial regeneration is under-scored when it is noted that long-term anastomotic patency is not necessary for many microsurgical procedures. The flap or replant is in an "all or none" survival situation initially, but at some point, the surrounding tissue will begin to support it by small vessel ingrowth. In animal experiments (19), it ap-pears to take at least 8 days before surrounding tissue will maintain the viability of the tissue. In the clinical setting, this phenomenon appears to vary with the vascular quality of the recipient site (20). With digital replantation, there may be problems with cold intolerance when circulation is marginal, but in most late free flaps, the maintenance of a patent microvascular anas-tomosis becomes irrelevant.

The Causes of Thrombosis

Since most microvascular thromboses begin at the site of endothelial injury or anastomosis within a circumscribed period of time, close monitoring for several days and prompt reoperation upon failure are indicated. With growing understanding of the etiologic factors in microvascular complications, it is becoming easier to predict the fate of initial operations as well as reexplorations. The causes of failure can be identified as those associated with previously damaged vessels, with conditions at the anastomotic site, and with extravascular factors (Table 2). Of these, problems at the anastomosis and in the extravascular environment can be corrected with the highest probability of success.

Table 2   Factors Associated with Microvascular Complications

Preoperative vascular damage
  Protracted warm ischemia
  Mechanical damage
    Crush injury
    Avulsion injury
    Cold injury secondary to improper storage
  Irradiation
  Metabolic
    Atherosclerosis
    Diabetes mellitus

Factors at the anastomotic site
  Vasospasm
  Inadequate debridement
  Technical errors
    Improper suture technique
    Poor tissue alignment
    Repair under tension
    Crush with clamps or instruments

Factors in the perivascular environment
  Edema
  Hematoma
  Compressive dressings
  Fascial tightness
  Tight skin closure

Preoperative Evaluation

Ischemia and the "No Reflow" Phenomenon

The transfer of tissue by microvascular anastomosis requires a period of time during which the tissue is isolated from the circulation. In the tightly controlled circumstances of free flap transfer, this period of time is short, and the tolerance to ischemia by the donor tissue is well defined. In the case of amputated parts, many hours may elapse before circulation can be restored, and the chances of a successful revascularization will vary with the type of tissue in the part and the temperature at which the part is preserved.

Skin and subcutaneous tissue are relatively resistant to the effects of anoxia, as are bone and cartilage; skeletal muscle and peripheral nerves are much less tolerant of ischemia, with irreversible changes evident within 4 hours (21). Cooling prolongs the tolerance to ischemia in all tissues by reducing the metabolic rate of the tissues, reducing the accumulation of toxic metabolic products, and inhibiting bacterial growth. While the duration of ischemia in a digit without cooling should not exceed 6 hours, this can be extended safely to at least 24 hours if immediate cooling to 4°C is instituted. The more proximal the amputation, the shorter the acceptable ischemic interval because of the increased muscle mass involved (22).

Clinically, tissue subjected to prolonged warm ischemia can be revascularized with good initial blood flow, but it has been observed that flow diminishes within a short period of time, the microcirculation becomes occluded with thrombi, and tissue death inevitably results. This phenomenon has been referred to as the "no reflow" effect, meaning the failure to reperfuse an ischemic organ despite restitution of an interrupted vascular supply (23). The explanations for the "no reflow" effect include ischemia-induced endothelial swelling due to malfunction of the sodium-potassium membrane pump and trapping of formed blood elements within the narrowed lumen of a microvessel. Stagnation and hemoconcentration are accompanied by endothelial slough, exposure of the subendothelial connective tissue, thrombus formation, and activation of the coagulation pathways. Seen in various organs with different degrees of ischemic insult, the phenomenon becomes irreversible after a tissue-specific ischemic period, and all subsequent revascularization efforts are doomed to failure. In clinical surgery, vascular anastomoses after a period of extended ischemia may be complicated by repeated and unexplained early thrombosis; the tissue may not be salvageable despite proper execution of all surgical measures (23).

Mechanical Damage and the "Zone of Injury"

Among the absolute contraindications to replantation surgery is severe crush-avulsion injury of the affected limb or part. Because the small vessels are damaged beyond salvage in these parts, revascularization is not possible. Yet, there are cases with lesser degree of crush or avulsion injury in which surgery may proceed despite the much higher risk of postoperative thrombotic complications. In these cases, the viability of the replant will depend on extensive debridement and resection of the damaged vessels in the zone of injury so that healthy intima is available for the vascular anastomosis. Vein grafts to bridge gaps are successfully employed in these situations.

Assessment of the zone of injury should include inspection of the vessels under magnification for segmental damage. The "red line sign" is extravasation of blood along the neurovascular bundle caused by trauma that shears tiny branches from the trunk of the digital arteries (24). This sign heralds a need for generous vascular resection, as does the "ribbon sign," which is a marked tortuosity of an artery after stretching and recoil (25). Again, because of intimal disruption, arterial resection and bridging of the resultant gap with a vein graft will be necessary if revascularization is to be attempted. Other clues to intimal damage include separation of the intima from the media of a vessel, separation of the media from the adventitia, hemorrhagic intima, spotty hematomas in the adventitia, and persistence of intraluminal clot adherent to the intima that cannot be irrigated away (26,27).

The same principles apply in the selection of recipient vessels in free flap surgery. The majority of free flaps are performed for the late sequelae of trauma, cancer resection, irradiation, and previous surgery. Dissection of the small vessels in the "zone of injury" is technically difficult and injurious to already abnormal vessels. To avoid injury and thrombosis, it is necessary to dissect beyond the "zone of injury" for recipient vessels. These undamaged vessels may lie at some distance from the defect, but experience has shown that a long vein graft into a normal recipient vessel will yield better results than anastomosis to a scarred vessel (6). It has been reported that the most critical judgment in the perioperative period of free flap surgery is selection of recipient vessels (7). A wrong decision generally will require correction with a revision of the anastomosis, but with reoperation, the success rate should be high.

Irradiated Tissue

Free flaps frequently are used to close large defects after cancer surgery where tissue healing is impaired by irradiation. Often, it is not possible, particularly in the head and neck area, to go beyond an extensive zone of injury to find recipient blood vessels outside the field of radiation. This occurs, for example, when a free skin flap to restore integument or a free jejunal flap to restore a mucosal surface is required. In these situations, the thrombosis rate is higher. Both clinical and experimental studies have shown that irradiated vessels have greater wall thickness and a higher incidence of intramural dissection, as well as more fibrin deposition, microthrombi, and endothelial cell dehiscence, than do normal vessels. To try to minimize the higher risk of thrombosis in these irradiated vessels, recommendations have included use of end-to-end anastomoses and passing surgical needles through the wall only from the inside to outside to prevent intramural dissection. Strict avoidance of electrocautery and minimal dissection and cross-clamping of the vessels are advocated. Reoperative recommendations include resection of the vessel in the event of thrombosis, rather than efforts at thrombectomy (28).

Preoperative Angiographic Evaluation

Preoperative magnification angiographic study of both the donor and recipient sites has been recommended (29), when handling tissues lying in the zone of injury, because of the potential for unexpected alterations in the vasculature. The studies permit orderly preoperative planning, particularly helpful where there has been extensive previous injury or surgery; there is no evidence for a deleterious effect of the radiographic contrast material on the microvessels (29).

Intraoperative Management

The basic criteria for successful microsurgery are: (1) normal vessels obtained by uncompromising resection of friable or damaged vessels; (2) avoidance of tension at the repair site, with plans for interposition vein grafting as necessary; and (3) gentle handling of recipient vessels since even limited handling can cause direct endothelial damage as well as vasospasm. Prolonged vasospasm induced by dissection can produce endothelial fragmentation and sloughing, which expose subendothelial elements and induce platelet aggregation, fibrin deposition, and resultant thrombus formation. Experimental studies (13) have demonstrated that microvessels subjected to vasospasm for

more than 2 hours become almost entirely denuded of their endothelial layer
(13).

However, even if the foregoing criteria are observed, failure can accompany
technical lapses where there is not meticulous attention to detail and adequate visualization of the lumen during anastomosis.

Suture Techniques

The most significant damage to vessel walls at the time of anastomosis is due
to needle and suture penetration and technique of placement. Large needles
and obliquely placed sutures can cause major endothelial lacerations, exposing subendothelium and inducing platelet aggregation. Repeat needle
puncture for suture placement produces platelet plugs at the bleeding site.
Unequal suture distance leaves endothelial gaps, distortion, constriction, and
exposed intimal flaps. Loosely tied sutures expose subendothelial elements to
the bloodstream and anastomotic bleeding with subsequent platelet plug
formation. Too many sutures or sutures tied too tightly can cause endothelial
slough (1,3).

Interrupted Versus Continuous Suture

Most microsurgeons use interrupted suture techniques. Some, however,
advocate a continuous suture technique, citing a reduction in anastomotic
time, fewer passes of the needle through tissue, and fewer suture line leaks
with a running suture (30). On the other side of the argument, breakage of
the suture while handling requires repeat anastomosis; furthermore, a greater
amount of suture material is used, which may narrow the lumen or expose
thrombogenic material to the bloodstream (31). Studies (14,32) have shown
little difference in microvascular anastomotic patency using either technique
in the laboratory setting.

End-to-End Versus End-to-Side Anastomosis

It is reasonable that in the early days of microvascular surgery, the end-to-end
anastomosis was used almost exclusively. It is a simpler technique and appears
to offer a hemodynamically efficient way of getting blood from one microvessel into another. It was not until the late 1970s that better results with
end-to-side anastomoses were reported (33), with three advantages proposed:
(1) avoidance of vessel retraction and contraction, with some subsequent
tension at the anastomotic site (often observed in the completely transected
vessel); (2) utility in extremities with only one recipient artery that is critical

to the survival of the extremity; and (3) utility when significant vessel size discrepancy exists (34). Subsequently, disadvantages of the end-to-side techniques have been pointed out: (1) less room for error or revisions with the inability to repeat or repair with vein grafts at reexploration; and (2) technical difficulties when recipient vessels are thick or atheromatous (34).

Several laboratory studies (35) have compared the hemodynamics of the two techniques in the microcirculation, and no statistical differences in peripheral resistance, blood flow, or tissue survival have been found. From this has developed the recommendation that the clinical choice of the type of anastomosis should be based on anatomic factors, such as size and availability of recipient vessels.

Nonsuture Anastomoses

Since each suture inflicts significant injury on the wall of a microvessel, a search for other methods of anastomosis has led to the development of microvascular couplers and other repair techniques that make use of tissue adhesives, electrocoaptation, and laser sealing. Most of these are not in clinical use because there is no consensus that their application is less traumatic than suturing.

Use of Vascular Clamps

Among the essential instruments for the microvascular surgeon is the double approximator clamp to bring the vessel ends into approximation with minimal handling. The closing pressures of these devices must be less than 30 mg/mm^2 to avoid damage to the small vessels. Moreover, there is some new evidence that the duration of clamp application is proportional to the incidence of late occlusion (36). Endothelial cell damage can be demonstrated in both settings, emphasizing a need to shorten the duration of arterial clamping and to consider using an extra-soft vessel approximator.

Use of Microvascular Grafts

Vascular repairs must be performed in undamaged vessels without tension. Meticulous inspection under the microscope will show the necessary level of vascular debridement and the resultant gap, be it 2 or 20 cm in length, must then be bridged by a microvascular graft (37). Because interpositional autogenous vein grafts are used most commonly, the question has arisen as to whether placing two anastomotic repairs in sequence will not predispose to turbulence and thrombosis greater than that seen in simple repairs. This question becomes especially meaningful for the surgeon considering reexploration of a thrombosed microsurgical repair site, since anastomotic revision without grafting rarely is possible.

Autogenous Vein Grafts

From a variety of laboratory studies has come the information that the size, length, and nature of autogenous grafts determine patency rates.

1. In vessels smaller than 0.9 mm, graft patencies may not be so good as with simple repairs for both arteries and veins (38), although some have obtained comparable results with grafts as small as 0.5 mm in diameter (36).

2. Discrepancies in size between host and graft vessels are tolerable, but when the ratio exceeds 1:1.5, patency rates of end-to-end anastomoses are decreased (38).

3. For grafts 1.0 mm in diameter, patency is equal with grafts 1.0 and 4.0 cm in length, but patency rates have not been evaluated in smaller diameter or other lengths of grafts (38).

4. Histologic studies have shown that vein-to-vein grafts and artery-to-artery grafts heal better than vein-to-artery grafts. This is consistent with the subintimal hyperplasia with narrowing of the suture lines and changes leading toward fibrosis (39), often observed when a vein graft is arterialized. The relevance of this is negligible in those microsurgical procedures where long-term patency is unimportant, but it must be weighed in cases such as digital replantation, where relative ischemia causes cold intolerance. Some recommend that vein grafts be obtained from the lower extremity or foot, where their walls are already thicker because they withstand higher hydrostatic pressures (38).

Synthetic Microvascular Grafts

A number of experimental investigations of synthetic materials for small vessel replacement have been made because obtaining vein grafts generally takes time and requires additional incisions. Polyurethane and microporous or expanded polytetrafluoroethylene small diameter grafts have been evaluated; these prostheses do not have patency rates comparable with those of vein grafts. At the 1.0 to 2.0 mm level, the anastomotic site tends to become occluded by circumferential clot, and when the prosthetic tube remains open, a thin layer of mural thrombus can be found lining the entire lumen (40).

Pharmacologic Management

Ten to 20 percent of microvascular repairs will thrombose despite having been performed well technically. Thus, interest exists in prophylactic and therapeutic use of pharmacologic agents that might control small vessel thrombosis. With increasing understanding of the dynamics of blood coagulation in the small vessel, recommended drug regimens have been aimed increasingly at the platelet, or platelet activity and release of products. Yet, despite this reasoned approach to the microcirculation and laboratory evidence of the efficacy of these agents, there is little indication that any one pharmacologic agent or program substantially improves clinical results.

A variety of anticoagulants, vasodilators, and fibrinolytic agents are used clinically (Table 3). In a 1982 worldwide survey (41) of anticoagulation practices, about 30% of both free flap and replant surgery was being done with no anticoagulation at all. For those using anticoagulants, some 21 different agents were recorded as being in routine use, the duration of therapy

Table 3   Pharmacologic Agents Used In Clinical Microvascular Surgery

Anticoagulants
  [a]Aspirin
  [a]Dextran
  [a]Heparin

Vasodilators
  Dipyridamole (persantine)
  Reserpine
  Chlorpromazine
  Stellate ganglion block

Topical agents
  [a]Heparinized saline irrigant
  2% Lidocaine (xylocaine)
  0.75% Bupivacaine (marcaine)
  20% Magnesium sulfate

Fibrinolytic agents
  Urokinase
  Streptokinase

[a]Agents used most commonly.

ran from 3 to 14 days, and there were no significant differences among the success rates with and without antithrombotic agents (41).

Aspirin is the most commonly used agent, followed by low molecular weight dextran. Heparin in either full anticoagulation or "mini-dose" regimens follows as a remote third. Topical irrigants are widely used in the operating room, with heparinized saline most commonly chosen.

Systemic Anticoagulants

Aspirin inhibits platelet aggregation occurring in response to collagen; moreover, it diminishes thromboxane-induced release of platelet enzymes by inhibiting thromboxane synthesis (12). Unfortunately, it also inhibits synthesis of prostacyclin, a strong antiaggregation agent. Since the dose for thromboxane inhibition is lower than that for prostacyclin inhibition, a low dose of aspirin is recommended, probably in the range of 3 mg/kg per day, although it should be noted that aspirin is not used at all in some major microsurgical centers (42).

Dextran markedly inhibits platelet adhesiveness, increases blood flow, decreases viscosity, and alters the fibrin structure of a clot, making it more susceptible to fibrinolysins. These actions are molecular weight-dependent, and the administration of 1 unit of dextran-70, daily for several days, to replantation patients has been recommended (12), with the infusion begun preoperatively or intraoperatively (43).

Heparin accelerates the action of antithrombin and its use in microvascular surgery is limited (although some years ago it was used extensively). Studies (18) have failed to show a higher patency rate for microvessels repaired with heparin compared with untreated controls, and almost all of the complications related to anastomotic bleeding and hematoma have occurred when heparin was used. Low dose heparin, 5000 units given twice daily, may have some place in microsurgery.

Topical Anticoagulants and Vasodilators

The use of heparinized saline irrigant during the course of a microsurgical procedure is commonplace, but other topical agents have been introduced for the treatment of vasospasm. Vasospasm is the tight vasoconstriction that develops in a microvessel before or after anastomosis, and it may be recalcitrant to mechanical dilation. Spasm retards proximal arterial inflow to the anastomosis and occurs both in veins and arteries. Although vasospasm is associated with dissection and handling of the vessel, it also occurs in the absence of these manipulations and may persist despite an apparently satisfactory vascular environment. Magnesium sulfate is a vasodilator and antiplatelet drug that will relieve vasospasm when applied topically to the vessel; it also may cause protracted bleeding at the anastomotic site (44). Topical anesthetic agents applied intraoperatively have been useful in treating vasospasm, and the effect appears to be concentration-dependent and related to a smooth muscle-relaxant effect (45). Vasospasm in replanted digits has been treated successfully with the prolonged infusion of local anesthetics via a catheter placed near the ulnar or median nerve in the forearm, thereby producing a pharmacologic sympathectomy (46).

Comments on Pharmacologic Management

While there is no uniformity in the use of anticoagulants in microvascular surgery, some trends do emerge. In general, anticoagulants are not used for free flap transfers or surgery where vascular and technical conditions are optimal. In clinical situations where unfavorable features cannot be avoided or improved, anticoagulants probably are indicated even though no clinical studies exist that firmly establish their efficacy.

Postoperative Monitoring

In light of the significant number of microvascular anastomoses that require reexploration and the high proportion of compromised anastomoses that can be salvaged, close postoperative monitoring is mandatory. In the past, repeated clinical observations by the same examiner at frequent intervals have been routine. Tissue color, capillary refill, tissue turgor, and temperature are useful in assessing perfusion (Fig. 1). However, these clinical methods of evaluating blood flow have limitations, perhaps the greatest being the lag between a vascular mishap and its manifestation. For example arterial compromise usually is characterized by a gradual slowing of capillary refill, rather than by its sudden cessation. Subtle changes in color are difficult to interpret, and peripheral vasoconstriction may be difficult to differentiate from venous thrombosis. Clinical observation is more difficult in the black patient where capillary refill is harder to judge, and clinical monitoring is impossible for free tissue tranfers that are buried, such as free jejunal grafts to the neck or free omental transfers to a chest defect.

These limitations in clinical assessment have led to the search for a reliable method of tissue transfer monitoring; one that is accurate, continuous, sensi-

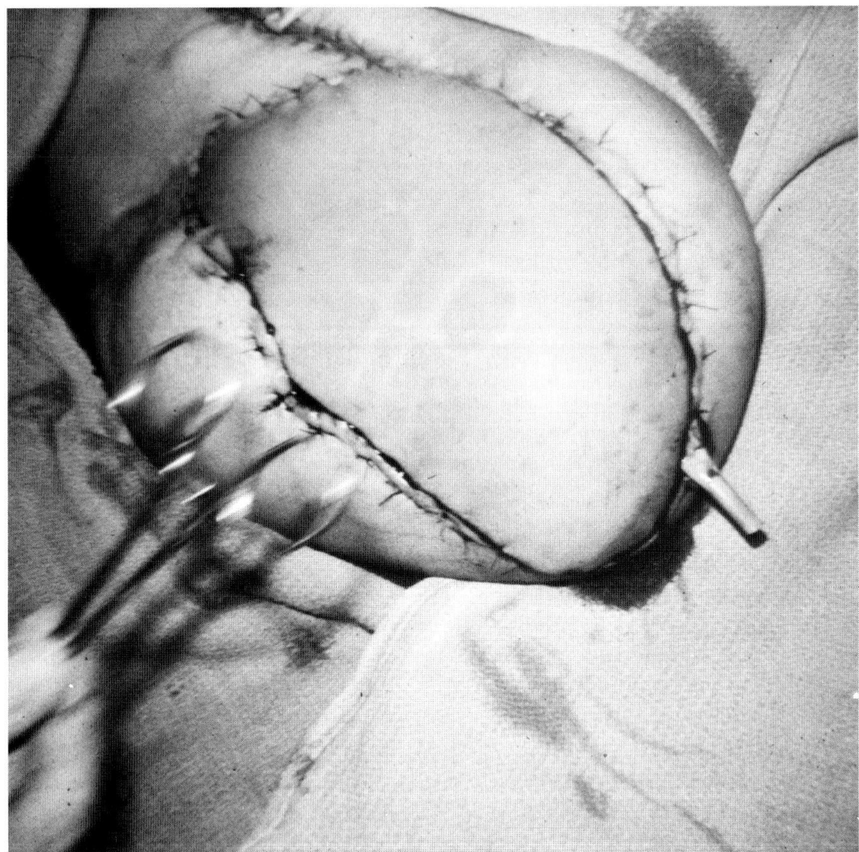

Figure 1   A free tissue transfer with the signs of arterial insufficiency (sluggish capillary refill after the application of pressure by the clamp, a mottled color, and cool temperature) in the postoperative period. The flap was reexplored, with revision of a thrombosed arterial anastomosis.

tive, portable, simple, and inexpensive (Table 4) (47). Devices that measure temperature in transplanted tissue are the most widely used at present, and surface thermocouples (48) and an implantable thermocouple probe (47) have both proven their reliability in clinical studies. For intraoperative and

Table 4 Modalities for Monitoring
the Patency of Microanastomoses

Doppler ultrasound flowmeter
  Laser Doppler probe

Surface temperature probe
  Implantable thermocouple

Fluorescein dye uptake
  Fluorescein dye clearance

Photoplethysmography

Percutaneous oxygen tension monitor

Radioisotope clearance

Evoked M-wave monitoring (muscle)

---

postoperative monitoring, the most commonly used instrument continues to
be the Doppler flowmeter (49). Other microsurgeons have found photoplethysmography (16), fluorescein dye uptake or clearance (50), and tissue
oxygen or tissue pH monitoring (51) helpful. For the postoperative monitoring of buried free muscle transfers, evoked M-wave monitoring appears to
be a sensitive indicator of muscle ischemia (52). With these more objective
monitoring systems, an early return to the operating room can be accomplished well before ischemia or relative ischemia can take their toll on the
endothelium. It will be of interest to see if the present salvage rate of 50 to
75% after reexploration will improve as objective monitoring is more widely
used.

References

1. Tebbetts JB. Microsurgery: free tissue transfer and replantation. Selected
   Readings in Plastic Surgery 3:1-21, 1985.
2. Shaw WW. Microvascular free flaps: survival, donor sites and application.
   In: Buncke HJ, Furnas DW (eds). Symposium on Clinical Frontiers in Reconstructive Microsurgery. St. Louis, CV Mosby Co. 1984, pp 3-10.
3. Morrison WA, O'Brien BM, MacLeod AM. Evaluation of digital replantation — a review of 100 cases. Orthop Clin North Am 8:295-308, 1977.

4. Schlenker JD, Kleinert HE, Tsai TM. Methods and results of replantation following traumatic amputation of the thumb in sixty-four patients. J Hand Surg 5:63-70, 1980.

5. Tamai S. Twenty years' experience of limb replantation — review of 293 upper extremity replants. J Hand Surg 7:549-556, 1982.

6. Shaw WW, Microvascular free flaps: the first decade. Clin Plast Surg 10: 3-20, 1983.

7. Daniel RK, Lidman D. Vascular complications in free flap transfer. In: Buncke HJ, Furnas DW (eds). Symposium on Clinical Frontiers in Reconstructive Microsurgery. St. Louis, CV Mosby Co, 1984, pp 387-396.

8. Jones BM. Predicting the fate of free tissue transfers. Ann R Coll Surg Engl 67:63-70, 1985.

9. Lineaweaver WC, Buncke HJ. Complications of free flap transfers. Hand Clin 2:347-351, 1986.

10. Weiland AJ, Villarreal-Rios A, Kleinert HE, Kutz J, Atasoy E, Lister G. Replantation of digits and hands: analysis of surgical techniques and functional results in 71 patients with 86 replantations. J Hand Surg 2:1, 1977.

11. Chang WHJ, Petry JJ. Platelets, prostaglandins, and patency in microvascular surgery. J Microsurg 2:27, 1980.

12. Ketchum LD. Pharmacological alterations in the clotting mechanism: use in microvascular surgery. J Hand Surg 3:407-415, 1978.

13. Weinstein PR, Mehdorn HM, Szabo Z. Microsurgical anastomosis: vessel injury, regeneration, and repair. In: Serafin D, Buncke HJ Jr (eds). Microsurgical Composite Tissue Transplantation. St. Louis, CV Mosby Co. 1979, pp 111-144.

14. Harashina T, Fujino T, Watanabe S. The intimal healing of microvascular anastomoses. Plast Reconstr Surg 58:608-613, 1976.

15. O'Brien BM, Morrison WA, Ishida H, MacLeod AM, Gilbert A. Free flap transfers with microvascular anastomosis. Br J Plast Surg 27:220, 1974.

16. Harrison DH, Girling M, Mott G. Monitoring the circulation in the free flap transfer. In: Buncke HJ, Furnas DW (eds). Symposium on Clinical Frontiers in Reconstructive Microsurgery. St. Louis, CV Mosby Co. 1984, pp 399-407.

17. Ketchum LD, Wennen WW, Masters FW, Robinson DW. Experimental use of pluronic F68 in microvascular surgery. Plast Reconstr Surg 53:288-292, 1974.

18. Hayhurst JW, O'Brien BM. An experimental study of microvascular technique, patency rates and related factors. Br J Plast Surg 28:128-132, 1975.

19. Black MJM, Chait L, O'Brien BM, Sykes PJ, Sharzer LA. How soon may

the axial vessels of a surviving free flap be safely ligated: a study in pigs. Br J Plast Surg 31:295, 1978.

20. McGrath MH, Adelberg D, Finseth F. The intravenous fluorescein test: use in timing of groin flap division. J Hand Surg 4:19-22, 1979.

21. Ericksson E, Anderson WA, Replogle RL. Effects of prolonged ischemia on muscle microcirculation in the cat. Surg Forum 25:254, 1974.

22. McGrath MH. Microvascular surgery in reconstruction of the hand. Surg Clin North Am 60:1105-1119, 1980.

23. May JW, Chait LA, O'Brien BM, Hurley JV. The no-reflow phenomenon in experimental free flaps. Plast Reconstr Surg 61:256-267, 1978.

24. Sixth People's Hospital of Shanghai. Replantation of severed fingers: clinical experience in 162 cases involving 270 severed fingers. Chin Med J 1:3, 1973.

25. VanBeek AL, Kutz JE, Zook EG. Importance of the ribbon sign, indicating unsuitability of the vessel, in replanting a finger. Plast Reconstr Surg 61:32-35, 1978.

26. Goldner RD. Postoperative management. Hand Clin 1:205-215, 1985.

27. Strauch B, Greenstein B, Goldstein R, Liebling RW. Problems and complications encountered in replantation surgery. Hand Clin 2:389-399, 1986.

28. Guelinckx PJ, Boeckx WD, Fossion E, Gruwez JA. Scanning electron electron microscopy of irradiated recipient blood vessels in head and neck free flaps. Plast Reconstr Surg 74:217-226, 1984.

29. May JM, Athanasoulis CA, Donelan MB. Preoperative magnification angiography of donor and recipient sites for clinical free transfer of flaps or digits. Plast Reconstr Surg 64:483-490, 1979.

30. Man D, Acland RD. Continuous-suture technique in microvascular end-to-end anastomosis. J Microsurg 2:238, 1981.

31. Hamilton RB, O'Brien BM. An experimental study of microvascular patency using a continuous suture technique. Br J Plast Surg 32:153, 1979.

32. Lee BY, Thoden WR, Brancato RF, Kavner D, Shaw W, Madden JL. Comparison of continuous and interrupted suture techniques in microvascular anastomosis. Surg Gynecol Obstet 155:353-357, 1982.

33. Godina M. Preferential use of end-to-side arterial anastomoses in free flap transfers. Plast Reconstr Surg 64:673-682, 1979.

34. Albertengo JB, Rodriguez A, Buncke HJ, Hall EJ. A comparative study of flap survival rates in end-to-end and end-to-side microvascular anastomosis. Plast Reconstr Surg 67:194-199, 1981.

35. Rao VK, Morrison WA, Angus JA, O'Brien BM. Comparison of vascular hemodynamics in experimental models of microvascular anastomoses. Plast Reconstr Surg 71:241-247, 1983.

36. Huang GK, Hu RQ, Pan GP. Influence of vessel clips on vascular patency

in microarterial grafts less than 0.5 mm in external diameter. J Hand Surg 10A:538-541, 1985.

37. Alpert BS, Buncke HJ, Brownstein M. Replacement of damaged arteries and veins with vein grafts when replanting crushed, amputated fingers. Plast Reconstr Surg 61:17-22, 1978.

38. Buncke HJ, Alpert B, Shah KG. Microvascular grafting. Clin Plast Surg 5: 185-194, 1978.

39. Biemer E. Autologous vein grafts as artery replacement in microsurgery. An experimental study of micro- and macromorphologic changes 3 weeks to 12 months postoperatively. Handchirurgie 13:108, 1981.

40. Ganske JG, Demuth RJ, Miller SH, Buck DC, Dolph JL. Comparison of expanded polytetrafluoroethylene microvascular grafts to autogenous vein grafts. Plast Reconstr Surg 70:193-201, 1982.

41. Davies DM. A world survey of anticoagulation practice in clinical micro-vascular surgery. Br J Plast Surg 35:96-99, 1982.

42. Kleinert HE, Jablon M, Tsai TM. An overview of replantation and results of 347 replants in 245 patients. J Trauma 20:390-398, 1980.

43. Kleinert HE, Tsai TM. Microvascular repair in replantation. Clin Orthop Rel Res 133:205-211, 1978.

44. Nomoto H, Buncke HJ, Chater NL. Improved patency rates in micro-vascular surgery when using magnesium sulfate and a silicone rubber vas-cular cuff. Plast Reconstr Surg 54:157-160, 1974.

45. Puckett CL, Winters RRW, Geter RK, Goebel D. Studies of pathologic vasoconstriction (vasospasm) in microvascular surgery. J Hand Surg 10A: 343-349, 1985.

46. Phelps DB, Rutherford RB, Boswick JA. Control of vasospasm following trauma and microvascular surgery. J Hand Surg 4:109-117, 1979.

47. May JW, Lukash FN, Gallico GG, Stirrat CR. Removeable thermocouple probe microvascular patency monitor: an experimental and clinical study. Plast Reconstr Surg 72:366-379, 1983.

48. Lu SY, Chiu HY, Lin T, Chen MT. Evaluation of survival in digital re-plantation with thermometric monitoring. J Hand Surg 9A:805-809, 1984.

49. Rossi LFA, Hoare MR, Greenhalgh RM. Peroperative proof of patency of microvascular anastomoses. Ann R Coll Surg Engl 63:189-191, 1981.

50. Friedman R, Gordon L, Buncke HJ, Alpert BS. Digital replantation: indi-cations and innovations. In: Buncke HJ, Furnas DW (eds). Symposium on Clinical Frontiers in Reconstructive Microsurgery. St. Louis, CV Mosby Co, 1984, pp 21-30.

51. Raskin DJ, Erk Y, Spira M, Melissinos EG. Tissue pH monitoring in microsurgery: a preliminary evaluation of continuous tissue pH moni-toring as indicator of perfusion disturbances in microvascular free flaps. Ann Plast Surg 11:331-339, 1984

52. Fasching MC, Van Beek AL. Monitoring muscle viability using evoked M
     waves. Plast Reconstr Surg 75:217-222, 1985.

17

Reoperations for Thoracic Outlet Compression Syndrome and Vascular Disorders of the Upper Extremity

HERBERT I. MACHLEDER and FRANZ L. MOLL[*]
UCLA School of Medicine, Los Angeles, California

Although the concept of thoracic outlet compression has been generally accepted as a clinical entity for almost three decades, progress has been encumbered by the lack of specific diagnostic tests having acceptable sensitivity and specificity (1). Expressions in the medical literature and in the transactions of national surgical meetings suggest that establishing a diagnosis of thoracic outlet syndrome involves considerable uncertainty, which often results in a diagnosis of exclusion rather than one arrived at by specific objective tests. As a consequence of this diagnostic imprecision, controversies regarding therapy and operative approach remain unresolved and tend to obscure other important issues, particularly those dealing with the incidence and management of *recurrent* thoracic outlet syndrome.

Incidence

Although scattered anecdotal experiences have been reported suggesting a substantial incidence of recurrent or incompletely relieved symptoms as well as adverse consequences of therapy, there are relatively few reports in the literature that clearly distinguish between the true incidence of therapeutic failure, residual symptomatology, and recurrence of thoracic outlet syndrome (2). The occasional reports describing experience with reoperation for thoracic outlet compression are generally derived from referral surgical practices, rendering it difficult to access the size of the population from which these cases are drawn.

*Present affiliation: Medical Center Alkmaar, Alkmaar, The Netherlands

On the University of California-Los Angeles (UCLA) services during the 15 year period from 1965 to 1980, attempts were made to formulate a specific diagnosis of the compressive elements in each case of thoracic outlet syndrome, with operations being tailored accordingly. In selected instances, scalenectomy, subclavius tendonotomy, and pectoralis minor tendonotomy were all employed in addition to transaxillary first rib resection. During that period, there was a 41% incidence of residual or recurrent symptoms. In this group of patients, subsequent reoperation by a more comprehensive approach resulted in a remaining incidence of recurrence or incompletely relieved symptoms of 9%, with 91% of these patients achieving long-term benefit.

In the 5 year period from 1980 to 1985, transaxillary first rib resection became the procedure of choice for the majority of patients presenting with symptomatic thoracic outlet compression who were unresponsive to conservative management. During this subsequent period, of 90 consecutive transaxillary first rib resections, eight patients developed recurrence of their symptoms, an incidence of 9%. It is often difficult to generalize about the actual incidence of complications from the specific reports of a few large series. Nevertheless, there are some representative reports in the literature that suggest the frequency with which the average surgeon in practice may encounter this situation (Table 1). In 1973, Sanders and co-workers (3) reported a 15% incidence of recurrence after transaxillary first rib resection. Using a similar approach, Alquist (4) reported a 12% incidence, Quarfordt and associates (5) reported a 20% incidence, and Urschel and colleagues (6),

Table 1   Recurrent Thoracic Outlet Syndrome: Incidence After First Rib Resection

Source	Year	No. of Cases	Interval	Incidence (%)
Sanders et al. (3)	1973	214	–	15
Urschel et al. (6)	1975	700	3 mo.	1
Alquist (4)	1975	48	2 mo.	12
Quarfordt et al. (15)	1984	97	15 mo.	20
UCLA	1984	90	14 mo.	9

using the posterior approach to first rib resection, reported a 1% incidence of recurrence. The "interval," or mean time to recurrence of symptoms, is skewed in several large series (7,8) by patients who had "immediate" or "early" recurrence (within 1 month). Our own experience with the UCLA series and with patients referred by others suggests that it is quite difficult to evaluate the results of therapy in the first 4 to 6 weeks after surgery. Operative pain, transient sensory deficits, analgesic requirements, and other factors make the diagnosis of recurrence hazardous in this setting. Truly recurrent thoracic outlet syndrome is more apt to be seen at 6 months to 2 years, with earlier symptom complexes more likely to be the consequence of incomplete decompression, iatrogenic injury, or inaccurate diagnosis.

Uncertain results with transaxillary first rib resection have generated renewed interest in transcervical scalenectomy as well as a combined approach of transaxillary rib resection and transcervical scalenectomy. In two separate surgical eras, Adson (9) and Sanders and co-workers (3) reported an approximate 18% incidence of recurrent symptoms after scalenectomy or scalenotomy (Table 2).

Diagnosis

When a diagnosis of recurrent thoracic outlet syndrome is suspected, careful distinction must be made between several important subgroups of patients who may present with similar complaints.

The first group is comprised of patients having residual symptoms after presumably adequate thoracic outlet decompression. These symptoms may be related to concurrent conditions such as cervical neuroforaminal disease, de-

Table 2   Recurrent Thoracic Outlet Compression Syndrome: Incidence After Scalenectomy

Source	Year	No. of Cases	Incidence (%)
Adson (9)	1947	53	19
Sanders et al. (3)	1979	239	17

generative disc disease, primary shoulder disease (arthritis, tendonitis, or bursitis), peripheral nerve entrapment syndromes (cubital tunnel or carpal tunnel syndrome), and myofascial pain. Included in this group would be patients who, in retrospect, may not have had clinically significant thoracic outlet syndrome.

The second group is made up of patients who sustained iatrogenic injury. Identification of this group is facilitated by the surgeon's familiarity with the common complications seen after various primary surgical approaches to thoracic outlet decompression.

A third group of patients has probably had inadequate thoracic outlet decompression and experience residual symptoms that may have been obscured by analgesics and postoperative restrictions, becoming manifest when the patient resumed work or normal activity.

A fourth group is represented by patients who experienced initial complete relief of symptoms, returned to work or usual activities, and then developed recurrence of a similar picture of neuromuscular disability and pain after this symptom-free interval. The most reliable evidence of recurrence is a symptom-free period usually lasting from 6 months to 2 years.

It should be evident from the foregoing that the initial step in evaluating a patient with presumed recurrent thoracic outlet compression syndrome is a careful reassessment of the diagnosis. Much has been written about the clinical presentation of thoracic outlet compression, and this still remains the foundation on which accurate diagnosis rests (10). The clinical picture has often been subdivided into symptoms that reflect predominantly upper plexus compression (C5,C6,C7), lower plexus compression (C8,T1), or a combination of these, with an important but numerically smaller group of patients having predominantly arterial or venous obstruction. The most reliable clinical feature, both historically and on examination, is positionally related dysesthesias or pain, predominantly in the ulnar or median nerve distribution, exacerbated by abducting the upper arm with external rotation of the forearm.

Specific laboratory studies can be useful in establishing the diagnosis and investigating the possibility of concurrent conditions. If not done previously, radiologic survey of the cervical spine should be reviewed to look for neuroforaminal encroachment or narrowed disc spaces. When abnormalities are detected, computed tomography (CT) scan or metrizamide myelography can be done to further clarify the possibility of nerve root compression or degenerative disc disease. These studies can be particularly useful in evaluating patients who are in the late fourth and fifth decades of life, which in our experience, is somewhat beyond the peak age incidence for thoracic outlet compression.

Chest radiography, including apical lordotic views, should be obtained to assess the length of residual first rib, or presence of recurrent calcification where periosteum has been incompletely removed (Fig. 1). During the transaxillary approach to first rib resection, retention of the posterior third of the first rib is quite common (Fig. 2).

Electrophysiologic tests are routinely evaluated. Although questions have been raised in the surgical literature regarding the importance of these tests, we feel their value to be considerable, particularly in the evaluation of recurrent symptoms and, specifically, by surgeons in their early years of experience with thoracic outlet compression syndrome. Nerve conduction times and electromyography aid in identifying cervical disc disease, neuroforaminal disease, and peripheral nerve entrapment syndromes. When properly done and interpreted, these tests provide definitive evidence of peripheral nerve entrapment or muscle denervation. Because carpal or cubital tunnel syndrome probably occurs coincident with thoracic outlet syndrome in 10 to 15% of patients, these entities must be identified when present. The most sensitive neurophysiologic evaluation is the somatosensory-evoked response test (11). This should be performed for both median and ulnar nerves in both upper extremities in the stressed (abducted externally rotated) and neutral positions. This test can be used intraoperatively to demonstrate when complete relief of compressive neuropathy has been achieved. Peripheral median and ulnar nerve peaks often return to normal immediately after compressive elements are removed. Figure 3 illustrates the somatosensory-evoked potential changes in a patient with bilateral thoracic outlet compression syndrome. Bilateral absence of normal post stimulation ulnar nerve peripheral peaks can be seen in Figures 3A and B. After left transaxillary first rib resection and scalenectomy, return of a normal left peripheral ulnar nerve voltage peak is illustrated, with no concomitant change in the peripheral peak on the uncorrected side. (Fig. 3C).

Occasionally, arteriographic or venographic studies will be useful, particularly when symptoms of arterial insufficiency or venous hypertension are part of the clinical picture. The accuracy of angiographic demonstration of thoracic outlet compression has been variable as reported in the literature. Even with clearly demonstrable clinical evidence of arterial compromise, arteriography in the supine position is often inconclusive. When a patient has a reduction in the radial pulse or an axillosubclavian bruit with Adson's maneuver or abduction and external rotation, arterial compression can gener-

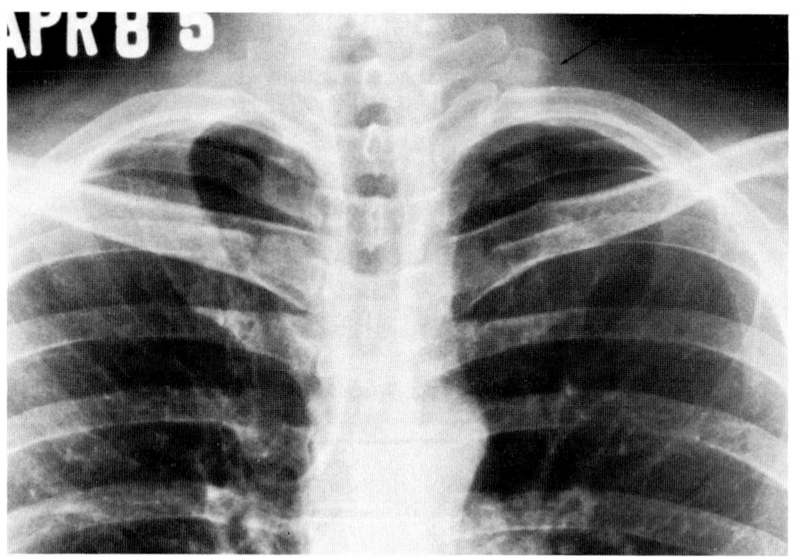

Figure 1 Chest x-ray of a patient after transaxillary left first rib resection. Note small residual stump of first rib.

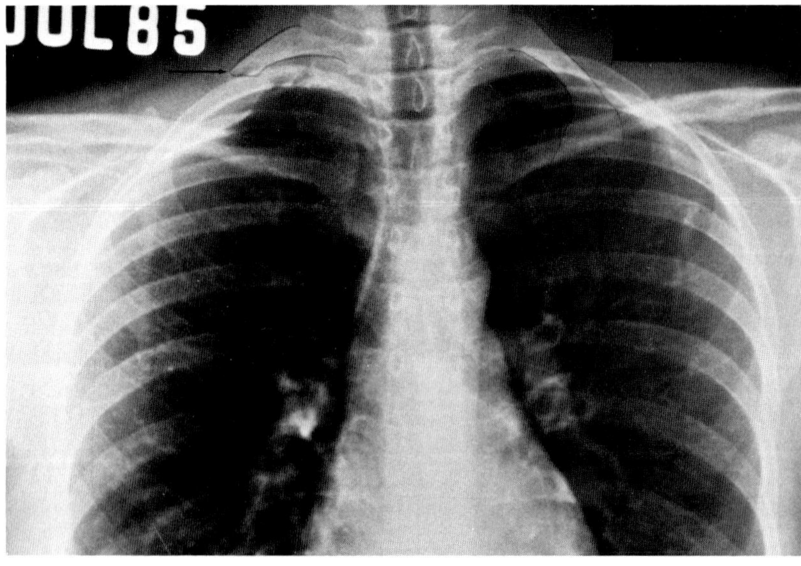

Figure 2 Chest x-ray of a patient after right first rib resection. Note the common finding of residual distal third of rib remaining.

ally be demonstrated if arteriography is performed with the patient in the sitting position (Fig. 4).

It is probably injudicious for the average well trained surgeon to expect that clinical judgment without the benefit of complete reassessment and ancillary tests will be sufficient to identify the patient with recurrent thoracic outlet compression syndrome and to indicate appropriate therapy. Experience dictates that in this particular entity, the liberal use of diagnostic tests may well protect the patient from injury and the surgeon from liability.

Iatrogenic Injury

Unfortunately, iatrogenic injury is not uncommon and must be distinguished from symptoms of recurrent thoracic outlet compression. Elements of the brachial plexus should be carefully assessed to establish the level of injury if this has occurred (12).

There are specific neuromuscular abnormalities that characterize brachial plexus injury at various levels. Traction injury to the roots of the brachial plexus is often accompanied by long thoracic nerve palsy (with consequent winging of the scapula). The long thoracic nerve arises from the C5, C6, C7, and occasionally C8 nerve roots, remaining in close proximity to these roots before piercing the scalenus medius muscle to descend posteriorly. The dorsal scapular nerve from the C5, -C6 nerve roots is also intimately associated with the proximal brachial plexus. Clinical or electromyographic evidence of rhomboid or levator scapulae denervation is commonly seen with injury to the upper brachial plexus roots.

The phrenic nerve, arising from C2, C3, C4, tends to travel with the C5 nerve root, and ipsilateral diaphragmatic paralysis can occur with proximal root injury. Injury to the brachial plexus at the C8, T1 nerve roots will often result in Horner's syndrome as a consequence of the gray rami communicantes arising from these two roots at a very proximal level. If such injury is suspected, myelography is often helpful and may show meningoceles associated with the nerve roots.

Interpretation of these findings must be cautious because isolated injury to the long thoracic and phrenic nerves is not uncommon in thoracic outlet surgery and does not signify concomitant injury to the branchial plexus nerve roots. The long thoracic nerve traverses the scalenus medius muscle before continuing down the posterior axilla closely related to the serratus anterior muscle, and can be injured during either the transaxillary or posterior approach to first rib resection or during the supraclavicular approach when the scalenus medius muscle is dissected from the first rib. Injury to the phrenic

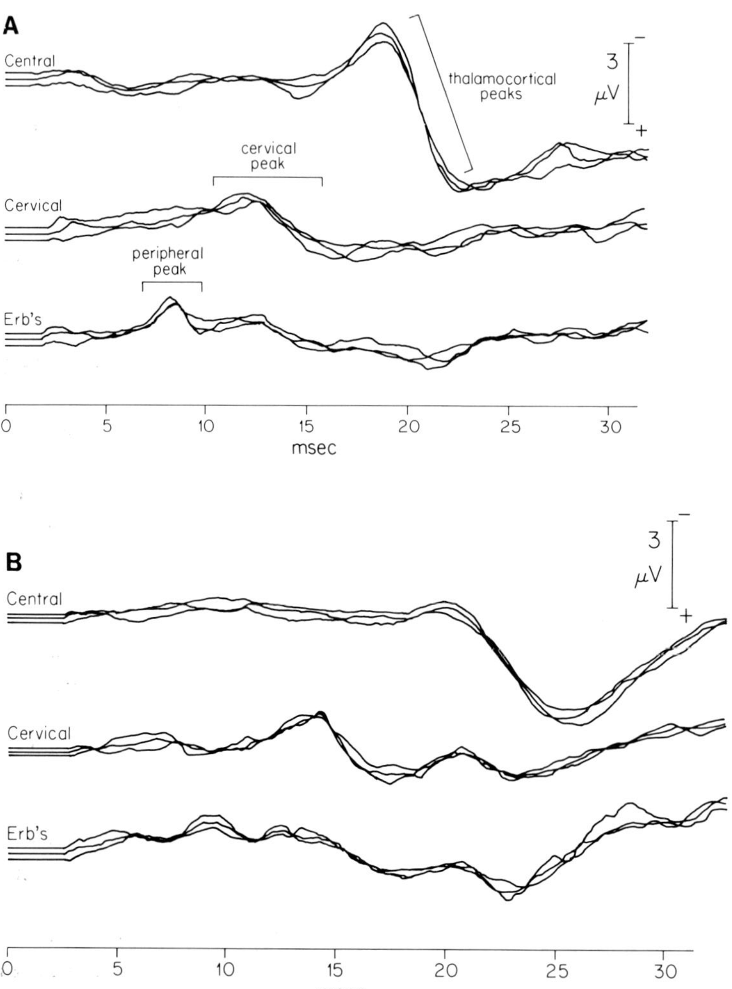

Figure 3 *A*: Somatosensory-evoked response of right ulnar nerve in patient with bilateral thoracic outlet compression syndrome. There is absence of the normal Erb's Point peripheral peak as calculated by voltage change from base line. *B*: Somatosenory-evoked response of left ulnar nerve in the same patient. Normal peripheral peak is absent in both stress and neutral positions. *C*: After left first rib resection and scalenectomy, somatosensory-evoked response has returned to normal, with peripheral peak seen at 9 ms (Erb's). *D*: Persistant attenuation of peripheral peak on the unoperated side.

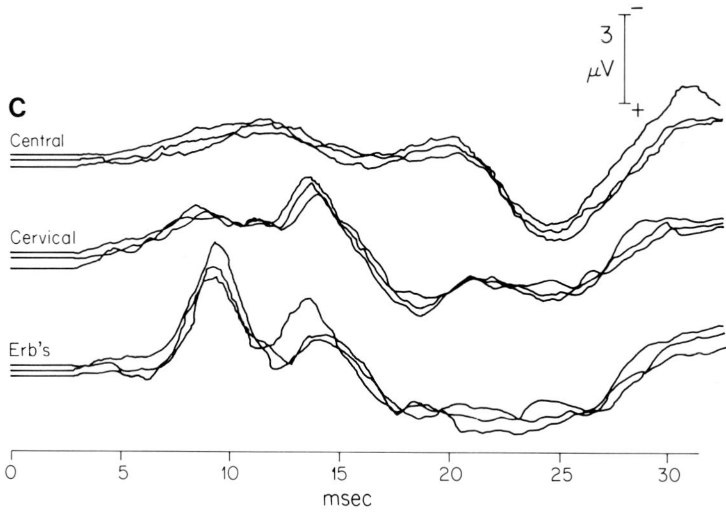

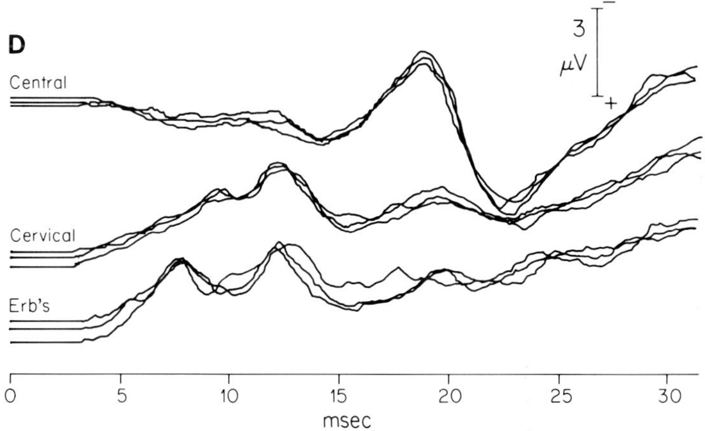

Figure 3 (Continued)

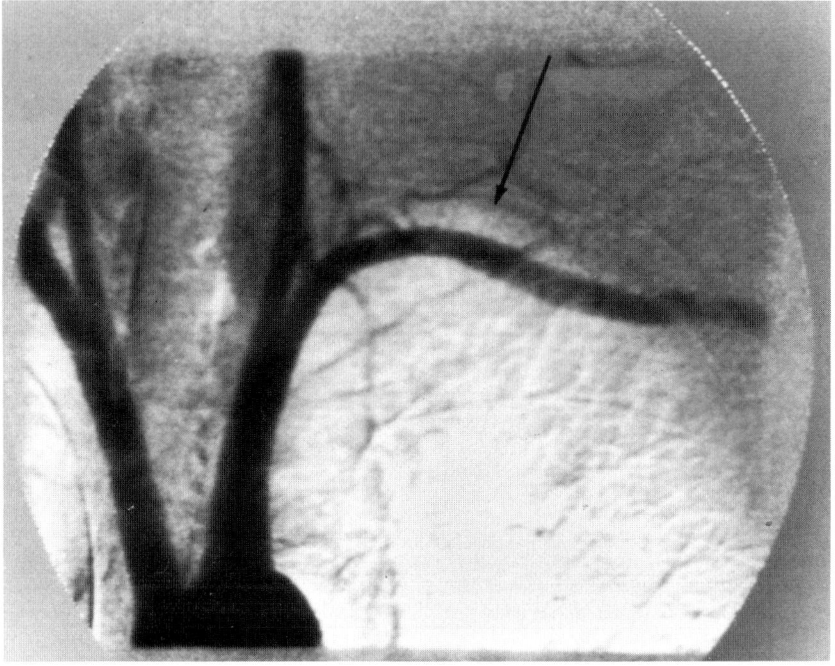

A

Figure 4 *A*: Supine position digital subtraction angiogram. Patient with thoracic outlet compression syndrome. *B*: Angiogram with the patient sitting and arm abducted.

nerve can likewise occur, either from the transaxillary or transcervical approach due either to traction or traumatic manipulation. The posterior approach to the first rib is associated with an 8 to 10% incidence of winging of the scapula due either to incomplete healing of the rhomboid muscles or actual injury to the long thoracic nerve.

Systematic assessment of any brachial plexus element deficiency will greatly facilitate diagnosis of injury and recognition of possible residual areas of compression. It should be emphasized that nerve continuity alone does not ensure proper nerve conduction. The internal architecture may be distorted such that regeneration cannot possibly take place. In cases of brachial plexus injury after thoracic outlet compression surgery, a 3 month period of time

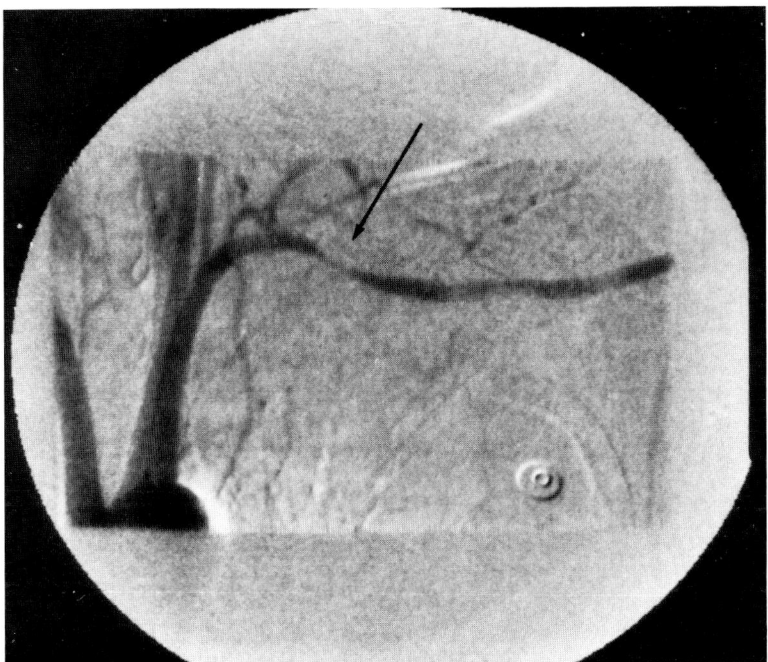

B

Figure 4 (Continued)

should be utilized for observation and assessment of the separate elements. If there is progress in reinnervation, further observation is appropriate. If there is no evidence of reinnervation, surgical intervention may be indicated. Motor function will generally return more rapidly than sensory function, and consequently a delay in sensory return alone is not a reliable indication for early intervention. If the lack of motor or sensory improvement indicates the need for surgical exploration, intraoperative nerve action potentials are assessed across injured areas, facilitating recognition of elements appropriate for resection and nerve grafting. When scar tissue involves the brachial plexus, external neurolysis can be helpful in restoring sensory and motor function.

Electromyography has limited usefulness in detecting reinnervation changes because the abnormalities (denervation potentials and fibrillation potentials with absence of insertional activity) will persist until axonal and neuronal regeneration reaches the end plates. Injuries to the brachial plexus at the trunk level (the distal margin of most thoracic outlet surgery) will usually require 7 to 8 months before electromyographic changes demonstrate reinnervation. When brachial plexus injury occurs during thoracic outlet surgery, it is most likely neuropraxic rather than disruption of nerve continuity.

After transaxillary first rib resection, hypoesthesia or dysesthesia of the inner aspect of the upper arm to the level of the elbow is not uncommon as a consequence of retraction of the intercostobrachial nerve. This should not be considered evidence of residual or recurrent symptoms from thoracic outlet compression.

Residual Symptoms

Residual symptoms occur most frequently in those patients having initial evidence of both upper and lower branchial plexus root compression. After transaxillary first rib resection, relief of hand and arm symptoms is generally prompt and enduring. With gradual return to normal physical activity, the patient may notice the onset or recrudescence of shoulder, neck, occipital, and midscapula area pain, which will result in various degrees of disability. These residual symptoms are most likely secondary to inadequate retraction of the anterior scalene muscle after transection at the level of the scalene tubercle of the first rib. Traction on the muscle during transaxillary first rib resection will often allow division of the muscle at a higher level and may obviate some of these residual symptoms.

Occasionally, inadequate resection of the posterior third of the first rib will result in residual C8, T1 ulnar nerve distribution sensory changes. Recurrent symptoms may also arise from this area as a consequence of postoperative changes, which will be further described.

Recurrent Symptoms

Occasional reports of recurrent thoracic outlet compression symptoms occurring immediately or within 1 month of operation appear in the surgical literature. In some series (4,7), this number may be as high as 20 to 25% of the group. It is unclear whether these cases represent true recurrence or are, in reality, manifestations of residual symptoms. The initial evaluation of patients who have undergone first rib resection is often difficult and inconclusive until at least several weeks after operation. Dysesthesia or hypoesthesia in the distribution of the intercostal brachial nerve secondary to retraction is not uncommon, nor is numbness and dysesthesia in the distribution of the medial, radial, or ulnar nerve, which may be seen for 3 to 4 days after operation, related most likely to traction on the arm or compression of the forearm during surgical manipulation. Testing of the latissimus dorsi, serratus anterior, and trapezius muscles is often restricted by postoperative pain in the cervical and back region. Adequate posterior resection of the neck of the first rib requires manipulation and retraction of the T1, C8 root, and patients will often have transient dysesthesia in that distribution in addition to transient weakness of the interosseous muscles with poor grip strength.

The vast majority of patients with excellent long-term results are significantly free of symptoms by the fourth to sixth week after operation. Patients who develop recurrent symptoms usually have a symptom-free interval of approximately 6 to 24 months, with the mean time to reoperation in our series being 14 months. This figure is quite close to the mean interval of 15 months reported by Quarfordt and associates (5). A report by Sessions (7) indicates a mean symptomatic recurrence time of 2 months, although 40% of these patients had symptoms returning either immediately after operation or within 1 month of surgery. At this interval, we suspect that these symptoms result from inadequate thoracic outlet decompression, rather than true recurrence.

Etiology

On reexploration of the thoracic outlet for recurrent symptoms, the most consistent finding is reattachment of the scalene muscle to either the bed of the first rib, the subclavian artery, Sibson's fascia, or the perineurium of the brachial plexus. Occasionally, we have found associated anomalies of the scalene muscle, which may include a scalenus minimus inserting into Sibson's fascia between the subclavian artery and the brachial plexus, or a tendinous band of scalenus medius muscle lying beneath the brachial plexus and causing a friction-type injury (particularly when trapped between a fibrotic and reattached scalenus anticus muscle). Interdigitations between the scalenus anterior and scalenus medius can occasionally be found at the level of the brachial plexus roots, and fibromuscular bands between the C7 transverse process and the periosteum of the first rib are described in 15 to 20% of the cases in some series. A fibrocartilaginous cervical rib may not be appreciated from the transaxillary approach and is likewise encountered in about 10% of recurrent cases. Fibrosis around the roots and trunks of the brachial plexus is occasionally encountered. As mentioned previously, inadequate resection of the first rib can be found when a patient's initial operation has taken place either from the transaxillary or transcervical route. It is common to see the posterior third of the first rib remaining after transaxillary resection. This portion of the rib is most completely removed via the posterior approach described by Claggett (13) and Martinez (14).

Regeneration of the first rib can be seen in cases where the rib has been removed subperiosteally, and can often be identified by calcifications seen in the bed of the first rib in the apical lordotic or reversed lordotic view of the chest. On occasion, when the posterior rib osteotomy has been irregular, a fibrocalcific scar can be seen binding the bony spike to the T1 nerve root, which is a condition also encountered in the smoothly transected but elongated rib stump. After scalenotomy alone, the muscle can often be found firmly reattached to the first rib by dense scar coursing over the subclavian artery.

Reoperation

Although several different approaches to reoperation have been widely practiced, the most frequent and perhaps most successful is transcervical scalenectomy and neurolysis of the brachial plexus. This approach is particularly useful if the initial operation has been a transaxillary first rib resection because it gives excellent access to the residual scalene muscle, allowing adequate resection. The anterior approach also enables resection of the scalenus medius muscle and division of fibrous bands that may be compressing the brachial plexus from the posterior position. Exposure of the roots and trunks of the brachial plexus (the most common areas of recompression) is likewise facilitated. Although the transaxillary approach has been utilized in cases where there is a large residual posterior segment of the first rib, the problem of scarring from previous transaxillary surgery poses formidable hazards.

The posterior approach probably allows the best exposure of the C8, T1 nerve roots and additionally allows the most complete resection of the posterior third of the first rib. Nevertheless, there is a fairly consistent though small incidence of winged scapula after this approach, and morbidity is generally more significant than from either the transaxillary or transcervical approach.

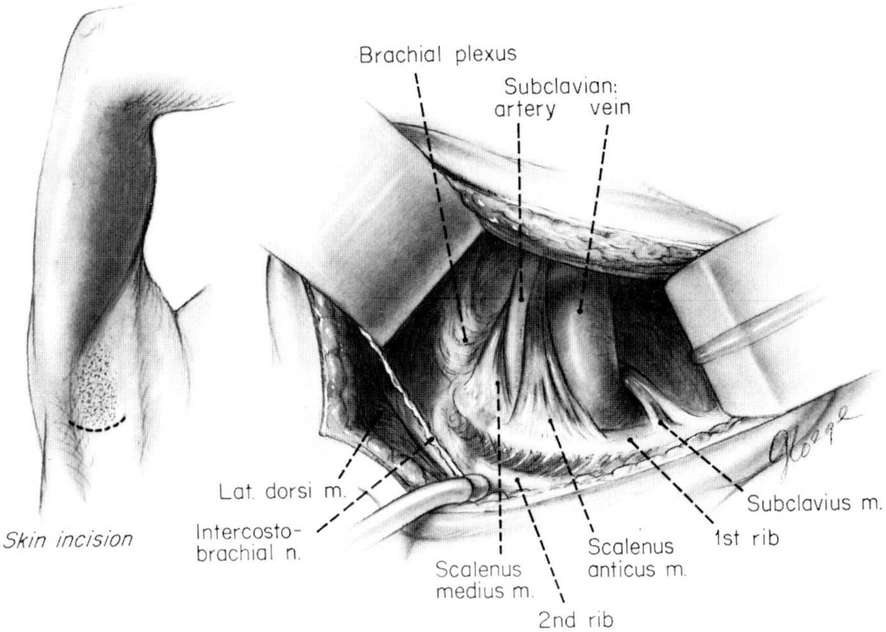

Figure 5 Perspective of thoracic outlet as seen from the transaxillary position. Note abnormal insertion of a portion of scalenus medius or scalenus minimus anterior to brachial plexus.

Technical Details

The transaxillary approach is performed with the patient in the lateral decubitus position (Fig. 5), and has been previously described in detail (12). If the patient retains sensation in the distribution of the intercostal brachial nerve, an effort should be made to identify and preserve this nerve where it traverses the axilla at the level of the second intercostal space. Injury to the long thoracic nerve is more common with secondary operations via the transaxillary approach, and the nerve will often be situated more medially than is usually encountered in the primary operation. The use of a nerve stimulator can be very helpful, and the anesthesiologist can be advised to avoid the use of neuromuscular blocking agents after initial induction. Generally, it is

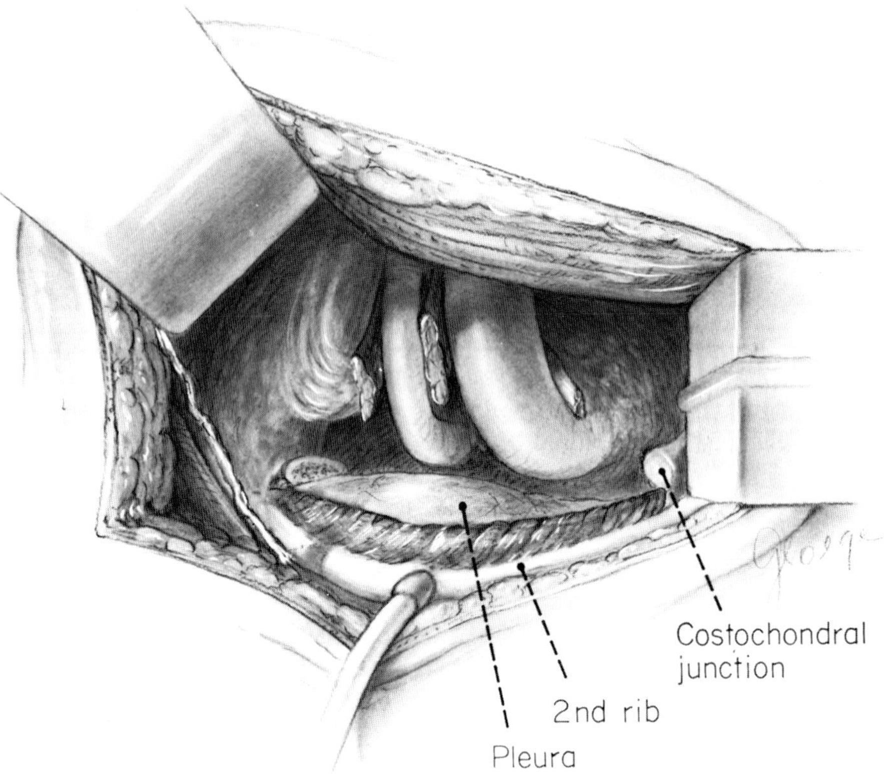

Figure 6 View of thoracic outlet after transaxillary resection of first rib showing the relationship of important structures.

easiest to locate the axillary artery, which lies anterior to the area of dense scar and adhesions (Fig. 6). When adhesions are particularly well developed between the neurovascular structures and the pleura, dissection can be facilitated by entering the pleural cavity. The T1 root will usually be found lying very close to the axillary artery and must be carefully separated from the stump of the residual first rib. In the technique described by Roos (8), a flap of axillary fat can be mobilized and sutured posteriorly to protect the exposed T1 nerve root from the dissected area.

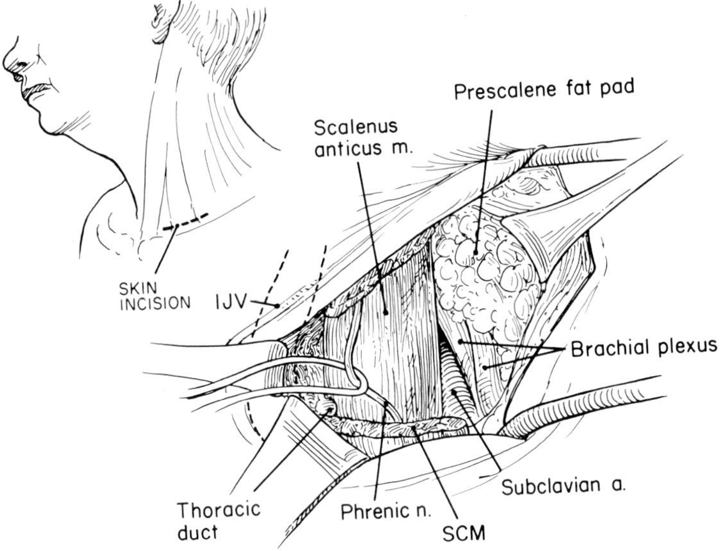

Figure 7 Transcervical approach to scalenectomy for treatment of recurrent thoracic outlet compression syndrome after transaxillary first rib resection.

Transcervical

Reoperation via the transcervical approach should be done under general anesthesia with the patient in the supine position. Two folded sheets are placed at the level of the scapula and the head turned to the contralateral side in hyperextension. An incision is made in the supraclavicular area from the medial border of the sternal head of the sternocleidomastoid muscle and carried laterally to the anterior jugular vein (Fig. 7). The clavicular head of the sternocleidomastoid muscle is divided, and care is taken to avoid trauma to the spinal accessory nerve. The omohyoid muscle will often be found traversing this field, and can be divided. The prescalene fat pad is dissected from the jugular vein, care being taken to avoid the thoracic duct on the left side and, occasionally (in 10% cases), on the right side at the jugular-subclavian vein junction. The fat pad is retracted laterally, exposing the scalene muscle and the brachial plexus emerging from its lateral margin. Surprisingly, the scalene muscle will often appear intact, hypertrophied, and taut at the level

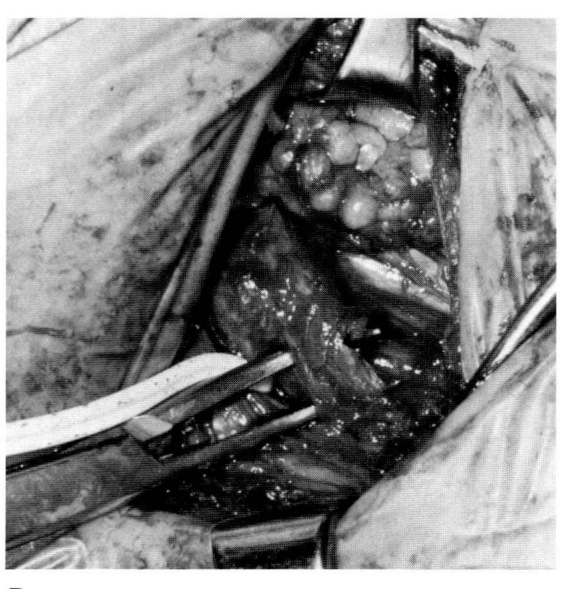

A

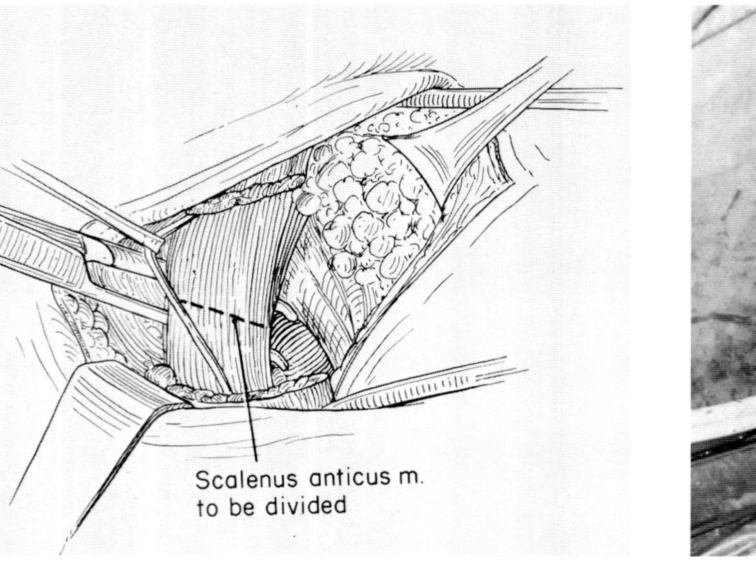

B

Figure 8 *A*: Initial division of anterior scalene muscle superior to subclavian artery. *B*: Operative view. Stepwise transection of anterior scalene muscle.

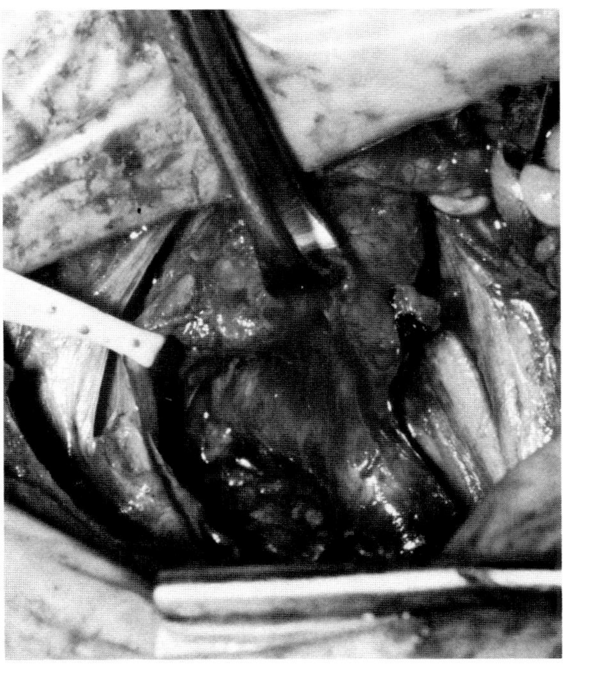

A

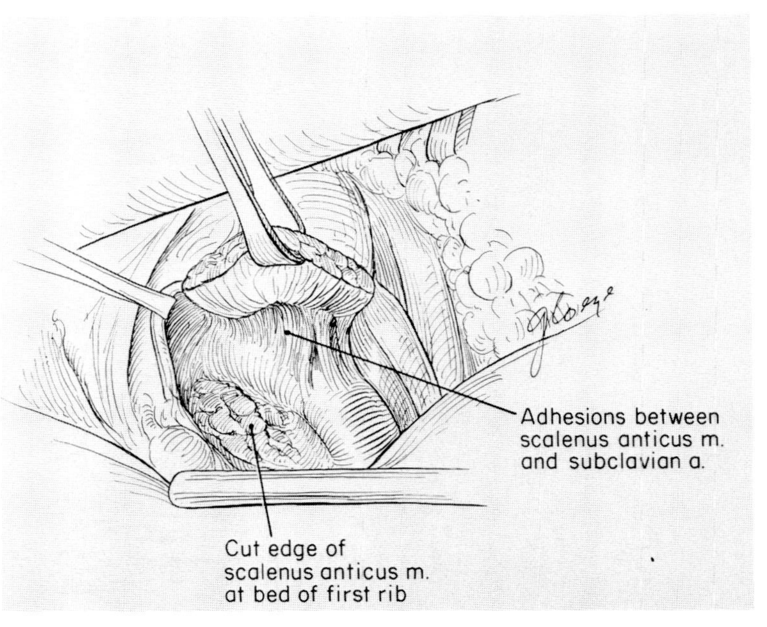

B

Figure 9   *A*: Operative view of anterior scalene adhesions to subclavian artery. *B*: Artist's drawing of *A*.

of the dissection. The phrenic nerve should be carefully identified and dissected free of the prescalene fascia so that it can be retracted medially, allowing complete resection of the scalene muscle. The medial and lateral borders of the scalene muscle are then developed, and palpation is used to identify the position of the subclavian artery. We have favored transecting the scalene muscle superior to the attachment at the bed of the first rib, thus limiting problems of dissecting the dense scar from the superior surface of the subclavian artery (Fig. 8). When the muscle has been completely transected, it is retracted superiorly such that adhesions to the subclavian artery can be identifed, as well as aponeurotic attachments to Sibson's fascia (Figs. 9 and 10). This phase of the operation is generally accomplished with 3X or 4X magnification to aid identification of the perineurium from fibrous scar tissue often found in this area. As the scalene muscle is retracted superiorly, a number of adhesive bands will be encountered traversing the under surface of the muscle to the perineurium of the brachial plexus (Figs. 11 and 12). To remove a sufficient portion of the scalene muscle the dissection is carried back to at least the first attachment to the transverse process. When extensive fibrosis is encountered around the roots and trunks of the brachial plexus, a careful external neurolysis is performed.

After meticulous hemostasis has been achieved, the area should be irrigated and tested for pneumothorax, and the brachial plexus carefully reinspected to determine whether any additional constricting fibrous bands are present. It is often necessary at this point to decide whether resection of a portion of the scalenus medius muscle is indicated. The long thoracic nerve pierces the body of the scalenus medius muscle before descending posteriorly, and great care must be exercised to avoid injuring this nerve. Occasionally, when a cervical rib has been previously excised, there will be residual bands of periosteum or fibrous adhesions which must be carefully excised.

When the dissection has been completed, the scalene fat pad is sutured over the brachial plexus with fine catgut sutures between the fat and fascia adjacent to the jugular vein. A silastic suction drain catheter is left in the scalene fossa and brought out through a separate incision beneath the wound. The sternocleidomastoid muscle is reapproximated using figure-of-eight sutures. The platysma muscle and subcutaneous tissue are closed with absorbable continuous suture and the skin with a subcuticular suture of absorbable material. Four to 6 weeks of recuperation is generally necessary before the patient can resume full physical activity. Restricted activity of the upper extremity is encouraged for at least 2 to 3 weeks after surgery.

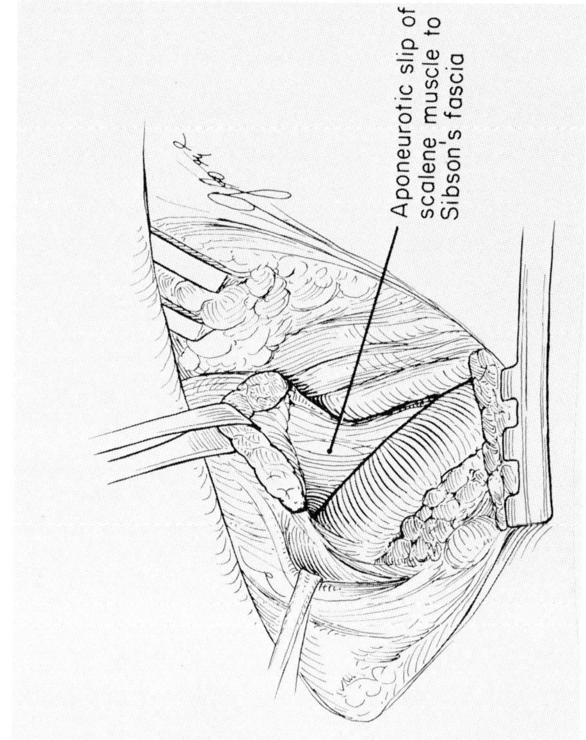

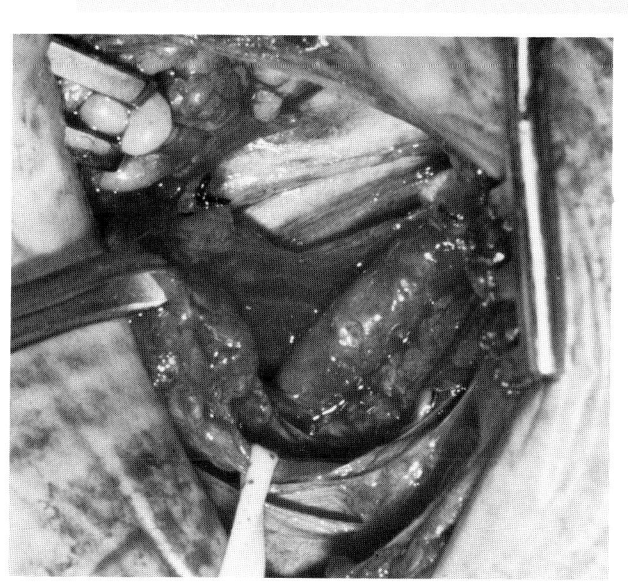

Figure 10 *A*: Muscle attachments between anterior scalene and Sibson's fascia. Occasional site of scalenus minimus muscle. *B*: Drawing of anatomic relationships in *A*.

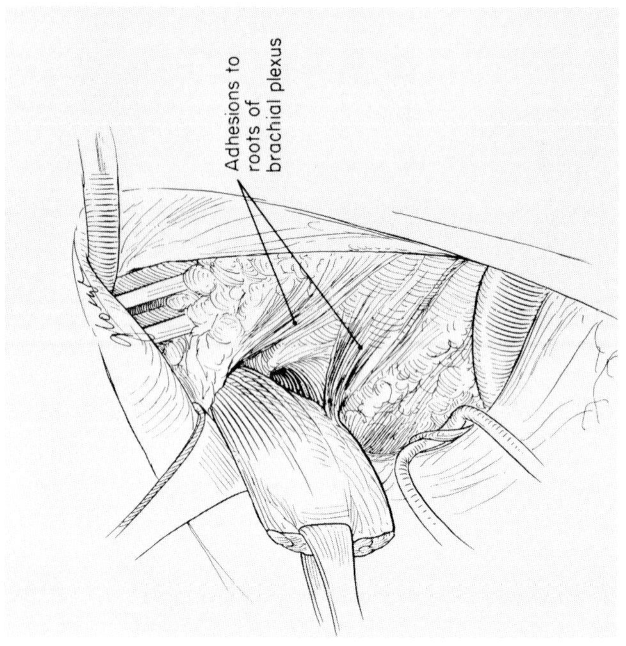

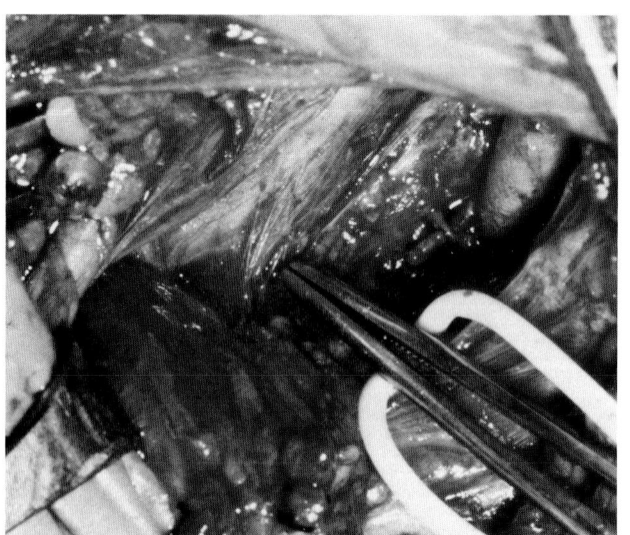

Figure 11 *A*: Adhesions between under surface of anterior scalene muscle and brachial plexus. *B*: Drawing of anatomic relationships in *A*.

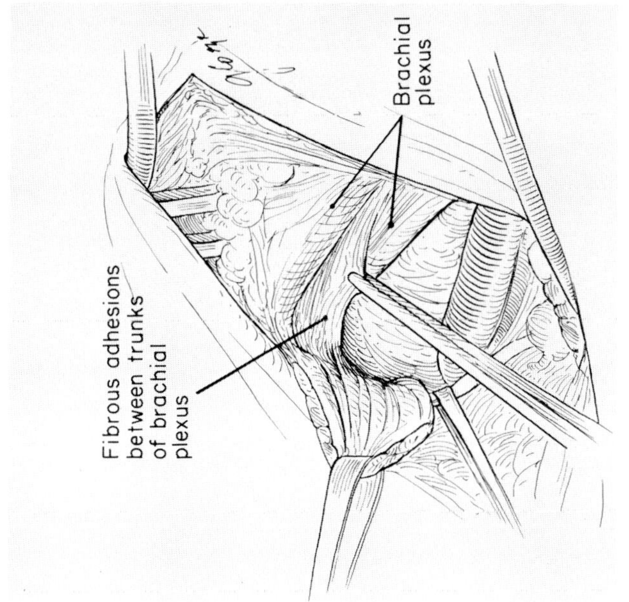

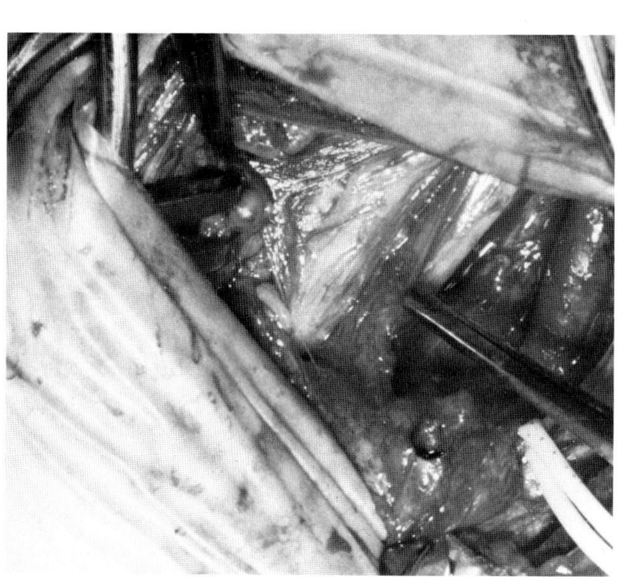

Figure 12 *A*: Fibrous adhesions from undersurface of anterior scalene muscle extending between trunks of brachial plexus. Interdigitations traversing brachial plexus from anterior scalene to middle scalene muscles are also seen in this region. *B*: Anatomic drawing of *A*.

Table 3   Recurrent Thoracic Outlet Compression Syndrome: Results of
Reoperation

		Results (%)			
Source	No. of Cases	Excellent	Good	(Total)	Poor
Alquist et al. (14)	6	83		(83)	17
Quarfordt et al. (5)	20	80	20	(100)	0
Roos (8)	76	60	35	(95)	5
Sessions (7)	29	14	68	(82)	18
UCLA	14	82		(82)	18
Urschel et al. (6)	30	91		(91)	9

Results

Reported results after reoperation for recurrent thoracic outlet syndrome are
generally quite satisfactory, with almost 80 to 90% of reported patients
achieving good or excellent results. Table 3 summarizes the results of representative series in the surgical literature.

Recurrent Obstruction and Occlusion of the Axillosubclavian Vein

The most common occlusive process seen in the major vessels of the upper extremity is recurrent obstruction and occlusion of the axillosubclavian vein.
The clinical presentation of patients who develop axillosubclavian vein thrombosis was first described by Paget (16) in 1875 and then by Von Schroetter
(17) in 1884. By 1949, the entity was called Paget-Schroetter syndrome, and
300 published cases were chronicled by Hughes (18).

Recurrent nonthrombotic occlusion of the axillosubclavian vein was first
reported by McLaughlin and Palma (19) in 1939, but it was not until 1959
that McCleery and co-workers (20) published five cases and suggested muscu-
lotendinous compression at the thoracic outlet, and advanced surgical approaches for relief of this syndrome. In 1969, Adams and associates (21) reported eight cases, of which five were treated surgically. Although one patient
treated by claviculectomy did well, four patients had recurrent symptoms

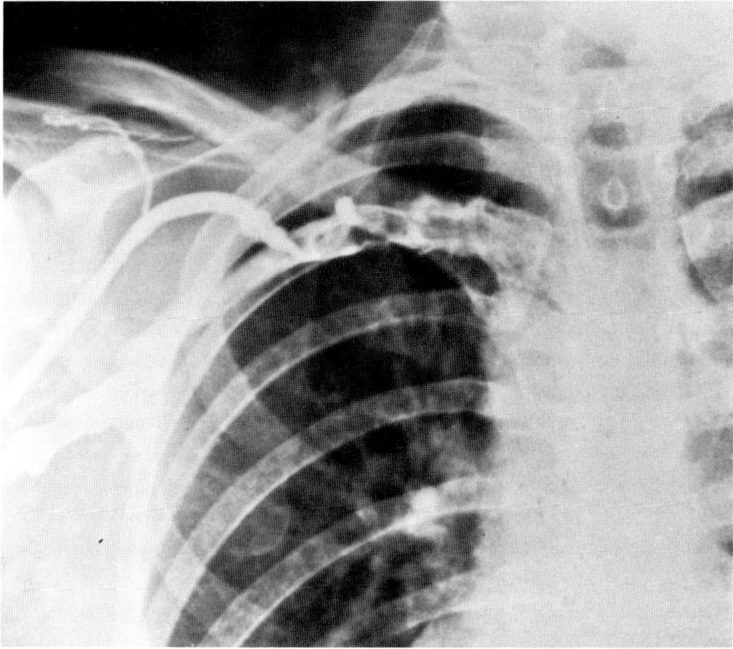

Figure 13 Axillosubclavian vein thrombosis at thoracic outlet as seen in right upper extremity venogram.

after three anterior scalenotomies and one pectoralis minor tenotomy. Resection of the first rib or subtotal claviculectomy as a secondary procedure gave excellent results in these patients.

The history of axillosubclavian vein thrombectomy is similar, with a high incidence of rethrombosis. It has gradually become evident that compression of the axillosubclavian vein at the thoracic outlet is common to both intermittent obstruction and "effort" thrombosis. Primary treatment of the venous thrombosis or decompression of the thoracic outlet by soft tissue excision alone has been associated with a high incidence of recurrence requiring reoperation. It has further become evident that venous obstruction or thrombosis is not the primary event, but a consequence of thoracic outlet compression syndrome.

Among 80 consecutive patients with transvenous pacemakers, it was noted that 35% had asymptomatic subclavian vein thrombosis and another 35% had asymptomatic high grade stenosis. This type of evidence has led to the belief that axillosubclavian thrombosis as a consequence of thoracic outlet compression syndrome is a highly symptomatic event, whereas primary axillosubclavian thrombosis secondary to other causes may be a bland asymptomatic clinical consequence (22).

In 1970, DeWeese and co-workers (23) added 6 cases of axillosubclavian thrombosis to 22 others collected from the literature. Only nine patients had pre- and postoperative venography, and the postoperation patency rate in this subgroup was 70%, with 30% documented reocclusion. In 1975, Glass (24) drew attention to the relationship of axillary venous thrombosis to thoracic outlet compression syndrome, observing a significant incidence of recanalization and relief of symptoms after transaxillary first rib resection without concomitant thrombectomy.

Our own approach has been to treat the acute axillosubclavian venous thrombosis with regional streptokinase infusion followed by heparinization and treatment with Coumadin if the posttreatment venogram demonstrates reestablishment of flow. Transaxillary first rib section has been performed at an interval without the use of subsequent anticoagulation. A variation of this approach, using systemic thrombolytic therapy, has recently been reported by Taylor and associates (25).

Reoperation for symptomatic axillosubclavian vein thrombosis should be directed at thoracic outlet decompression unless other etiologic mechanisms have been clearly demonstrated.

References

1. Robb CG, Standeven A: Arterial occlusion complicating thoracic outlet compression syndrome. Br Med J 2:709-712, 1958.
2. Dale WA: Thoracic outlet compression syndrome, critique in 1982. Arch Surg 117:1437-1445, 1982.
3. Sanders RJ, Monsour JW, Gerber WF, Adams WR, Thompson N: Scalenectomy versus first rib resection for treatment of the thoracic outlet syndrome. Surgery 85:109-121, 1979.
4. Alquist RA: Discussion in Quarfordt: supraclavicular radical scalenectomy and transaxillary first rib resection for thoracic outlet syndrome. Am J Surg 148:111-116, 1984.
5. Quarfordt PG, Ehrenfeld WK, Stoney RJ: Supraclavicular radical scalenectomy and transaxillary first rib resection for thoracic outlet syndrome. Am J Surg 148:111-116, 1984.

6. Urschel HC Jr, Razzuk MA, Albers JE, Wood RE, Paulson DL: Reoperation for recurrent thoracic outlet syndrome. Ann Thorac Surg 21: 19-25, 1976.
7. Sessions RT: Recurrent thoracic outlet syndrome: causes and treatment. South Med J 75:1453-1461, 1982.
8. Roos DB: Recurrent thoracic outlet syndrome after first rib resection. Acta Chir Belg 79:363-372, 1980.
9. Adson AW: Surgical treatment for symptoms produced by cervical ribs and the scalenus anticus muscle. S.G.O. 85:687-700, 1947.
10. Roos DB: In Machleder HI (Ed): Vascular Disorders of the Upper Extremity. Mount Kisco, New York, Futura, 1983.
11. Glover JL, Worth RM, Bendick PJ, Hall PV, Markland OM: Evoked responses in the diagnosis of thoracic outlet compression syndrome. Surgery 89:86-93, 1981.
12. Kline DG, Judice DJ: Management of selected brachial plexus lesions. J. Neurology 58:631-649, 1983.
13. Claggett OT: Research and prosearch. J Thorac Cardiovasc Surg. 44: 153-166, 1962.
14. Martinez NS: Posterior first rib resection for total thoracic outlet decompression. Surgery 173:429-442, 1971.
15. Roos DB: Experience with first rib resection for thoracic outlet syndrome. Ann Surg 173:429-442, 1971.
16. Paget J: Clinical Lectures and Essays. London, Longman's, Green and Company, 1875.
17. vonSchroetter L: Erkrankungen de Gefasse. Nothnagal Handbuch der Pathologie und Therapei. Win, Holder, 1884.
18. Hughes ESR: Venous obstruction in the upper extremity (Paget-Schrotter's syndrome). International Abstracts of Surgery 88:89-125, 1949.
19. McLaughlin, CW Jr, Palma AM: Intermittent obstruction of the subclavian vein. JAMA 113:1960-1963, 1939.
20. McCleery RS, Kesterson JE, Kirtley JA, Love RB: Subclavius and anterior scalene muscle compression as source of intermittent obstruction of subclavian vein. Ann Surg 133:588, 1951.
21. Adams JT, DeWeese JA, Mahoney EB, Rob, CG: Intermittent subclavian vein obstruction without thrombosis. Surgery 63:147-165, 1968.
22. Parsonnet VN: Discussion in Campbell CB, Chandler JG, Tettmeyer CJ, Bernstein EF: Axillary, subclavian and brachiocephalic vein obstruction. Surgery 82:816-826, 1977.
23. DeWeese JA, Adams JT, Gaiser AL: Subclavian venous thrombectomy., Suppl. II to Circulation 41/42 (suppl II):II-158-164, 1970.
24. Glass BA: The relationship of axillary venous thrombosis to the thoracic outlet compression syndrome. Ann Thorac Surg 613-621, 1975.

25. Taylor LM, McAllister MD, Dennis DL, Porter JM: Thrombolytic therapy
    followed by first rib resection for spontaneous ("effort") subclavian
    vein thrombosis. Am J Surg 149:644-647, 1985.

18

Reoperation on the Inferior Vena Cava After Previous Ligation or After Insertion of Interruption Devices

ANTON N. SIDAWY
VAMC, Washington, D.C.

Because primary operations on the inferior vena cava are infrequent, reoperations will be rare but, nonetheless, sometimes will be necessary. This chapter describes direct reoperations on the inferior vena cava to correct complications after caval interruption devices have been inserted. In addition, management options for control of the consequences of severe lower extremity venous hypertension due to ligation or complete thrombosis of the vena cava will be reviewed.

Direct Reoperations on the Inferior Vena Cava to Correct Complications After Filter Insertion

Incidence and Etiology

The use of intracaval devices to protect against pulmonary embolism in patients with deep vein thrombosis is increasing for a number of reasons. The frequency of diagnosis of deep vein thrombosis is more frequent because of the increased awareness of this entity. Caval interruption devices are easy to insert, require only local anesthesia, and are effective in protecting against the lethal effects of pulmonary emboli. In particular, the Greenfield filter is effective and has a low complication rate.

"

The first intracaval device popularized was the Mobin-Uddin umbrella (1). This device offered excellent protection against pulmonary embolism; however, it had a high rate of inferior vena caval thrombosis of about 50 to 70% within a 1 to 5 year period (2,3). In 1973, Greenfield and co-workers (4) described a new intracaval device that was found to be effective as protection against recurrent pulmonary emboli, with only 2 to 5% recurrent emboli 1 to 3 years after insertion (2,5). This device resulted in excellent long-term patency of the inferior vena cava of about 95% and, due to its design, proximal migration of the filter has only rarely been reported (2,5,6). Messmer and Greenfield (7-8) noticed uncomplicated minimal distal migration of the filter in 29% of their patients. Wingred and co-workers (9) found two uncomplicated distally migrated filters that did not require removal. We (10) reported a distally migrated and deformed filter in a quadriplegic patient in whom the so-called "quad cough" maneuver was a necessity. This maneuver is a forceful compression of the rib cage done to help clear secretions in patients with neurologic injuries. We postulated that this forceful compression resulted in a sudden increase in intrathoracic pressure that raised the pressure in the inferior vena cava, resulting in distention of the vena cava and causing release and distal propulsion of the filter.

Technical Considerations

Operations on the inferior vena cava to remove intracaval devices or to correct their complications are rarely necessary. If required within 7 days of a Greenfield filter insertion, a transjugular device for removal has been described (11). After 7 days, and with other devices, a direct caval approach can be employed (12). A celiotomy is performed with a midline incision, and the inferior vena cava is exposed. Although the Greenfield filter struts will often penetrate the cava wall, this is almost always without sequelae (2). Nonetheless, when removing a Greenfield filter, a wire cutter may be necessary to remove protruding struts to obtain adequate exposure of the anterior vena cava. If the struts are easily removed from the wall of the vena cava, Stewart and co-workers (12) suggest covering them with polyethlene tubing (PE240, internal diameter 0.066 inch) to prevent the pointed hooks from snagging on tissues or penetrating the gloves of the operating team. In the patient we reported (10), the filter had been deformed (Fig. 1) and the struts had penetrated overlying bowel (Fig. 2). The cava is approached by reflecting the duodenum and ascending colon to the left (Fig. 3). Once the cava is exposed anteriorly, the lumbar veins are controlled posteriorly using clips or ligatures. The vena cava should then be encircled for control proximal and distal to

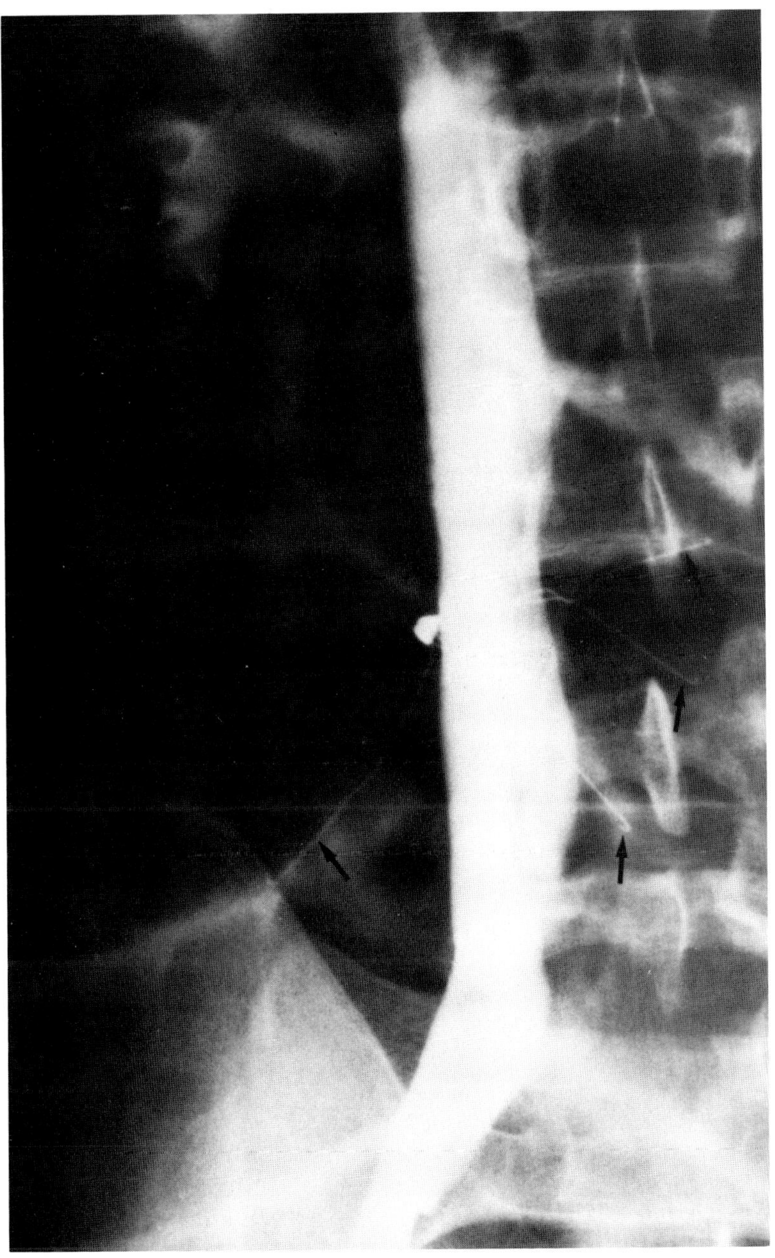

Figure 1 Inferior vena cavagram showing deformed Greenfield filter with struts penetrating cava wall.

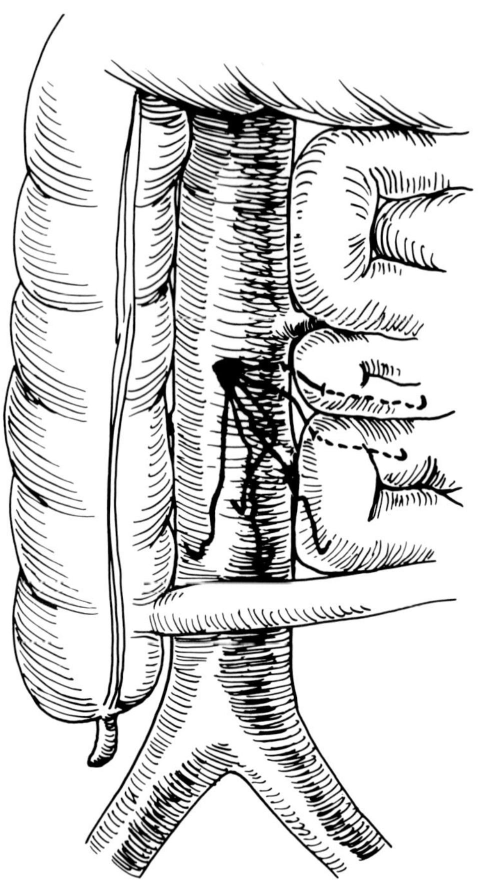

Figure 2 Struts penetrating overlying bowel.

the filter (Fig. 4). A longitudinal venotomy is made and the filter extracted, again with the aid of a wire cutter. Fragments of extracaval struts left behind should present no subsequent problems. The cava is then closed directly with restoration of blood flow cephalad. Regardless of whether there is a continued need for a vena cava filter, we believe the risk of partial or complete caval thrombosis is increased after operative manipulation. As a consequence, after filter extraction, another Greenfield filter should be inserted through the

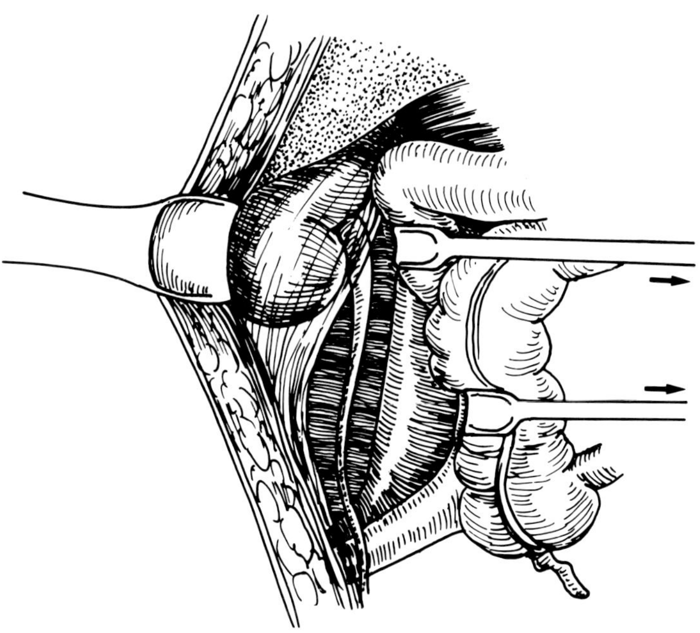

Figure 3 Exposure of anterior surface of vena cava, with reflection of duodenum and ascending colon to the left.

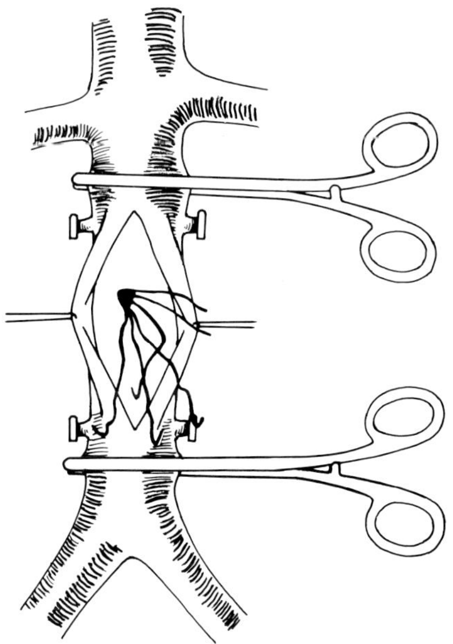

Figure 4 Lumbar veins clipped and control of inferior vena cava proximally and distally, with deformed filter in place.

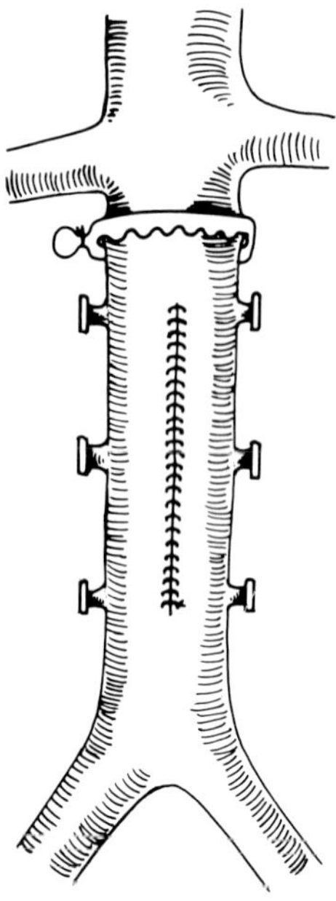

Figure 5   The Adams-DeWeese clip just below the renal veins.

caval opening using the femoral carrier. As an alternative, an external device
such as an Adams-DeWeese clip can be placed on the vena cava just below the
left renal vein (Figs. 5 and 6) (13). Postoperatively, the patient is maintained
on anticoagulation for at least 3 to 6 months and perhaps longer. Recurrent
problems such as emboli or limb swelling constitute indications for repeat
venography to visualize the caval segment.

Bypass of Completely Occluded Inferior Vena Cava

Incidence and Etiology

Inferior vena cava occlusion may result from deliberate ligation or the use of
external vena caval clips or intracaval devices — especially the Mobin-Uddin
umbrella (50 to 70% long-term occlusion) (2) or the Hunter-Sessions balloon
(100% occlusion) (14,15). Though its performance is superior, even the
Greenfield filter is associated with a thrombosis rate of the inferior vena cava

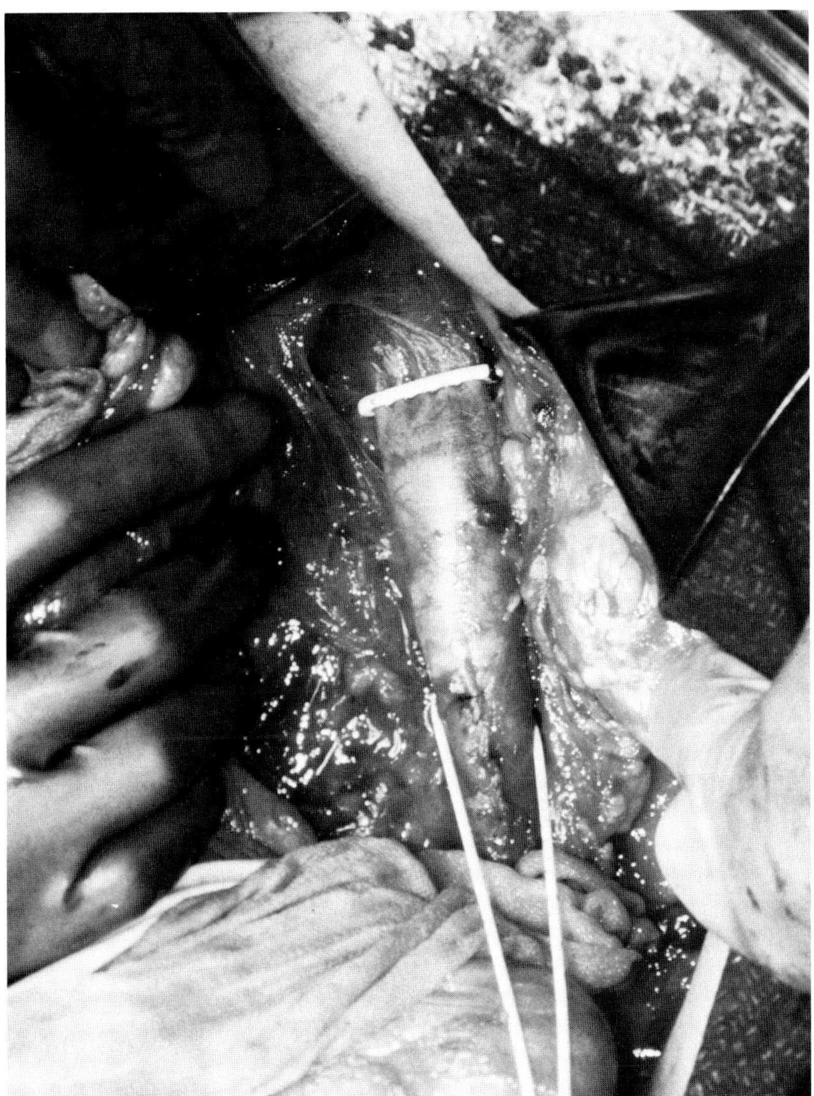

Figure 6 Adams-DeWeese clip in place.

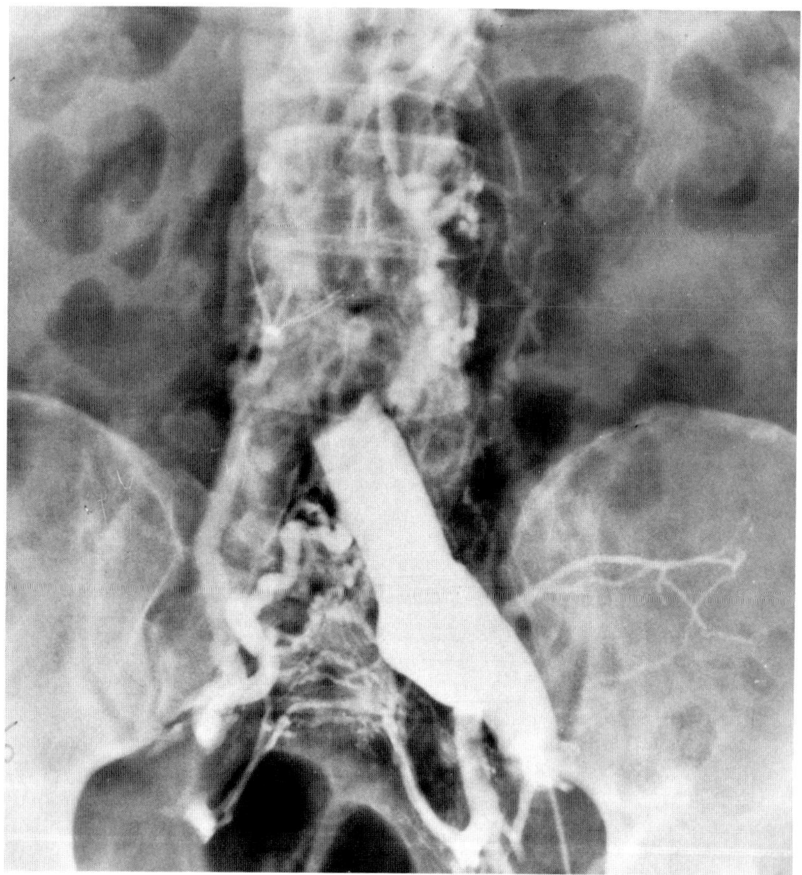

Figure 7   Occluded inferior vena cava by venogram.

of about 2 to 5% (2,4). Depending on the adequacy of venous collateral vessels, thrombosis of the inferior vena cava causes venous hypertension of the lower extremities, with resulting symptoms ranging from mild unilateral lower extremity edema to extensive bilateral postphlebitc syndrome.

Though some (16) have discounted the long-term consequences of vena caval ligation, others (17) have observed that over 50% have severe stasis changes in at least one lower extremity. Five patients in this latter study

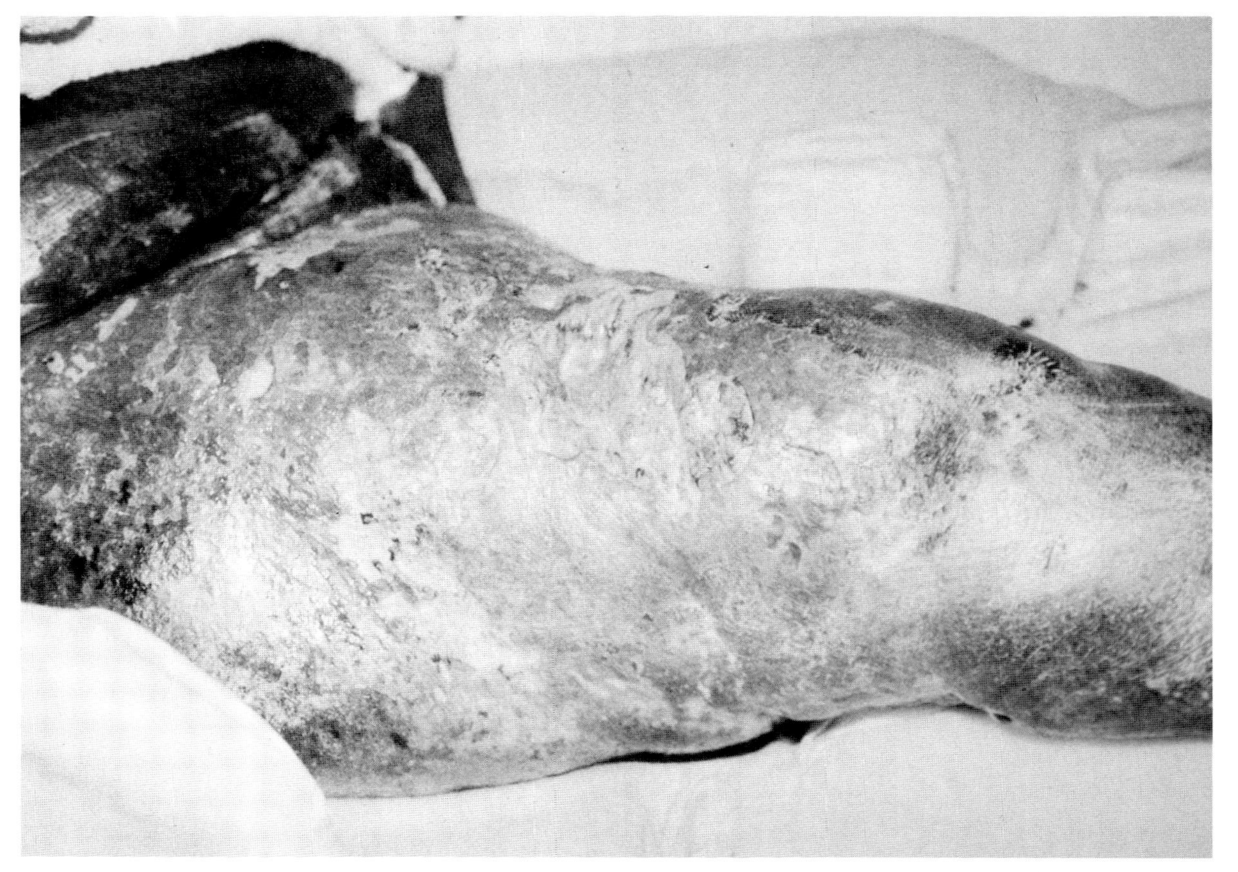

Figure 8 Gangrenous right lower extremity secondary to a thrombosed inferior vena cava.

developed phlegmasia cerulea dolens. In some instances, as Haimovici (18) has
noted, phlegmasia cerulea dolens may progress to gangrene of the extremities
secondary to venous occlusion. An example of this "venous gangrene" is a
50 year old woman who had a Mobin-Uddin umbrella 1 year before admission. Her inferior vena cavogram (Fig. 7) showed venal caval occlusion; unfortunately, her lower extremities were already gangrenous (Fig. 8) and she
subsequently died. Other complications of vena caval occlusion such as renal
vein thrombosis, hepatic vein thrombosis (Budd-Chiari syndrome), or recurrent pulmonary emboli through collateral channels (or from fresh thrombi
formed on the cephalad portion of the established caval thrombus) may occur
as well, although the incidence of these complications is not known.

Technical Considerations

Maintaining the patency of peripheral venous bypasses has been one of the
most vexing problems for the vascular surgeon. Replacement of a thrombosed
inferior vena cava is an especially difficult challenge. Some of the approaches
to this problem will be considered.

Bypass Materials

Many types of materials have been used as bypass prostheses for the inferior
vena cava. These include venous autograft and homograft, aortic homograft,
orlon, nylon, and freeze-dried venous and arterial homografts. Fresh venous
autografts have been the most successful as many have reported (19-22).
Other reports (23-26) have confirmed the failure of prosthetic materials to
maintain patency of the inferior vena cava. The cause of postoperative failure
of vena caval reconstruction is postulated to be inadequate flow rates in the
inferior vena cava (27). In 1972, Soyer and co-workers (28) reported the use
of polytetrafluoroethylene (PTFE) grafts as venous bypasses in different
locations in animals. The least successful position was the infrarenal inferior
vena cava, which exhibited a patency of only 33%. In 1974, Scherck and associates (29) reviewed the current status of the vena caval replacement. They
concluded that grafts in the superior vena cava were more likely to remain
patent compared with inferior vena cava grafts, and that the type of material
used for bypass was important.

In 1974, Fujiwara and his colleagues (30) reported the use of PTFE in both
the superior and inferior vena cava in dogs. They postulated that this material
was superior to other available materials for large vein replacement because of
minimal pseudointimal formation and tissue reaction around the graft.
They achieved a success rate in the inferior vena cava of 60%. Other reports

(31,32) have confirmed the success of PTFE grafts in the caval position, with acceptable patency rates.

In 1984, Dale and co-workers (33) reported the successful use of PTFE to replace the inferior vena cava in three patients; one of these was an inferior vena caval bifurcation graft. In 1963, Todd and associates (25) were among the first to advocate the external rigid support for venous grafting. The importance of the rigid support is thought to be the prevention of prosthesis collapse due to the combination of low venous pressure and the weight of viscera over the graft. In the arterial system, the externally supported PTFE graft has no known superiority over the nonsupported PTFE graft. In contrast, in the venous system, the externally supported PTFE grafts have been reported (34) to have a high patency rate, particularly where a distal temporary arterial venous fistula was added to the bypass.

Methods to Increase the Patency of Prosthetic Venous Grafts

1. *Use of externally supported PTFE grafts.* As discussed, the externally supported PTFE graft has given the best results yet achieved with prosthetic materials.
2. *Use of anticoagulation.* In 1956, Blum and co-workers (35) used an aortic bifurcation homograft to replace the infrarenal vena cava. For 3 days, the patient was given an intravenous heparin drip in both saphenous veins. At 11 months, the graft was confirmed patent by venography. Long-term anticoagulation after vena caval bypass may well be indicated, although no firm data yet exist to confirm this impression.
3. *Use of distal arteriovenous fistula.* Because of the low patency of venous grafts, attributed to low flow rate and low pressure, some (35-39) have advocated adding a distal arteriovenous fistula to increase the pressure and flow in the venous system. Again, though no hard evidence is currently available to confirm this hypothesis, the concept is sound and merits consideration and trial.

Results

Though reports in humans are anecdotal, it seems at present that in this challenging field of venous replacement, externally supported PTFE grafts, supplemented with a distal arteriovenous fistula and the use of anticoagulation, offer a potential for reconstruction.

References

1. Mobin-Uddin K, McLean R, Bolooki H, Jude JR. Caval interruption for prevention of pulmonary embolism: long-term results of a new method. Arch Surg 99:771, 1969.
2. Cimochowski GE, Evans RH, Zarins CK, Lu CT, DeMeester TR, Greenfield filter versus Mobin-Uddin umbrella: the continuing quest for the ideal method of vena caval interruption. J Thorac Cardiovasc Surg 79:358, 1980.
3. McIntyre AB, McCready RA, Hyde GL, Mattingly W. A ten year follow-up of the Mobin-Uddin filter for vena cava interruption. Surg Gynecol Obstet 158:513, 1984.
4. Greenfield LJ, McCurdy JR, Brown PP, Elkins RC. A new intracaval filter permitting continued flow and resolution of emboli. Surgery 73:599, 1973.
5. Greenfield LJ. Current indications for and results of Greenfield filter placement. J Vasc Surg 1:502, 1984.
6. Gomez GA, Cutler BS, Wheeler HB. Transvenous interruption of the inferior vena cava. Surgery 93:612, 1983.
7. Messmer JM, Greenfield LJ. Greenfield caval filters: long-term radiographic follow-up study. Radiology 156:613, 1985.
8. Greenfield LJ. Use and abuse of intracaval devices. Surgery 99:383, 1986.
9. Wingred M, Bernhard VM, Maddison F, Towne JB. Comparison of caval filters in the management of venous thromboembolism. Arch Surg 113:1264, 1978.
10. Sidawy AN, Menzoian, JO. Distal migration and deformation of the Greenfield vena cava filter. Surgery 99:369, 1986.
11. Greenfield LJ, Crute SL. Retrieval of the Greenfield vena cava filter. Surgery 88:719, 1980.
12. Stewart JR, Loughlin V, Crute SL, Greenfield LJ. Operative removal of misplaced Greenfield vena caval filters. Am J Surg 145:406, 1983.
13. Blumenberg RM, Gelfand ML. Long-term follow-up of vena caval clips and umbrellas. Am J Surg 134:205, 1977.
14. Hunter JA, Dye WS, Javid H, Najafi H, Goldin MD, Serry C. Permanent transvenous balloon occlusion of the inferior vena cava. Ann Surg 186:491, 1977.
15. Hunter JA, DeLaria GA. Hunter vena cava balloon: rationale and results. J Vasc Surg 1:491, 1984.
16. Ochsner A, Ochsner JL, Sanders HS. Prevention of pulmonary embolism by caval ligation. Ann Surg 171:923, 1970.
17. Piccone VA, Vidal E, Yarnoz M, Glass P, LeVeen HH. The late results of caval ligation. Surgery 68:980, 1970.

18. Haimovici H. Gangrene of the extremities of venous origin: review of the literature with case reports. Circulation 1:225, 1950.
19. Sauvage LR, Wesolowski SA, Anastomoses and grafts in the venous system with special reference to growth changes. Surgery 37:714, 1985.
20. Bryant MF Jr, Lazenby WD, Howard JM. Experimental replacement of short segments of veins. Arch Surg 76:289, 1958.
21. Bower R, Frederici V, Howard JM. Continuing studies of replacement of segments of the venous system. Surgery 47:132, 1960.
22. Earle AS, Horsley JS, Villavicencio JL, Warren R. Replacement of venous defects by venous autografts. Arch Surg 80:119, 1960.
23. DeMeitz A, Philips LL, Habif DV, Jacobson JH. Use of fibrinolysin in inferior vena caval replacement. Arch Surg 83:883, 1961.
24. Hambraeus G, Anderson MN. Experimental vena cava replacement with Teflon prostheses. Arch Surg 85:220, 1962.
25. Todd RS, Sive EB, DeJode LR, Danese C, Howard JM. Replacement of segments of the venous system. Arch Surg 87:998, 1963.
26. Dale WA, Scott HW. Grafts of the venous system. Surgery 53:52, 1963.
27. Najafi H, Battung V, Sarfatis P, Hirose M, DeWall RA. Experimental inferior vena cava replacement. J Thorac Cardiovasc Surg 53:243, 1967.
28. Soyer T, Lempinen M, Cooper P, Norton L, Eiseman B. A new venous prosthesis. Surgery 72:864, 1972.
29. Scherck JP, Kerstein MD, Stansel HC Jr. The current status of vena caval replacement. Surgery 76:209, 1964.
30. Fujiwara Y, Cohn LH, Adams D, Collins JJ Jr. Use of Goretex grafts for replacement of the superior and inferior venae cavae. J Thorac Cardiovasc Surg 67:774, 1974.
31. Smith DF, Hammon J, Anane-Sefah J, Richardson RS, Trimble C. Segmental venous replacement: a comparison of biological and synthetic substitutes. J Thorac Cardiovasc Surg 69:589, 1975.
32. Wilson SE, Jabour A, Stone RT, Stanley TM. Patency of biologic and prosthetic inferior vena cava grafts with distal limb fistula. Arch Surg 113:1174, 1978.
33. Dale WA, Harris J, Terry RB. Polytetrafluoroethylene reconstruction of the inferior vena cava. Surgery 95:625, 1984.
34. Bernstein EF, Chan EL, Bardin JA. Externally supported grafts for inferior vena cava bypass. In Bergan JJ, Yao JST (Eds): In Grune & Stratton, 1985.
35. Blum L, Medl WT, Keefer EBC. Aortic homograft substitution for the postrenal inferior vena cava. Arch Surg 72:567, 1956.
36. Gerbode F, Yee J, Rundle FF. Experimental anastomoses of vessels to the heart: possible application to superior vena caval obstruction. Surgery 25:556, 1949.

37. Kunlin J. Le retablissement de la circulation veineuse par greffe en cas d'obliteration traumatique ou thrombophlebitique. Greffe de 18 cm entre la veine saphene interne et la veine iliaque externe. Thrombose apres trois semaines de permeabilite. Memoires de L Acad de Chirurgie 79:109, 1953.
38. Stansel HC Jr. Synthetic inferior vena cava grafts, influence of increased flow. Arch Surg 89:1096, 1964.
39. Steinman C, Alpert J, Haimovici H. Inferior vena cava bypass grafts. Arch Surg 93:747, 1966.

Index

About the Editors

HUGH H. TROUT, III is Clinical Professor of Surgery at the Uniformed Services University of Health Sciences and at George Washington University Medical Center in Washington, D.C. In addition, he serves as a consultant in vascular surgery at the Washington Veterans Administration Hospital and at the National Cancer Institute of the National Institutes of Health in Bethesda, Maryland. He was professor of surgery at George Washington University until entering private practice in 1986. He remains on part-time faculty there and, in addition, is an attending surgeon now at Sibley, Holy Cross, and Surburban Hospitals in the metropolitan Washington area. His clinical interests focus on vascular surgery and he has published numerous articles in this field, many of which address problems presented by patients requiring reoperation. Dr. Trout received the B.S. degree (1963) from Washington and Lee University and M.D. degree (1967) from Duke University School of Medicine. He completed his internship and residency at UCLA Medical Center in Los Angeles, California, and a vascular fellowship under Dr. Jesse E. Thompson in Dallas, Texas.

JOSEPH M. GIORDANO is Professor of Surgery, Director of the Clinical Vascular Laboratory, and Chief of the Division of Vascular Surgery at George Washington University Medical Center in Washington, D.C. He is also a consultant in vascular surgery at the National Institutes of Health and the Washington Veterans Administration Hospital. His major clinical and research interest is vascular surgery, on which he has published many articles. He is a member of the International Society for Cardiovascular Surgery, American College of Surgeons, and Southern Association for Vascular Surgery. In addition, he is a founding member of the Chesapeake Vascular Society and Eastern Vascular Society. Dr. Giordano received the B.S. degree (1963) from Georgetown University and M.D. degree (1967) from Jefferson Medical College. He completed his residency at George Washington University Medical Center.

RALPH G. DePALMA is Professor and Chairman of the Department of Surgery at George Washington University in Washington, D.C. He is also Chief of Surgery at George Washington University Medical Center and a consulting surgeon at the Veterans Administration Medical Center in Washington, D.C. The author or co-author of over 120 publications mainly focusing on his clinical interest, vascular surgery, he conducts research in new techniques in vascular surgery and in the pathogenesis of atherosclerosis. Dr. DePalma received the A.B. degree (1953) from Columbia College and M.D. degree (1956) from New York University College of Medicine. He completed his internship at Presbyterian Hospital in New York City and his residency at University Hospitals of Cleveland in Cleveland, Ohio.